Praise for *Our Earth, Our Species, Our Selves*

"You'll see things differently after reading this book. I hope everyone will read it and thrive while advancing the health and environmental revolution we so urgently need. If you are concerned about our world and our prospects for addressing environmental and health problems, I prescribe *Our Earth, Our Species, Our Selves.*" —*Mark Hyman, MD, ten-time #1* New York Times *bestselling author, Director of the UltraWellness Center and The Cleveland Clinic Center for Functional Medicine, and Chairman of the Board of the Institute for Functional Medicine*

"Through science and stories, Moyer convinces us that we can create a sustainable world—if we act immediately. And she tells us how. What's more, we can thrive while making positive change. *Our Earth, Our Species, Our Selves* is a must-read for anyone who cares about the environment or personal well-being." —*Marci Shimoff, #1* New York Times *bestselling author of* Happy for No Reason, Love For No Reason, *and* Chicken Soup for the Woman's Soul

"Wisdom is making the right decisions today that will benefit and protect us decades from now. Our modern world must learn and embrace the wisdom in Dr. Moyer's book. We all share this marvelous planet and what could be more important than protecting it for our children and theirs." —*Joel Fuhrman, MD, six-time* New York Times *bestselling author, including* The End of Diabetes *and* The End of Heart Disease

"Ellen Moyer, PhD, is a brilliant and powerful voice for the healthy survival of our planet. What makes Ellen's book so compelling is that she is not a demagogue with a political or personal agenda but a woman who has passionately devoted the last thirty years conducting in-depth research and cleaning up the contamination caused by our current way of life. This book was not written to scare us but to provide us with the factual evidence that will inspire us to action. Ellen clearly lays out why there is still time to change course and implores us to not only work with existing institutions but to individually do our part as integral contributors to future outcomes." —*Debra Poneman, Founder and President of Yes to Success, Inc. and Co-founder of Your Year of Miracles, LLC*

"As we face the greatest crisis in human history, Ellen Moyer's book is exactly what we need. It not only brings us face-to-face with the breadth and depth of the crisis we face, but also provides great encouragement. Encouragement that the solutions are available to us, and that taking on the challenge of bringing about the solutions will enrich us, rather than impoverish us. Moyer brings an amazing breadth of knowledge to this topic, which illuminates the complexity and interrelatedness of the challenges we face. If we have the wisdom to follow the course she lays out for us, this book will stand beside a handful of others that have inspired people to transform our world." —*Paul Severance, Co-Chair, Elders Climate Action*

"This is an easy to read and well-written book about the planetary emergency we find ourselves in today. Ellen has very skillfully demonstrated how the current challenge can be converted into an opportunity by transforming ourselves and our institutions for a healthier, prosperous, peaceful, and sustainable world. Issues like climate change, pollution, and human tragedy have been covered. Ellen has explained, with good reasons, that human behavior must change along with the way we think. This would be accompanied by restructuring institutions around us. A lot will depend on our collective action, as everybody is a part of the problem and also the solution. This book is a must read by President-elect Donald Trump, his team, and all of us." —*Kamal Meattle, CEO of Paharpur Business Centre, New Delhi, and Trustee of The Climate Reality Project, India, set up by Nobel Laureate Al Gore*

"In this well-researched book Ellen Moyer shares how we can use our heads, our hearts, our hands, and our connections in community to create a more sustainable and enjoyable life on planet Earth. Her words take on a special significance because she has personally been on the front lines of positive change." —*Joan Maloof, PhD, author of* Nature's Temples: The Complex World of Old-Growth Forests *and Founder of the Old-Growth Forest Network*

OUR EARTH, OUR SPECIES, OUR SELVES

How to THRIVE While Creating a SUSTAINABLE WORLD

ELLEN MOYER

GREENVIRONMENT

Print ISBN: 978-1942936282
E-book ISBN: 978-1942936275
Library of Congress Control Number: 2016961034

Art by Ellen Moyer
Cover design by Brenda Mihalko

Greenvironment Press is an imprint of Chris Kennedy Publishing.
Greenvironment Press
2052 Bierce Drive, Virginia Beach, VA 23454
chris@chriskennedypublishing.com
http://chriskennedypublishing.com/

Ordering Information: Special discounts are available on quantity purchases by corporations, associations, and others. For details, contact the Special Sales Department at the address above.

Printed on paper with 30 percent post-consumer waste recycled material.

    Moyer, Ellen E., author.
    Our Earth, our species, our selves : how to thrive while creating a sustainable world / by Ellen Moyer.
    Includes bibliographical references and index.
    LCCN 2016961034
    ISBN 978-1942936282 (print)
    ISBN 978-1942936275 (e-book)
    1. Sustainability. 2. Environmentalism.
    3. Sustainable living. 4. Environmental responsibility.
    5. Environmental health. 6. Environmental economics.
    I. Title.
    GE196.M69 2017   333.72   QBI17-900012

For our Earth, and all who live upon it

CONTENTS

FOREWORD

I FIRST BECAME INTRIGUED WITH Ellen Moyer's work in 2012, when she attended a workshop I presented. At a break, she handed me a paper that listed my keys to "ultrawellness." Alongside my keys she had listed two additional sets of keys, relating to environmental health and the health of our society. We both thought the parallels were striking. Ellen told me she was writing a book about transforming our health, our environment, and our society. Now that the book has arrived, I can tell you, it was worth the wait.

For those unfamiliar with my work, I'm a practicing family physician, *New York Times* bestselling author, and internationally recognized leader, speaker, educator, and health advocate. I direct The UltraWellness Center and the Cleveland Clinic Center for Functional Medicine and chair the board of the Institute for Functional Medicine. You may have seen one of my public television specials or other television appearances in which I teach viewers how to achieve better health.

My specialty, Functional Medicine, focuses on keeping the whole patient healthy and treating the root causes of illness, if it occurs. Functional Medicine often successfully treats patients after conventional medicine has failed. One reason for Functional Medicine's effectiveness is its consideration of the impacts of the patient's environment, which can be considerable. *Our Earth, Our Species, Our Selves: How to Thrive While Creating a Sustainable World* emphasizes the ways in which humans literally *are* their environment. It explains how optimal human health depends on healthy air, water, soil, plants, animals, climate, consumer products, and much more.

Ellen Moyer is the right person to write this book. A registered professional engineer, she has more than three decades of experience assessing and cleaning up contaminated waste sites. She is a US Green Building Council Leadership in Energy and Environmental Design (LEED)–accredited professional and has been actively involved in designing the green systems we will need for the future. She has studied the problems we're facing and brings extensive experience in developing solutions to overcome and prevent them. Her background in anthropology allows her to take a big-picture view of our situation and borrow ideas from other cultures.

People often feel trapped in the status quo, believing that changing course will be difficult or unpleasant. *Our Earth* dispels these beliefs. It shows that we can transform our health and environment—along with our economy, democracy, and society—more easily than we might think. And we can thrive while we are doing it.

When we improve one area of life—our health, environment, or economy—the other areas improve as well, due to the interconnections between them. *Our Earth* shows how humans in the past have repeatedly responded to environmental and health crises by creating epic change, and it explains why we can successfully do so again. Our current challenges present us with a great opportunity to dramatically ramp up our way of life for the better. It's an incredible time to be alive because change is coming, and you and I can help shape that change.

Ellen Moyer pulls together a remarkably wide range of topics, drawing from diverse perspectives, and presents them in a fresh, straightforward, and accessible style. *Our Earth* inspires us with its hopeful and empowering message and motivates us to take enjoyable actions that help our planet, our species, and ourselves.

You'll see things differently after reading this book. I hope everyone will read it and thrive while advancing the health and environmental revolution we so urgently need. If you are concerned about our world and our prospects for addressing environmental and health problems, I prescribe *Our Earth, Our Species, Our Selves: How to Thrive While Creating a Sustainable World.*

Mark Hyman, MD
November 17, 2016

INTRODUCTION

The best way to predict the future is to design it.

—*Buckminster Fuller*

WE'RE ALL INVITED TO PARTICIPATE in a radical transformation unfolding before our eyes. At this critical decision point in the human story, will we

- Create a sustainable way of life?
- Stay the course and flame out as just another evolutionary "nice try," a tiny, forgettable blip in the Earth's timeline?
- Continue on, but in a diminished state after a half-hearted attempt?

We must choose.

Our Earth, Our Species, Our Selves: How to Thrive While Creating a Sustainable World is about stories—stories we tell ourselves about who we are, who we can be, and what we can do. We can change our stories and our systems whenever we want, though we tend to forget this. Environmental crises signal that it's now time for our species to create a new story and a new path. Our new story says we absolutely *can* create a sustainable world, and we'll thrive on the path of doing so.

WHY I WROTE THIS BOOK

One day in 2010, I sat in my parents' kitchen talking with my mother. We were discussing my latest efforts to defeat proposed wood-burning power plants in Massachusetts.

"We really need another environmental movement," I said to her.

"What would it take to have one?" she asked, ever the practical problem-solver.

"It would take another book like *Silent Spring,*" I replied. The outcry that followed the publication of biologist Rachel Carson's book in 1962 spurred revolutionary changes in the laws affecting our air, land, water, and fellow species.

"Why don't you write it?" she asked.

I didn't answer, changing the subject, but I gave the idea a lot of thought afterward. I knew my mother's question was serious because her father, my grandfather, was Pulitzer Prize–winning author and civil rights activist Paul Green. Being blessed with many advantages and, unlike countless others on this Earth, able to speak freely, I could not think of any good reason *not* to write the book.

Why did I tell my mother we need another environmental movement? Despite practicing environmental engineering for the past thirty years, events outside my day job drove me to the conclusion. For the past five years, I had been fighting proposals to construct four large, wood-burning biomass plants near my home in western Massachusetts. (Biomass is organic matter burned as fuel to generate electricity.) At first, when I heard about the plans, I thought "cool, Massachusetts is leading the way once again." But as I read up on the proposed projects, I became horrified by how devastating they would be. They would wreck the climate, clear-cut forests, dry up rivers, pollute the air, and rip off ratepayers and taxpayers—while generating a paltry amount of electricity, due to their rock-bottom inefficiency.

Regulatory agencies and environmental nonprofit organizations had been taken in by project developers' insupportable "green-washing" claims that they could produce clean and renewable energy. Regulators were green-lighting these projects without scrutiny and despite dangers that couldn't have been more obvious. I almost fainted one afternoon to find myself at a meeting arguing against representatives from my once-favorite environmental nonprofit organization, who, surreally, were all for these biomass plants. The realization that no one was protecting citizens or the environment from this potential devastation came as a shock and changed my life.

I was also surprised to learn how one action, burning wood to generate electricity, can generate many negative impacts in diverse areas of life, and how when we harm the environment we harm ourselves directly. I wondered whether positive actions, such as planting trees instead of destroying them, could be equally powerful. I marveled at how human health, the environment, politics, and the economy are deeply intertwined.

I also learned of the individual and collective power of ordinary citizens. One of the main reasons I wrote this book is to remind you that we are powerful and have the capacity to create the change we want, even when our institutions fight us.

Although citizens won the battle over the biomass plants, I saw the victory as temporary and shallow because I knew developers would be back with other damaging schemes. Also, it had taken years of intense effort to achieve this one victory. Citizens simply don't have the time, energy, or resources to fight every destructive project or program thrown at them, when there are so many.

I realized we need a comprehensive approach that addresses root causes and prevents bad schemes from popping up, like mushrooms, in the first place. We need a sustainable way of life that will allow generations of humans, and the living environment on which we depend, to continue on Earth far into the future.

Our Earth offers this big-picture approach and calls for widespread and accelerated change to help pull us out of the broad environmental, health, and economic crisis in which we find ourselves today. (Biomass burning is just one symptom of the crisis.) Species go extinct when they can't adapt fast enough, and we are at risk of not responding quickly enough to the environmental changes we ourselves created. Responding successfully involves transforming ourselves, our technology, and our social, political, and economic systems. But here's the good news: Changing course is not only doable, but it is also not so difficult as we may think—and it can be fulfilling.

I wrote the book because I had to. We are in a state of emergency, with everything on the line—our life-support system, health, economy, and democracy. I can't put it better than Rachel Carson, who penned this line to a friend: "There would be no future peace for me if I kept silent."[1]

WHAT THIS BOOK OFFERS

Our Earth is intended to illuminate, reassure, and inspire you.

- It shows how humans can create a health and environmental revolution. This revolution can pull us out of the downward environmental, health, and economic spiral we find ourselves in and put us on an upward spiral instead. This book inspires and assures us, "We can do this. Now is the time. We *want* to do this."

- It synthesizes anthropology, environmental science, and self-empowerment perspectives. It takes a 40,000-foot view and dives deep into how everything in our world is connected in a web of relationships.

- Whereas many books explain the problems in our world without offering practical solutions—leaving readers feeling overwhelmed and blue—*Our Earth* shows we have what it takes to manage our problems and that challenges are natural and even necessary for our evolution. It honestly says, "Yes, we are heading straight for the rocks" but then shows us how we can change course, using solutions we already have. *Our Earth* tends to be United States–centric, because I live in the United States and am most familiar with this country, but also because of the United States' role as a world leader. However, this book is relevant to people living in other parts of the world too.

- It shows why right now might be the most exciting and important time to be alive in all of human history.

- Whereas other books typically focus on one or the other, *Our Earth* comprehensively merges two topics: personal growth and creating a sustainable world. It shows the parallels and interconnections between individuals and our world and describes how we can simultaneously transform both.

- It advises how we can begin immediately to help ourselves—and the world at the same time—by taking practical, manageable, and enjoyable steps.

Challenges are natural and even necessary for our evolution.

METAPHOR FOR OUR TIME

The analogy of a caterpillar metamorphosing into a butterfly aptly characterizes the frightening yet exhilarating process we're undergoing today. An egg hatches into a caterpillar, which feeds ravenously on leaves, beginning with the leaf on which it was born, and grows rapidly. One day, it stops eating, hangs upside down from a twig or leaf, and forms a hard chrysalis. Within this protective casing, the caterpillar transforms into a butterfly. During this energy-intensive process, the chrysalis loses nearly half of its weight, and waste products accumulate.

The caterpillar releases enzymes that cause its body to disintegrate. Certain cells that are different from the rest of the caterpillar cells and had lain dormant in the caterpillar—"imaginal cells"—survive this process. Imaginal cells contain the genetic blueprint for a butterfly. These cells multiply and connect to construct the butterfly, reusing the components of the former caterpillar.[2]

Just when it seems the life of the caterpillar is coming to an end, the beautiful butterfly is created, with the freedom to fly from flower to flower, providing the essential service of pollination while non-destructively sipping nectar. This miracle occurs routinely, like clockwork, generation after generation, going back eons.

The human species now finds itself in a crisis stage. We are like the once-gorging caterpillar disintegrating as imaginal cells begin constructing the butterfly. Will we transform quickly enough, or will we run out of resources and die in our own waste? The answer is up to us. The future of the human species hinges on what you and I do at this point in human history. For this reason, we may be the most important humans who ever walked the Earth.

Our Earth celebrates the vision of the future butterfly. It inspires you to live like an imaginal cell that creates the butterfly. In fact, this book itself attempts to serve as an imaginal cell.

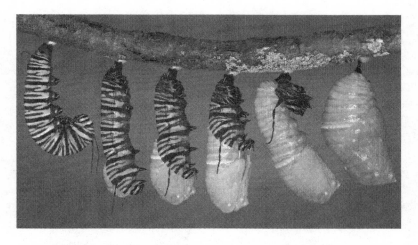

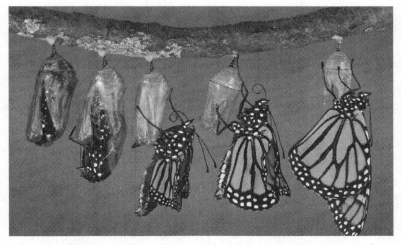

Caterpillar becoming a chrysalis (top photo) and butterfly emerging from a chrysalis (bottom photo). Photo credits: ©Istockphoto.com/Cathy Keifer.

PROGRESSION OF THIS BOOK

Part I, "World Out of Whack" (chapters 1 through 4), describes how we evolved to our present state and, in so doing, inadvertently created massive problems. A brief status report summarizes our challenges and shows how we could be enjoying greater health and happiness. We stand on a knife edge where we cannot remain. Part I also reveals the interconnections between us, our environment, our economy, and our problems and solutions. Because of interconnections, change in one area of life affects other areas, facilitating transformation on several fronts.

Part II, "Our Selves" (chapters 5 through 7), shows we have far greater capacities than we typically know or actualize. We can grow as individuals more easily than we might think, developing healthy bodies, hearts, minds, spirits, vocations, wealth, and actions—both for our own sake and to promote the wider good. We'll be ill equipped to make the heavy lift that's called for if we're malnourished, tired, stressed, depressed, or impoverished or if we feel powerless, overwhelmed, disconnected, or purposeless. Playing big is much more fulfilling and better for the world than allowing limiting beliefs to constrain our lives. Part II suggests actions we can take in our daily lives to help steer ourselves, our species, and our environment onto a healthy and sustainable path.

Part III, "Our Species" (chapters 8 through 12), shows how we can transform our technology and our collective economic, political, and social systems. Individual actions alone are insufficient to create a sustainable world. Success also requires group actions to transform our institutions and policies. Our crises provide the opportunity for epic change and participation by people everywhere.

Many strategies for individual development also apply to our collective development as a populace. One example is setting ambitious goals. Just as a sick patient with a compelling reason to live recuperates faster, we will more effectively improve our collective situation if we share goals loftier than merely surviving.

Part III shows that by making a manageable number of important changes, we can create an exponentially increasing upward spiral of solutions. These solutions will address many interconnected problems affecting individuals, humankind, and the environment, and they will ultimately create better lives for all. Our problems have become too large for our institutions and politicians to solve on their own. Plus, as citizens, we need to ensure our interests are served. As the saying goes, "If you're not at the table, you're on the menu." Ordinary citizens fuel the upward spiral by demanding protection of human and environmental health through governmental regulation.

In medieval London, life was miserable and short due to sanitation problems that led to the Black Death, a severe epidemic of plague. Ordinary people—without the benefit of democracy, cell phones, the Internet, or much in the way of education—demanded and manifested lasting, positive change that propelled London into a state of prominence that continues today. We look upon Londoners who endured the horrific conditions before this transformation and think, *Those poor bastards. If only they had known not to throw their wastes in the streets, they could have saved themselves from so much misery and had much better lives.* People in the future may similarly look upon us with pity, thinking, *Those poor bastards. If only they had known not to throw toxic chemicals and greenhouse gases all over the place, they could have saved themselves from so much misery and had much better lives.* Well, now we know. Now we can change our situation.

In 1963, Rachel Carson wrote, "I think we're challenged as mankind has never been challenged before to prove our maturity and our mastery, not of nature, but of ourselves."[3] Her words still ring true today as we undertake another, more powerful, environmental movement to finish the job she started.

WHY THIS AUTHOR?

I grew up close to nature. My family lived on a road that crossed a floodplain in eastern Massachusetts, a place teeming with wildlife. Plus, we had lots of pets. But this beautiful nature was marred by human impact. People would dump refrigerators, stoves, and other unwanted items right next to the river and the road. They threw papers, bottles, and other trash out of their car windows. My parents paid us kids five cents for each grocery bag of litter we collected from the roadside. Thus began my environmental career, at the age of eight.

In college, I studied anthropology, the science of human beings. I wanted to know how we arrived at our current state and whether people in other times and places disrespected nature as "developed" societies do. I was heartened to learn that other societies have lived harmoniously and respectfully with nature, a fact that suggests we can change our ways and attitudes.

I went back to school to study environmental engineering, a specialty within civil engineering that uses engineering, biology, chemistry, and soil science to develop solutions to environmental problems. For several decades, I worked fairly quietly for environmental consulting firms, cleaning up sites that had soil and groundwater contamination. I knew the environment was in deep trouble but thought our institutions and policies were up to the job of solving the problems. Everything suddenly changed for me with my involvement in the "biomass wars." I spoke out in comments and letters to regulatory agencies and newspaper editors, on radio and television, at public hearings, and at the Massachusetts State House. Working "in the trenches" on this issue revealed to me the fundamental ways in which our institutions and policies are failing to protect us, our environment, and our economy.

As principal of my own consulting practice, Greenvironment, LLC, since 2004, I have worked for clients on all sides of environmental contamination issues, from corporations to state and federal agencies to citizens who have suffered contamination impacts. Three decades of assessing and remediating contaminated sites have shown me the exorbitant health, environmental, and economic costs of our toxic way of life. On the other hand, my consulting work in the areas of green design, resource conservation, and pollution prevention has shown me that sustainable solutions are less expensive and easier than many people think.

Our unsustainable predicament, and the ways out of it, are complex. My love for the environment and my background in anthropology, environmental cleanup, sustainability, economics, and personal development provide the diverse perspectives needed to "put it all together." If you're like me, you want to create a sustainable world—for both humans and other species, now and stretching far into the future—as quickly as possible. We can accelerate this process by acting collectively as well as individually.

Please feel free to communicate with me, about anything in this book, through my website, www.ellenmoyerphd.com. We are all in this together.

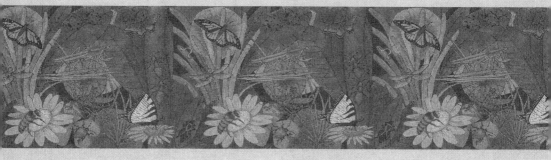

PART I
WORLD OUT OF WHACK

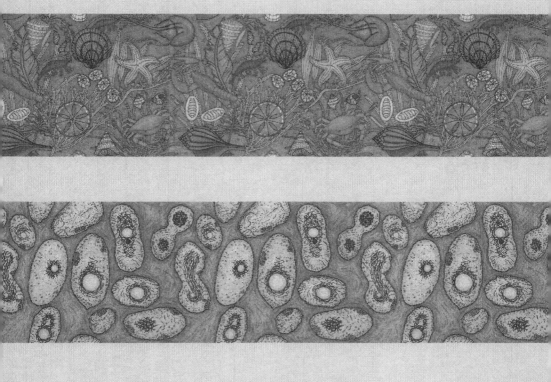

CHAPTER 1
TIME AND CHANGE

It was the best of times, it was the worst of times, it was the age of wisdom, it was the age of foolishness, it was the epoch of belief, it was the epoch of incredulity, it was the season of Light, it was the season of Darkness, it was the spring of hope, it was the winter of despair, we had everything before us, we had nothing before us.

—*Charles Dickens,* A Tale of Two Cities

THE TRAJECTORY OF LIFE ON Earth may not be so much smooth and gradual as punctuated by jumps.[4] Monumental leaps include transitions from nonlife to life, from bacteria to complex cells, from single cells to multi-celled organisms, from water to land, and, through a series of jumps, eventually to humans, with mass extinctions along the way. We tend to assume future change will unfold gradually and we'll have plenty of time to find ways to respond effectively. However, exponential changes in recent years have brought us up short with lethal threats that don't allow time for a leisurely approach. This book is about responding successfully by quickly overcoming inertia and implementing comprehensive changes. The first step is to take stock of our situation.

HOW DID WE GET HERE?

It helps to look at our place in the broad context of the history of Earth. The timeline below summarizes the history of Earth since the time of the "Big Bang" that created our universe fifteen billion years ago (BYA). This was followed much later by the formation of Earth and the rest of our solar system. The timeline stretches into the future, when the sun will expand into a red giant star and engulf Earth seven billion years from now.[5] We have the option of extending our time on Earth as long as possible into this vast future.

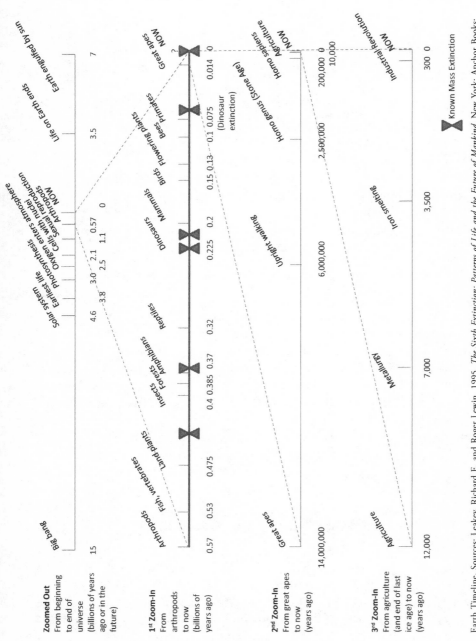

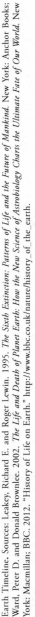

Earth Timeline. Sources: Leakey, Richard E. and Roger Lewin. 1995. *The Sixth Extinction: Patterns of Life and the Future of Mankind.* New York: Anchor Books; Ward, Peter D. and Donald Brownlee. 2002. *The Life and Death of Planet Earth: How the New Science of Astrobiology Charts the Ultimate Fate of Our World.* New York: Macmillan; BBC. 2012. "History of Life on Earth." http://www.bbc.co.uk/nature/history_of_the_earth.

The numbers on the timeline are approximate, and they change as new discoveries are made. Debate swirls around some of the dates. Notably, science has yet to agree on a formal description for our genus, *Homo*, or our species, *sapiens*. Consequently, scientists disagree over when they began.[6]

The earliest forms of life on Earth (prokaryotes) emerged 3.8 BYA. Much later, microorganisms began performing oxygen-producing photosynthesis, converting light energy from the sun into chemical energy the microorganisms used to fuel their activities. This was followed by the appearance of complex cells (having nuclei) and, later, by sexually reproducing organisms.

Among arthropods, invertebrate (backbone-less) animals—shrimp, crabs, lobsters, and the like—were the first animals to leave water for land. Arthropods were followed by the emergence of fish, land plants, insects, amphibians, reptiles, mammals, birds, flowering plants, and primates.[7]

The Earth timeline includes five known mass extinctions, in which more than 65 percent of animal species died in a "brief geological instant." We may be entering a sixth one, one for which we would be entirely responsible.[8] Over just the past 20 years, humans have eliminated 10 percent of the Earth's wilderness.[9] Biologist E. O. Wilson estimates that 30,000 species—more than three per hour—are disappearing each year.[10]

Great apes—chimpanzees, gorillas, humans, and orangutans—first appeared 14 million years ago (MYA). Genus *Homo*, to which we belong, entered the scene beginning about 2.5 MYA. *Homo sapiens*—that's you and me—appeared about 200,000 years ago.

We hunted and gathered food from complex ecosystems, living, by necessity, attuned to the natural world and showing up at the right place and time for various foods to be available. It wasn't until 12,000 years ago that agriculture began, leading to accumulation and storage of food and development of population centers, complex social and political institutions, increased division of labor, and specialization.[11]

The start of the Industrial Revolution—in England, with the textile industry in the mid- to late 1700s—is like only yesterday. For the first time, people were freed from reliance on local sources of human or animal muscle, wood, wind, or water for power. The Industrial Revolution was powered by fossil fuel energy, beginning with coal in the 1700s, oil in the mid-1850s, and natural gas in the early 1900s. Industrial agriculture began around the time of the Industrial Revolution with the use of synthetic fertilizers and, later, pesticides, antibiotics, and hormones.

The timeline shows that humans are extremely new to Earth, here for only a microscopic fraction of a blink of an evolutionary eye, and our high-tech way of life occupies an infinitesimally small span of time. The timeline also shows that change is the norm, and new life forms continually arise. Our long pre-human lineage, as well as the long lineage of other life forms with which we currently share the Earth, suggests that although humans arrived recently, our life-support system is long established and our roots go way back. We are part of nature and the natural progression of evolution. We have a long and impressive resumé of survival, and a look at the big picture leads us to wonder: What comes next?

Until the advent of agriculture, we lived on Earth in a relatively sustainable way. Sure, we affected things here and there, but our population was far too small to impact the long-established and resilient Earth ecology, and our lifestyle was fairly benign. With agriculture, our powers increased, and civilizations sometimes degraded regional environments. Deforestation for farmland and wood, and the soil erosion that followed, may have been at least partially responsible for the collapse of the Mayan civilization in Central America.[12]

With the advent of Western science and the onset of the Industrial Revolution just a few hundred years ago, human impacts exploded, becoming global in scale. The human population skyrocketed due to expanded food supplies and transportation and improved public health and living standards.[13] Energy use—the foundation of our wealth, power, and modern life—ramped up drastically. Today, inhabitants of industrialized countries use up to one hundred times more energy than our preindustrial ancestors. Unintended impacts of our way of life now threaten us, in the form of climate change and other dire environmental problems.[14]

Changes: Examples from My Lifetime. Changes just within my lifetime—good and bad—have been profound, and as a baby boomer (someone born between 1946 and 1964), I'm not all that old:

- Space travel and putting a man on the moon
- Computers
- The Internet
- Cell phones
- The modern environmental, civil rights, antiwar, and feminist movements
- Modern contraceptives
- Job security and career predictability replaced by multiple jobs and careers and alternative work arrangements (including teleworking)
- Mom-and-pop local stores and shops replaced by chain stores devoid of local identity and character
- Changes in plant and animal populations; we have lost and are losing so much— elephants, monarch butterflies, and others, some of which we haven't even identified. Meanwhile, invasive species such as zebra mussels, brown recluse spiders, and the Lyme disease bacterium increase.

- Widespread use of plastics
- Genetically modified organisms (GMOs) and ramped-up use of synthetic pesticides
- Loss of dark night skies full of stars, light pollution cutting us off from the cosmos
- Climate change

ENVIRONMENTAL CONCERNS

The consequences of uncontrolled resource exploitation and waste generation were noticeable even before the Industrial Revolution. In 1739, Benjamin Franklin and other Philadelphia residents petitioned the Pennsylvania Assembly to put an end to waste dumping and to remove tanneries from the city's commercial district. In 1775, around the time the Industrial Revolution began, the observation was made that chimney sweeps developed cancer from contact with soot.[15] John Muir, Henry David Thoreau, John James Audubon, and others promoted concern for protecting natural resources in the 1800s.

An environmental movement in the United States emerged in the late nineteenth and early twentieth centuries. The world's first national park, Yellowstone, opened in 1885. John Muir founded the Sierra Club in 1892. In 1899, the United States passed the Refuse Act, which prohibited the dumping of refuse into navigable waters except by permit. The first national wildlife refuge, Pelican Island, opened in Florida in 1905. Environmental awareness grew, and President Woodrow Wilson founded the National Park Service and the US Forest Service in 1916.

Los Angeles created the first air pollution agency in the United States in 1947. The next year, the United States passed the Federal Water Pollution Control Act. In 1952, 4000 deaths in London were attributed to smog. Similarly, around that time, some parts of the United States experienced pollution episodes like those now occurring across parts of China.[16] In 1975, the United States passed the National Air Pollution Control Act.

Public reaction to Rachel Carson's *Silent Spring* led to the ban of the pesticide DDT for agricultural use in the United States in 1972. DDT, a probable human carcinogen, was the first synthetic pesticide of the modern age, used as such beginning in the 1940s.[17]

What I Was Up To When Silent Spring Was Published. When I was in elementary school, the DDT trucks rumbled through our neighborhood on hot summer evenings to spray the pesticide for mosquito control. We kids begged to go outside to play in the mist. Thankfully, our wary parents said no.

Silent Spring heightened awareness of both the severity of our environmental problems and their impacts on human health. Gaylord Nelson, then–US Senator from Wisconsin, founded Earth Day on April 22, 1970 after the massive 1969 oil spill in Santa Barbara, California. He announced the idea for a "national teach-in on the environment" to the national media and promoted events across the country. On the first Earth Day, twenty million Americans from all walks of life—Republicans and Democrats, rich and poor, urbanites and farmers—took to streets, parks, and auditoriums to rally for a healthy environment. Later that same year saw the creation of the US Environmental Protection Agency (USEPA) and the Occupational Safety and Health Administration and passage of major environmental legislation. Earth Day went global and now is celebrated by more than a billion people each year.[18]

> *On the first Earth Day, twenty million Americans from all walks of life—Republicans and Democrats, rich and poor, urbanites and farmers—took to streets, parks, and auditoriums to rally for a healthy environment.*

Environmental legislation passed between 1970 and 1980 laid out requirements for protecting air, water, endangered species, and worker and consumer safety and for managing hazardous substances. As a result of these laws, many of the "in your face" environmental problems (such as rivers catching on fire) have been mitigated; however, many environmental problems have worsened because they have not been addressed.[19] And additional problems have emerged.

Environmental regulations left a big gap with regard to the control of synthetic chemicals, which currently number well over 85,000 and increase by thousands each year.[20] The USEPA has tested only a small fraction of them and has restricted the use of very few.[21] By putting into use inadequately tested chemicals, we are engaged in a huge, uncontrolled experiment. Many chemicals end up in living things. Almost every animal in the world has polychlorinated biphenyls (PCBs), which are known to cause a variety of adverse health effects, in its body.[22] Contaminants can travel long distances and move between air, water, and soil. Health effects of various synthetic chemicals range from asthma, cancer, and neurological problems (including attention deficit disorders), to reproductive problems (including infertility), obesity and diabetes, and autoimmune diseases.[23] Of safety testing done on chemicals, psychiatrist Kelly Brogan says, "Get your tissues ... we're in big trouble."[24]

As just one example of our reckless approach, bisphenol A (BPA)—a widely used chemical found in some plastic water bottles, food-can linings, airline tickets, and store and automatic teller machine receipts—absorbs into your blood rapidly and has been linked to diabetes, obesity, and coronary artery disease.[25] Despite concerns and a petition to eliminate BPA from the US food supply, the US Food and Drug Administration ruled there was insufficient information to prohibit BPA. Furthermore, a closely related alternative, bisphenol S, was rolled out before it was even tested for the problems BPA has been found to cause.[26]

Because synthetic chemicals have not been well controlled on the front end, we end up with contaminated air, water, and soil requiring cleanup to protect human and environmental health.

From Assessing and Cleaning Up Environmental Contamination to Practicing Green Design. My experience in dealing with soil and groundwater contamination has spanned much of the period since the first major modern environmental legislation was passed, in the 1970s, up to the present. Looking back over my career, I realize how little we knew at the beginning of it and how little we know even now.

Historically, it was common practice to discharge untreated waste on the ground, into water bodies, or into the air. The general approach to assessing a site with suspected contamination is to first research the current and historical uses of the site to deduce the most likely types and locations of contaminants. Site assessment practitioners then collect samples of soil, surface water (from streams, ponds, and the like), and/or groundwater (water beneath the ground surface) and analyze them for suspected contaminants. From this and other information, we judge whether the site poses an "unacceptable risk" to humans or ecosystems.

If it does, we identify and evaluate potential ways to clean up the site. Remediation methods generally involve destroying, moving, or isolating the contaminants. The most complex sites can cost billions of dollars and take decades to assess and remediate. At some sites, high cleanup costs are used to justify not cleaning them up completely, leaving contamination for future generations to worry about.

Most people are doing the best they can. Site owners have their profits and shareholders to protect. Regulators work within their political and economic constraints. Consultants try to negotiate solutions that will satisfy their clients and regulators while protecting human health and the environment.

Site assessment and remediation is thus far from perfect, and negative, on many levels. Contaminated sites sicken and kill people and wildlife and drive site owners into bankruptcy. Sometimes taxpayers get stuck paying for cleanups. Workers who originally worked at these sites often suffered horrendous impacts. At the site of an electroplating plant I assessed, a worker had fallen into an acid bath and died. While assessing former tannery sites where waste animal hides—containing powerful pesticides—had been buried, I could only imagine the plight of the workers who had handled these materials.

We're learning an ounce of prevention is worth tons of cure. Green designers strive to prevent contamination and other environmental problems by using benign rather than hazardous materials and processes, and by recycling to eliminate waste altogether.

BACKSLIDING AND MONEY

In the decades since many of the environmental laws were passed, special interest groups have done their best to erode them. Former US Representative Sherwood Boehlert, a career Republican, wrote, "Those bedrock protections we all rely upon have come under a withering partisan assault, as some have sought to turn environmental protections into an issue to divide us, red and blue. We've seen commonsense air pollution and water quality rules attacked. We've seen funding for enforcement slashed. We've seen the authority of the USEPA undermined…. We need to rebuild the environmental majority that has served us so well for so long."[27]

The American Legislative Exchange Council (ALEC), a nationwide consortium of elected state legislators, works side by side with some of America's most powerful corporations. Journalist and public commentator Bill Moyers reports, "They have an agenda you should know about, a mission to remake America, changing the country by changing its laws, one state at a time. ALEC creates 'model legislation,' pro-corporate laws that its members push in statehouses across the nation … somehow, ALEC managed to remain the most influential corporate-funded political organization you'd never heard of."[28]

In another tactic known as "regulatory capture," a regulatory agency created to act in the public interest is made to advance the interests of the industry or sector it is charged with regulating. One method of capture is via a "revolving door," whereby people easily switch their employment back and forth between government and industry, sometimes repeatedly, shaping regulatory agencies to industry's liking and advising industry how to get around regulations. A former vice president of public policy at Monsanto Company worked several stints in government, most recently serving as the US Food and Drug Administration's "food safety czar."[29]

Some large environmental groups have also been tainted by corporate influence by entering into "partnerships" with corporations. Journalist Christine MacDonald, in *Green Inc.,* writes: "If anything, the big conservation organizations seem more like 'enablers' that are slowing down the corporate awakening to environmental and social responsibilities by providing the companies with easy ways to appear green without making significant changes.... Not only do the largest conservation groups take money from companies deeply implicated in environmental crimes; they have become something like satellite PR offices for the corporations that support them."[30] Not all environmental organizations are "in bed with corporate." It's important for donors and volunteers to thoroughly vet environmental organizations, even the oldest and most venerable, and support good ones for the amazing work they do.

A trick called "astroturfing" masks the sponsors of a message or organization to make it seem "grassroots." Astroturfing is used to manipulate public opinion, fulfill corporate agendas, create enough doubt to inhibit action, and harm scientific research. (The term *astroturfing* is derived from AstroTurf, a brand of synthetic carpeting designed to look like natural grass, a play on the word *grassroots*.) A classic example is the National Smokers Alliance, which tobacco companies created in 1993. More recently, an organization called Citizens for Fire Safety that promoted flame-retardant chemicals described itself as "a coalition of fire professionals, educators, community activists, burn centers, doctors, fire departments and industry leaders, united to ensure that our country is protected by the highest standards of fire safety." Yet the (now defunct, after being exposed) Citizens for Fire Safety had only three members: the three largest flame retardant manufacturers.[31]

In a tactic known as strategic lawsuits against public participation (SLAPP suits), industry tries to censor, intimidate, or silence critics by suing them, thereby draining their financial resources for legal defense. Yet another tactic is spreading "disinformation" about tobacco, climate change, evolution, and other subjects.[32]

An 1886 Supreme Court ruling gave corporations certain rights as "persons"—"corporate personhood"—allowing corporations' interests to trump citizens' interests in some situations.[33] A series of decisions beginning in the 1800s culminated with the *Citizens United v. Federal Election Commission* decision in 2010, which allows outside groups to anonymously pour unlimited sums of money into political campaigns, thereby influencing elections. Bill Moyers calls the *Citizens United* decision "grotesque," and at least 16 states and 680 localities have passed referenda to roll back this decision.[34]

In 2012, Moyers interviewed David Stockman, former President Ronald Reagan's budget director, who said our situation has become much worse over the last two to three decades. "The Federal Reserve is basically working on behalf of Wall Street, not Main Street," Stockman said. "The Congress is owned lock, stock, and barrel by one after another after another special interest.... I think we have to eliminate all contributions above $100 and get corporations out of politics entirely." He calls for a constitutional amendment "to cleanse our political system on a one-time basis from this enormously corrupting influence that has built up."[35]

> *The Congress is owned lock, stock, and barrel by one after another after another special interest. —David Stockman, former budget director for US President Ronald Reagan*

Reporter, editor, and producer Hedrick Smith writes that approximately fifty US multi-national corporations over the last decade legally dodged taxes through a merger with a foreign firm called a "corporate inversion." Smith describes an American corporation "gaming the system" for handouts ($300 million) and bailouts ($100 million) "and then walking out on Uncle Sam and all of us," thereby saving $150 million in taxes each year and handsomely rewarding the CEO for making the deal. In 2014, US companies were hoarding $2.1 trillion in profits offshore, which would have generated $620 billion in US taxes.[36]

These developments concentrate wealth and power in the hands of a few, with the rich getting ever richer. Political economy professor Gar Alperovitz says that "the top 400 people own more of this country than the bottom 180 million Americans taken together."[37] The graph below compares after-tax income in 1979 and 2007, in the lead-up to the Great Recession, for different income groups. In summary, the richer you were, the more your income grew. The income of the poorest fifth of the population grew by 16 percent during that twenty-eight-year period. The richest 1 percent of the population enjoyed a 281 percent increase during that same period.[38] Study coauthor Paul Pierson said, "If you really want the show stopper you have to go one step further because ... the real action is inside the top 1 percent. If you go to the top tenth of 1 percent or the top hundredth of 1 percent, you know, you would need a much bigger graph to show what's happening to incomes for that more select group. Because they've gone up much faster than have incomes for just your average top 1 percent kind of person."[39]

In 2012, economist Robert Reich pointed out that of all the developed nations, the United States has the most unequal distribution of income "and we're surging toward even greater inequality." He said that peak years of income inequality were 1928 and 2007, the years preceding the Great Depression and the Great Recession, and the parallels between these times are "breathtaking."[40] Subsequently, in 2013, income inequality increased even more.[41]

Many US citizens—from hard left to hard right—are deeply dissatisfied with both the government and the economy. They are suffering from income inequality, job insecurity, and financial losses from the Great Recession.

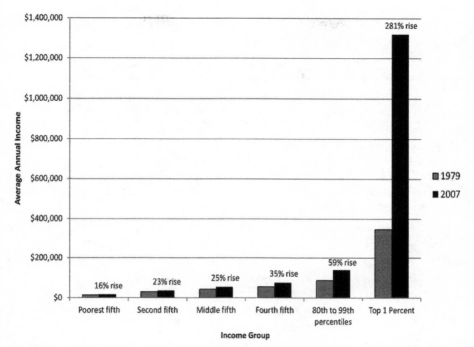

Lead-up to the Great Recession: Average Household After-Tax Income, Including Public and Private Benefits, in 1979 and in 2007. Used with permission. Hacker, Jacob S. and Paul Pierson. 2010. *Winner-Take-All-Politics*. New York: Simon & Schuster. Calculated from Congressional Budget Office. 2009. *Historical Effective Tax Rates, 1979–2006*. Washington, DC: Congressional Budget Office.

Some developed countries have more upward mobility than the United States, where 42 percent of children born into poverty will still be in poverty as adults. And middle class people are worried about falling into poverty as their incomes shrink. Reich says people are concluding something is fundamentally wrong with the economy—that the game is rigged by collusion between government, big business, and Wall Street.[42] Creating barriers to voting, through voter ID laws and other hassles, and gerrymandering, the manipulation of electoral district boundaries in order to provide a political advantage to a particular party or group, further entrench the status quo.[43]

HEALTH

Health outcomes go hand in hand with degradation of environmental and health safeguards and growing corporate power and income inequality. The World Health Organization estimates 1 in 4 human deaths globally is caused by living or working in an unhealthy environment, with environmental risk factors such as air, water, and soil pollution; chemical exposures; climate change; and ultraviolet radiation contributing to more than one hundred disease and injury types.[44]

> *The World Health Organization estimates 1 in 4 human deaths globally is caused by living or working in an unhealthy environment.*

Furthermore, physician and educator Mark Hyman, MD, writes, "The injustices that violate our health as a human right occur not just in impoverished countries like Haiti, but are embedded in twenty-first century America. And we are exporting disease across the globe, where the overweight—now 1.7 billion large—outnumber the malnourished. I would argue not only that health is a neglected human right, but that it is a right that has been taken from us. Our health has been hijacked—slowly, quietly, and often deliberately over the past century. Our social, political and economic conditions support obesity and disease. Almost three-quarters of Americans are overweight, and 1 in 2 Americans has one or more chronic diseases."[45]

In 1900, the global average lifespan was thirty-one years, and it was less than fifty years in even the richest countries. By 2005, the global average lifespan had increased to sixty-six years, and to more than eighty years in some countries, thanks to public health measures that include water and wastewater treatment and antibiotics.[46] However, according to a *New England Journal of Medicine* special report about life expectancy in the United States, "As a result of the substantial rise in the prevalence of obesity and its life-shortening complications such as diabetes, life expectancy at birth and at older ages could level off or even decline within the first half of this century."[47] Problems can start early. A third of nine-month-old American babies are already overweight or obese.[48]

Concurrently, health-care expenditures, in constant dollars, have increased dramatically, which is no surprise given our unhealthy lifestyles.[49] Dr. Hyman calls chronic lifestyle disease "an epidemic that now kills twice as many around the world every year as infectious disease. Chronic disease is a slow motion disaster, a tsunami of suffering whose global cost will be $47 trillion over the next 20 years." He writes that in less than 30 years, from 1983 to 2011, worldwide cases of diabetes increased ten-fold, with further increases projected in future decades. "When the collective cost of diabesity-related disease—heart disease, cancer, dementia, strokes, infertility, depression, and more is accounted for, it is the single biggest contributor to our health-care expenditures and our national debt."[50] (Diabesity is the continuum of health problems ranging from mild insulin resistance and being overweight to obesity and diabetes.)

Americans spend 18 percent of their gross domestic product—which is the monetary value of all goods and services produced in the United States—on health care, a percentage that may reach 30 percent.[51] Unhealthy lifestyles and chronic disease are not the only problems. Another is medical error, which, if it were considered a disease, would be the third leading cause of death in the United States, behind only heart disease and cancer.[52] The practice of medicine is beginning to change as health-care costs go through the roof and as progressive doctors—some having cured their own illnesses using alternative methods after conventional methods failed—become more prevalent and their successes become more widely known.

OVERCONSUMPTION

According to scientist David Suzuki, "we try to overwhelm nature with the power of our crude technologies." And we overwhelm nature by overconsuming. Suzuki explains the historical roots of our overconsumption. What got us out of the Great Depression after the stock market crash of 1929 was World War II, "and by the middle of the war, the American economy was blazing, white hot, pumping out guns and tanks and planes and weapons." When it became clear by the mid-1940s the Allies were going to win the war, people began to wonder how to keep the economy going in peacetime. The US President established a council of economic advisors to plan. "And the answer came back—consumption.... We've got to make consumption an American way of life. Get people to buy stuff, use it up, throw it away, and buy more stuff."[53] Planned obsolescence, the policy of designing products—light bulbs, clothes, and more—so they will become unfashionable or no longer functional after a limited period of time, became standard practice. The economy boomed as Americans expended resources like crazy, taking what we wanted from the Earth and dumping back what we didn't want. Economic advantage went to those who went through more resources and thus sold more products. This mode of operation can only continue for a finite period of time, until natural resources become depleted or degraded. Then what?

The ultimate engineering challenge presents itself now: How can we surmount the array of problems we've created and advance to the next level of technological sophistication, creating products, services, and systems that support rather than degrade our life-support system?

RATES OF CHANGE

In nature, change can be huge and sudden rather than gradual. Caterpillars become butterflies, eggs hatch, chicks fly, and seeds germinate. Vegetarian, aquatic tadpoles transform into carnivorous, amphibious frogs.

Sudden changes are often preceded by a long period of tension buildup. An earthquake abruptly shakes the Earth after pressure between tectonic plates has intensified over long periods of time.

Often, our perception is capricious. We tend to assume that change occurs over time in a linear way: 1, 2, 3, 4, 5, 6. But sometimes change is exponential: 1, 2, 4, 8, 16, 32, 64. Exponential change—both desirable and undesirable—can occur shockingly quickly and can take us by surprise. If you take a penny and double it every day, in a month you have $10 million.

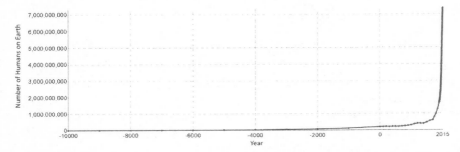

Growth of the Human Population in the Last 12,000 Years. Credit: Our World In Data. https://ourworldindata.org/world-population-growth/.

The graph above shows that the global human population did not change much over millennia—until the advent of the Industrial Revolution in the 1700s, when the population exploded. Similarly, atmospheric carbon dioxide concentrations in the atmosphere held fairly steady until around the same time, when they began to skyrocket—and most especially during the last century. Carbon dioxide concentrations in the atmosphere are much higher than before the Industrial Revolution and higher than at any time in at least the last 800,000 years.[54] And the rate of global carbon emissions is higher than at any time in fossil records, stretching back sixty-six million years to the age of the dinosaurs.[55]

Computer, Internet, and cell phone use has followed the model of exponential change. People are suddenly much more able to access information, express themselves, and connect with people all over the globe.

Running Out of Time

It's not too late for us to turn our situation around. Nature tends to self-heal once damaging activity ceases, just as a person's body tends to heal when he or she quits smoking cigarettes. The bald eagle population began to bounce back after the pesticide DDT was banned in the United States. If we appreciate our situation for the near-death situation it truly is, we will act now. Nobel

Prize–winning physicist Max Planck wrote, "A new scientific truth does not triumph by convincing its opponents and making them see the light, but rather because its opponents eventually die, and a new generation grows up that is familiar with it." In medicine, it can take more than 20 years for scientific findings to be incorporated into most physicians' practices.[56] Well, we don't have that kind of time.

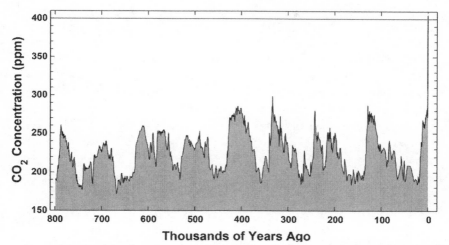

Atmospheric carbon dioxide concentrations during the last 800,000 years showing the rises and falls associated with several ice ages and the dramatic spike of the last 100 years to more than 400 parts per million (ppm). Credit: Scripps Institution of Oceanography, University of California, San Diego. Based on numerous data sets referenced at https://scripps.ucsd.edu/programs/keelingcurve/2015/05/12/what-does-this-number-mean/.

On the other hand, we can't allow opportunists to push ill-considered and damaging projects through hurriedly because we're "running out of time." Some alternative-energy projects—wind and solar power developments sited on pristine forestland—are hastily approved by gung-ho regulatory agencies without careful environmental review.[57] Intelligence is called for, even if we are in a hurry. *Especially* if we are in a hurry.

Although the human population has exploded since the Industrial Revolution, the more than seven billion people alive now are only a small fraction of all the people who have ever lived. An estimated one hundred billion people have lived on Earth over the last 50,000 years, many sacrificing mightily so we could be here.

Some Native Americans traditionally thought and planned ahead in terms of seven generations, choosing actions that would benefit seven generations to follow them. That is a pretty good approximation of thinking sustainably, and far preferable to the short-term "grab the resources and run" mentality that drives our way of life now.

Short-Term Thinking. In 2007, I sat on a committee to develop a "master plan" for my town. We solicited input from town residents and reviewed a number of plans other towns in our area had developed. One specified a planning horizon of one hundred years. Most did not specify a planning horizon at all. When I suggested adopting a hundred-year planning horizon for our town, a committee member was aghast and said ten years was long enough.

With a rapid and major course correction, we can create a sustainable world and better lives for ourselves and others. We have a long legacy of evolutionary success and have invented language, mathematics, and incredible art and music. We've put rovers on Mars. We have miraculous technologies—computers and the Internet—that empower and connect us. We absolutely can succeed again.

CHAPTER 2
OUR WORLD

Only to the white man was nature a wilderness and only to
him was the land "infested" with "wild" animals and "savage"
people. To us it was tame, Earth was bountiful and we were
surrounded with the blessings of the Great Mystery.

—*Black Elk, Oglala Lakota Sioux (1863–1950)*

HUMAN HEALTH UTTERLY DEPENDS ON environmental health. We
incorporate the environment into our bodies every minute of every day—air
with every breath we take and water with every sip we drink. We ultimately
take in soil with every bite of food we eat (except possibly seafood). We
take in information from the environment through our senses. What's more,
our bodies host ecosystems comprised of hundreds of nonhuman species.
Our entire body is composed of the environment. The environment *is* us,
not something out there, not a place where we go on vacation. By the same
token, humans shape the environment, for better or worse. So, in a sense,
environmental health expresses the health, intelligence, and actions of
humans. Environmental health and human health represent two sides of the
same coin.

This chapter focuses on the current status of our world and shows how
each of us is affected by damages to our life-support system. I am like the
doctor who says, "You know, if you don't do something about your high
blood pressure now, it's going to kill you, and soon." Please do not become
disheartened by this information. Later chapters show our world includes a
lot that is good and we can create the future we want.

METALS

Metals are substances with high electrical conductivity, luster, and malleability. Elements, including metals, are formed when stars die. Earth is made up of elements formed deep within the cores of dead stars.

People began mastering the use of metals around 7000 years ago, after the advent of agriculture. Prehistoric peoples used gold, silver, copper, tin, lead, and iron. The Iron Age began around 3500 years ago.[58] Iron was a key ingredient in the Industrial Revolution. Today, we use iron, steel, and other metals for buildings, transportation, piping, energy generation, appliances, electronics, and many types of equipment, machines, and weapons.

Some radionuclides (but not all) are metals. A radionuclide is an atom with an unstable nucleus that undergoes radioactive decay, emitting gamma rays and/or subatomic particles ("ionizing radiation"). Some radionuclides occur naturally; we artificially produce others in nuclear reactors, particle accelerators, and radionuclide generators. The world's first full-scale nuclear reactor for weapons production, at the Hanford Nuclear Reservation in Washington, produced plutonium for the atomic bomb dropped on Nagasaki in 1945.[59] The first nuclear reactor to produce electricity did so in 1951.[60]

Use of radionuclides leaves radioactive waste behind for future generations to deal with. The radioactive isotope strontium-90, which can cause cancer, did not exist before the nuclear era. Now, all humans have measurable amounts of strontium-90 in their bones.[61]

We have too much metal in our lives. We contaminate our bodies and ecosystems by bringing too much metal from relatively deep beneath Earth's surface up to the surface. Metals contamination in the environment typically results from mining and ore processing; industrial operations (metal recycling, recovery, smelting, finishing, and plating); agricultural pesticides containing lead and arsenic; burning coal, wood, and trash; and leaded fuels and paints. US government scientists tested fish in 291 streams throughout the United States and found mercury in every one.[62]

Mercury is implicated in many severe neurologic disorders. Fifteen percent of child-bearing women in the United States have toxic concentrations of mercury in their blood, exposing 600,000 American children each year before they are even born. Americans still allow mercury fillings ("amalgam") in children's teeth, although some other countries have banned this practice. The United States allowed mercury in children's vaccines until 2001.

Lead, another neurotoxin, is linked to an array of severe cognitive and behavioral problems in children. Lead is also linked to heart disease, heart attacks, strokes, and death. One study estimates that almost 40 percent of American adults have lead concentrations high enough to cause these problems. Bones of Americans today contain a thousand times as much lead as bones of preindustrial humans. Banning lead from gasoline and paint has helped, but lead remains a significant problem.[63]

Other heavy metals include arsenic, hexavalent chromium, and cadmium, all of which are known human carcinogens. Some heavy metals are linked to learning problems, attention deficit disorders, and violent behaviors in children.[64]

In many ways, metals bring us together by enabling transportation and communication. By the same token, they tear relationships apart by facilitating mobility. Family members often live very far apart and don't stay put. All this mobility tends to make us lose a sense of attachment to place. "This is my home, where I am from and where I live" is an alien concept to many.

WATER

Water is life. Yet most Americans take for granted that unlimited quantities of high-quality water—that finite and 100 percent necessary resource with zero substitutes—will always be available, right where we want it. When one day you turn the faucet handle and clean water does not come out, complacency will instantly change to respect for water.

Water comprises approximately 60 percent (women) and 66 percent (men) of the human body. Since we are more than half water, perhaps we should pay more attention to it!

Water arrived during Earth's formation, aboard meteorites and small bodies called "planetisimals."[65] The finite amount of water on Earth is constantly recycled. The vast majority of water at the Earth's surface is salt water, and of the remaining 2.5 percent, more than half is frozen. Much of the rest is groundwater. Far, far less than 1 percent of all water is fresh water in lakes, rivers, and streams. "Every drop of water that's here has seen the inside of a cloud, and the inside of a volcano, the inside of a maple leaf, and the inside of a dinosaur kidney, probably many times," writes journalist Charles Fishman.

Water has amazing and unique properties. Pure water is transparent, with no taste or smell and neutral pH. It is the only natural substance found on Earth in all three states (solid, liquid, and gas) at normal temperatures. The solid form (ice) is less dense than the liquid form, which is unusual (and causes ice to float). Most of Earth's water is actually in a fourth form, hydrated minerals ("watery rocks"), thought to be in a 150-mile thick layer from 250 miles deep to about 400 miles deep.[66]

My Attitude Toward Water. As a kid, I experienced both extremes, of too much and too little water. During the school year, we lived on a road that flooded periodically. I have surreal memories of canoeing through the rooms of our house. By contrast, at another place, before we got a well, utilities, or a house, we camped out and hauled all our water in large containers from a spring. I learned just how much energy it takes to move water.

Water is so pervasive that it is almost invisible and many of us take it for granted. I know I did. When I worked for an environmental nonprofit organization after college, the executive director was very concerned about water issues. I thought to myself, Get a life, dude! But as I learned more about the nature and extent of our water problems—or rather, mismanagement— my attitude changed completely. So much so that I pursued a career in water, a career that still continues.

In the United States, we frequently mismanage water. We employ inefficient irrigation practices or pricing policies that encourage increased water use. Water is lost via leaks in water distribution systems. Perverse agricultural policies promote the squandering of water resources even where they are scarce.[67] Globally, human consumption is rapidly depleting one-third of the largest groundwater basins.[68] In response, we keep drilling deeper wells in a "race to the bottom."[69]

Wetlands have not fared well either. Wetlands perform flood control, erosion control, water filtration, and groundwater recharge, and they provide wildlife habitat and recreation. From the time of European settlement in the early 1600s until the mid-1980s, the area that was to become the 48 contiguous United States lost more than half of its wetland acreage. The federal government historically encouraged land drainage and wetland destruction through a variety of legislative and policy instruments. The loss of wetlands continues today, even though we now appreciate their importance.[70]

We have allowed water to become contaminated with sewage, trash, pesticides, fertilizers, petroleum products, solvents, heavy metals, plasticizers, pharmaceuticals, radionuclides, and countless other contaminants. By 2050, there may be more waste plastic in the oceans than fish (by weight), if current trends continue.[71] Water can always be cleaned, but at what cost? And who pays? In many cases, no one—in which case the water isn't cleaned.

The Cuyahoga River in Ohio was so polluted with oil, trash, and other wastes that it caught on fire thirteen times from 1868 to 1969. The latest fire helped spur the environmental movement and passage of the Clean Water Act in 1972.[72] In New York, General Electric legally discharged more than one million pounds of PCBs into the Hudson River from 1947 to 1977, turning a 200-mile stretch of river into a Superfund site.[73]

Half of all fresh and saline water consumed in the United States is for cooling power plants.[74] Power plants typically evaporate much of the water and return the rest of it, contaminated and heated, to rivers and oceans—a practice that harms aquatic life.

We also allow air pollution to degrade water, for example, in the form of acid rain. We spend almost as much on bottled water as on maintaining our water systems as a whole, leaving behind mountains of waste plastic containers.

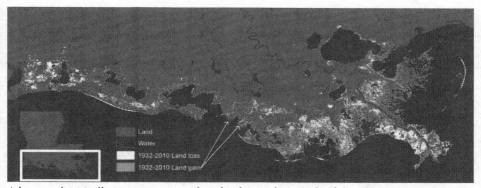

A large and critically important coastal wetland near the mouth of the Mississippi River serves as a breeding ground and nursery for fisheries in the Gulf of Mexico, an important stopover location for migrating birds, and a critical buffer of inland locations against storm damage. Between 1932 and 2010, 1883 square miles of wetland have been lost. This is approximately equal to the land area of Delaware. Some of the major causes of wetland loss, among others, include land subsidence, sea level rise, storms, sediment deprivation, and oil and gas extraction and infrastructure. Data provided courtesy of USGS. Couvillion, B.R., J.A. Barras, G.D. Steyer, William Sleavin, Michelle Fischer, Holly Beck, Nadine Trahan, Brad Griffin, and David Heckman. 2011. Land Area Change in Coastal Louisiana from 1932 to 2010: USGS Scientific Investigations Map 3164, Scale 1:265,000, 12 p. pamphlet.

More than 1 in 7 people on Earth lack access to clean water, and more than 1 in 5 have to walk an appreciable distance to get it. (Wildlife face similar challenges.) The job of hauling water in many countries falls on women and girls, often keeping them out of school. A plane crash makes front page news, while many people are unaware that 1.8 million children—the equivalent of 3500 Boeing 747 airplanes fully loaded—die each year from lack of water or from diseases contracted from drinking contaminated water.[75]

Toxic chemicals from our modern lifestyle get into our water supplies and our blood. Laboratory analysis of human umbilical cord blood shows infants are exposed to contaminants before they even draw their first breath. The Environmental Working Group detected 287 toxic chemicals in cord blood, 217 of which are toxic to the brain and nervous system, 180 of which cause cancer in humans or other animals, and 208 of which cause birth defects or developmental problems in nonhuman animals. The detected chemicals include mercury, BPA, flame retardants, dioxins, organochlorine pesticides such as DDT and chlordane, and PCBs, among others.[76]

SOIL

Soil is a thin layer of disintegrated rock and organic material on the Earth's surface in which plants have their roots. Healthy soil teems with life that includes bacteria, fungi, protozoa, algae, nematodes, mites, springtails, spiders, millipedes, beetles, earthworms, flies, snails, and slugs, not to mention plants, and vertebrates such as mice, moles, voles, chipmunks, and ground squirrels.

Soil, like water and air, is something we industrialized citizens typically take for granted and grossly mismanage. We derisively call it "dirt," as if it were something bad rather than the source of over 99 percent of our food.

Geographer Jared Diamond, in his book *Collapse: How Societies Choose to Fail or Succeed*, documents the role of soil problems—erosion, fertility loss, and salt accumulation—in the demise of civilizations in different times and places around the globe.[77] Recently, industrialized agriculture has degraded soil through the use of pesticides and synthetic fertilizers and has allowed soil to erode, much of it ending up in rivers, lakes, streams, and oceans.

Mounting evidence shows how our health depends on the health of the soil in which our food is grown. Soil teeming with diverse life is more likely to produce nutrient-dense food. Children raised on ecologically managed farms in Central Europe have much lower rates of allergy and asthma than children raised on industrial farms or in urban areas. This is attributed to the larger numbers of beneficial soil microbes and other microbes on the ecologically managed farms.[78]

Human flesh is contaminated with hundreds of synthetic chemicals, which we take up via ingestion, inhalation, and skin contact. Just in our food, the average American each year consumes pounds of hormones, antibiotics, food chemicals, additives, artificial sweeteners, and monosodium glutamate.[79] Data on toxic chemicals in human body fats provide definitive evidence that humans are now exposed to hundreds of synthetic pollutants—pesticides, plasticizers, PCBs, chlorinated solvents, benzene, and many others.[80]

PLANTS

We assume plants have been on Earth for a long time. Actually, plant life has been on land only for about the last tenth of Earth's 4.6-billion-year life, arriving about 475 MYA. Before that, plant life was limited to marine algae, and the land surface looked more like Mars than the Earth we know today.

Plants evolved from algae through liverworts, ferns, seed ferns, horsetails, gymnosperms (such as conifers), and, finally, angiosperms (flowering plants). Flowering plants have been here for only about 130 million years, arriving after amphibians, reptiles, mammals, and birds. They remain dominant today and account for 95 percent of vascular plant species.

Plants paved the way for land animals to evolve by increasing oxygen concentrations in the Earth's atmosphere. Plants have astounding abilities. They make their own food from sunlight, carbon dioxide, and water; defend themselves from attack by other organisms; keep from freezing in winter; and pump water against the force of gravity, sometimes long distances. We're even learning that trees are social beings that actively communicate and share nutrients with other trees who are sick or struggling.[81]

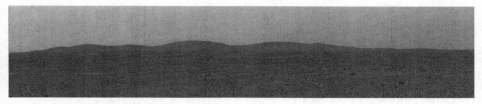

Bleak Mars. Photo credit: NASA. http://nssdc.gsfc.nasa.gov/planetary/mars/mars_exploration_rovers/mera_images.html.

Plants help the climate by removing carbon dioxide from the atmosphere and storing it in the plants themselves and in soil (from decomposing leaves and other plant matter).[82] The only other significant carbon dioxide removal mechanism is dissolution into oceans, a process that acidifies the water, damaging and killing marine life. Forests serve as Earth's heat shield; they lower ambient temperatures. We often think of rain forests as being the key players in helping the climate, but temperate and boreal forests are likewise critically important.

Plants purify the air by taking up air pollutants. They hold the soil together, preventing erosion, and they enrich the soil by recycling nutrients such as nitrogen through the shedding of leaves and seeds. Plants, especially trees, regulate the water cycle, preventing flooding and enhancing the recharge of surface water and groundwater, and purifying the water in the process. They provide habitat and food for wildlife. For humans, they provide medicine, food, and wood, and planted landscapes provide spiritual, aesthetic, and recreational opportunities.[83]

Humans have been cutting down forests for centuries, for agriculture and pasture land, lumber, and land area to colonize. Immediate effects of deforestation include loss of plant and animal life. Deforestation also impoverishes the soil by removing from the ecosystem the nutrients in the trees, nutrients that would otherwise be recycled back into the soil. When the forest is no longer there to absorb rainwater and hold the soil surface together, flooding and soil erosion can occur, washing away nutrients and other essentials for life. What was once forest may become desert, as has occurred in Ethiopia and Haiti.

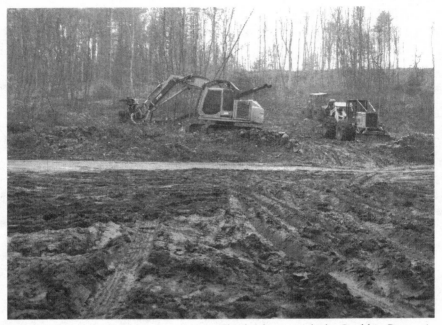

Deforestation at the Quabbin Reservation. This land surrounds the Quabbin Reservoir, which is the drinking water supply for the metropolitan Boston area in Massachusetts. Photo credit: Chris Matera.

Deforestation is a "double whammy." It accounts for at least 10 percent of global greenhouse gas emissions, while simultaneously reducing the future ability of forests to remove carbon dioxide from the atmosphere.[84] This ability is considerable; US forests remove and store 12 percent of total US greenhouse gas emissions.[85] Undisturbed, mature forests store more carbon than do forests that have been logged, and trees can continue to take up carbon and store it in wood and soil for 400 years or more.[86]

Destructive logging practices, such as clear-cutting, are often justified by dubious, quasi-scientific rationales that may sound plausible but on inspection turn out to be false.[87] Forestry academics generate copious literature in support of destructive logging; however, much of their funding comes from the forest products industry. Taking their advice is like taking financial advice from someone who makes commissions on selling financial products. Forest ecologists, who don't have such vested interests, often say forests are better off when left alone.[88]

The Earth has lost 46 percent of its trees since human civilization began, and rapid deforestation has occurred in recent decades.[89] Boreal, temperate, and rain forests alike are being butchered, and all are ecologically crucial.[90] Today's global deforestation is driven largely by the production of palm oil, timber and paper products, soybeans, cattle, and bioenergy.[91] Bioenergy is energy made available from biological materials; primary bioenergy technologies include burning wood for heat and electricity and using plants to make biofuels.

We are killing plants of all types, not just trees. As many as 68 percent of the world's flowering plants are now threatened or endangered—due to habitat loss and degradation and competition from invasive species—thanks to humans.[92]

As many as 68 percent of the world's flowering plants are now threatened or endangered.

Plants provide health-promoting chemical micronutrients—vitamins, minerals, and phytochemicals. (Phytochemicals are chemical compounds produced by plants.) Joel Fuhrman, MD, says strawberries contain about 700 micronutrients and broccoli contains about 1000, whereas processed food and meat contain very few. He writes, "Low levels of phytochemicals in our modern diet are largely responsible for the common diseases seen with aging, especially cancer and heart disease. These are diseases caused by nutritional ignorance and, in the majority of cases, can be prevented."[93]

ANIMALS

Simple animals evolved on Earth about 600 MYA, starting with the amoeba. Simple animals evolved to arthropods (ancestors of insects, arachnids, and crustaceans) and then to fish, amphibians, reptiles, and mammals.

Approximately 99.9 percent of all plant and animal species that have ever lived on Earth are extinct.[94] We don't have a comprehensive catalog of species currently on Earth and don't even know how many there are. To date, two million species have been classified. Estimates of the total number of species range up to one hundred million.[95] Animals serve critical functions in Earth's web of life—fertilizing soil and helping plants reproduce by spreading pollen and seeds, among others.

Like plant species, the number of animal species is decreasing. The World Wildlife Fund reports that between 1970 and 2010, populations of mammals, birds, reptiles, amphibians, and fish around the globe dropped by 52 percent. Earth's terrestrial wildlife population declined by 39 percent, Earth's marine wildlife population declined by 39 percent, and Earth's freshwater wildlife population plummeted by 76 percent, all while Earth's human population increased by 185 percent.[96]

> Between 1970 and 2010, populations of mammals, birds, reptiles, amphibians, and fish around the globe dropped by 52 percent.

Many Americans are ignorant of the wonders of the animal world. Take ants, which collectively weigh as much as Earth's humans. Ants began farming about fifty million years before humans did. Biologists Bert Holldobler and E. O. Wilson go so far as to call the most advanced insect societies "civilized." Leaf-cutter ants cultivate fungi in hygienic, air-conditioned nests that feature waste-disposal systems. They communicate mainly via smell, with "staggering" efficiency—a milligram of pheromone they use to mark their paths would lay a trail sixty times around Earth. Many ant species live in communist-like societies because the ants lack reproductive independence; worker ants are sterile and are forced to live in centralized societies with their queen.[97]

Another example of an amazing insect species is the monarch butterfly. Over three (or so) generations, they make the 2500-mile trip from Mexico to Canada. Then the fourth generation of these seemingly flimsy bits of life makes the arduous trip back. These remarkable creatures are threatened by logging in their southern homeland in Mexico and by industrial agriculture along their migratory route.[98]

Dolphins have been declared the world's second most intelligent animals after humans. Bottlenose dolphins can recognize themselves in a mirror and learn a rudimentary symbol-based language. They can solve difficult problems and "cooperate in ways that imply complex social structures and a high level of emotional sophistication."[99]

Humans' strong affinity for other animals is abundantly evident in our household pets, zoos, mascots, names of sports teams and rock bands, stuffed animals, cartoon characters, and totems. Our dependence on domesticated animals is obvious, for food, transportation, and labor. Dogs, a form of the gray wolf, may have been the first animal humans domesticated. Americans spend more on pets than the gross domestic products of many countries in the world.[100]

Most people in the United States eat industrially produced meat and dairy from animals typically raised in unspeakably inhumane and unhealthy crowded conditions in which no cameras or cell phones are allowed. Industrial animal products can contain pesticides, administered hormones, and antibiotics.

Our relationships with other animals are clearly out of whack. We're growing too many of some (for food) in too little space, killing off others with poison, and, in the course of our activities, destroying others unintentionally (manatees, to name just one species in a depressingly long list).

AIR

Earth's atmosphere (air) constitutes a thin veneer around Earth. There is no clear boundary between Earth's atmosphere and "outer space," because the atmosphere gradually thins out as the force of gravity weakens with distance.

Earth's original atmosphere was likely just hydrogen and helium. Earth's volcanoes then released water vapor, carbon dioxide, and ammonia.[101] Oxygen, first produced by cyanobacteria (blue-green algae), did not appear on Earth until about 2.7 BYA, and oxygen took up residence in the atmosphere later, about 2.5 BYA.[102] As oxygen concentrations in the atmosphere increased, carbon dioxide concentrations decreased. It took about a billion years for oxygen concentrations to increase to levels high enough for the evolution of animals. In addition, ultraviolet rays split some of the oxygen (O_2) molecules high in the atmosphere into single oxygen (O) atoms, which subsequently combined with oxygen (O_2) molecules to form ozone (O_3) molecules, which shield Earth from irradiation by ultraviolet rays. This protective ozone shield is thought to have formed by 600 MYA, enabling organisms to live on land rather than just in water. Dry air consists of 78 percent nitrogen, 21 percent oxygen, and 1 percent other gases. Other gases include carbon dioxide, which constitutes 0.04 percent of dry air, a number that is growing. Air also includes variable amounts of water vapor.

Combustion not only damages the climate with greenhouse gases, but it also releases other air pollutants that directly harm health. Coal-burning power plants produce fine particulates estimated (in 2011) to kill about 10,000 people each year in the United States alone.[103]

The USEPA designates six air pollutants as "criteria pollutants": fine particulates, ground-level ozone, carbon monoxide, sulfur oxides, nitrogen oxides, and lead. Other air pollutants include volatile organic compounds (VOCs), radionuclides, chlorofluorocarbons, and other heavy metals besides lead. Air pollution damages the heart, lungs, and brain and is a leading risk factor for stroke worldwide.[104]

Increasing concentrations of greenhouse gases—carbon dioxide, methane, nitrous oxide, and fluorinated gases—are changing our climate. Climate change threatens just about everything we depend on: land (from sea-level rise, among other effects), forests, oceans, terrestrial and marine species, food, cities, infrastructure, and human health.[105] The World Health Organization estimates that climate change will cause 250,000 deaths per year between 2030 and 2050 and that by 2030 the direct damage costs to health will be $2 billion to $4 billion per year.[106]

> *The World Health Organization estimates that climate change will cause 250,000 deaths per year between 2030 and 2050.*

The UN Food and Agriculture Organization warns of "potentially catastrophic" impacts on food production.[107] Public health professor Dickson D. Despommier says that for each 1 degree Celsius increase in temperature, Earth loses 10 percent of its arable land, and that "if climate change and population growth progress at their current pace, in roughly 50 years farming as we know it will no longer exist."[108]

Predicted impacts on water supplies are equally dire. Mountain snowpacks become increasingly unreliable as water supplies for dependent population centers downhill. Sea levels may rise by six feet by 2100 as snow and ice disappear and water expands as it becomes warmer, threatening coastal nations and cities.[109]

Diseases and deadly insects expand their territories, and ocean acidification threatens coral reefs, the marine food chain, and all who depend on that chain. All of these factors make climate change potentially the greatest economic threat imaginable. Consider the costs of having to recover from ever more numerous or more serious weather disasters, repeatedly reconstructing buildings and infrastructure or retreating inland. How about the costs to produce fresh water using expensive and energy-intensive desalination plants, or of dealing with increased epidemics of infectious diseases or millions of displaced environmental refugees?

Climate change also threatens our social fabric. Journalist Christian Parenti argues that climate change is already responsible for a degree of political and economic breakdown in the world due to competition over impacted resources such as water. He believes that some crises are exacerbated by climate change, if not caused by it.[110]

Clearly, we can't continue using the atmosphere as a sewer, as tempting as that is since air pollutants seem to go "away" quickly and often are invisible and difficult to trace back to their source.

FIRE

Humans' use of fire sets us apart from other organisms. It allows us to cook, greatly expanding our repertoire of edible foods, and provides warmth, protection, and light. We use fire for social purposes—at ceremonies, bonfires, and campfires—and antisocial ones—burning towns and villages, crops, and bridges. We use fire to incinerate wastes. We use fire to put to work the energy in coal, oil, natural gas, and wood.

Satellite photographs taken at night around the globe show large areas in flames from intentional fires, slash and burn agriculture, and unintentional forest fires.[111] The cityscape is a myriad of smokestacks of all sizes discharging carbon dioxide and other air pollutants from the burning of fossil fuels.

Inflammation is part of the body's response to injury. While familiar signs of inflammation are heat, pain, redness, and swelling, we don't sense some forms of inflammation. Fine particulates, caused mainly by combustion, are one cause of inflammation and can be linked to high blood pressure, diabetes, obesity, and brain problems.[112] Other triggers of inflammation include sugar, refined flours, food allergens, digestive problems, environmental toxins, infections, stress, inactivity, insufficient sleep, and nutritional deficiencies. Our addiction to sugar and flour for quick internal energy is analogous to our addiction to fossil fuels (and bioenergy) for quick external energy; both lead to inflammation.

Inflammation affects twenty-four million Americans with autoimmune diseases, fifty million with allergy diseases, thirty million with asthma, sixty million with cardiovascular and heart disease, ten million with cancer, and fourteen million with diabetes. Inflammation is connected to almost every known brain disease, from depression to anxiety and from schizophrenia to sociopathic behavior. Plus, the two-thirds of Americans who are overweight are also inflamed. "You might say we're all on fire" and we are facing an "epidemic of broken brains," concludes Dr. Hyman.[113]

Tobacco kills up to half its users, six million people each year worldwide.[114] Yet despite the undeniable harm, American taxpayers until 2014 were forced to subsidize tobacco farming.[115]

Nature Corrects Imbalances

This chapter explored how our health and environment suffer from exposure to too much metal and fire at the expense of water, earth, plants, animals, and air. These imbalances we have created will be corrected one way or another. While we have no choice in *whether* rebalancing occurs, we do have a choice in *how* rebalancing occurs.

In the case of climate disruption, one potential pathway is no human behavior change. That scenario likely ends in disaster for humans—droughts and floods ruining food crops, rising sea levels drowning cities, severe weather destroying infrastructure, and dealing with this chaos ravaging economies and escalating political strife over dwindling resources. Human health suffers, and greenhouse gas emissions eventually decrease as the human population shrinks. Vegetation and soil recover, removing carbon from the atmosphere. Though it could take eons, the climate stabilizes. In an alternative scenario, humans change their behavior and take less of a hit—putting out our fires, regenerating soil and the biosphere, and reducing our numbers to stabilize the climate. We choose—the hard way, or the easy way?

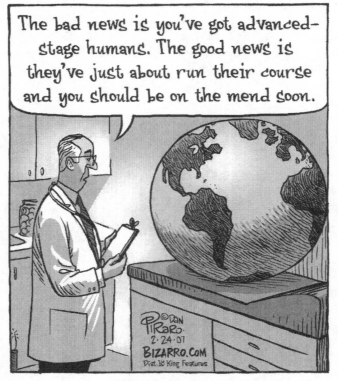

Earth at the Doctor's Office. Reprinted by permission of Dan Piraro.

Similarly, with regard to groundwater supplies, the "no action" alternative depletes the resource until water tables become too deep to access economically. As food becomes scarce and expensive, people die. Eventually, with less pressure on water resources, water tables rebound. Similar alternative pathways exist with soil and other resources we exploit unsustainably—presenting us with the choice of changing to sustainable resource use now or continuing on as is until we hit a wall.

The Gaia hypothesis, formulated by scientist James Lovelock and co-developed by biologist Lynn Margulis in the 1970s, holds that Earth's physical and biological processes evolved together and are tightly interconnected to form a self-regulating system that maintains conditions favorable for life on Earth.[116] We will either get with the program or Earth will get rid of us pesky humans. The difference between the human infestation and other infestations—say, by pathogens or insects—is that we have the ability to consciously change course.

CHAPTER 3
No Separate Existence

Human beings depend on Earth and its life-forms for every aspect
of their survival and life. It is impossible to draw lines that delineate
separate categories of air, water, soil, and life. You and I don't end at our
fingertips or skin—we are connected through air, water, and soil; we are
animated by the same energy from the same source in the sky above. We
are quite literally air, water, soil, energy, and other living creatures.

—*David Suzuki*

IN WESTERN WORLDVIEWS, WE SEE ourselves as sharply defined individuals,
each totally separate from everyone and everything else. This view is especially
pronounced in the United States, with its ideals of "rugged individualism"
and people "pulling themselves up by their own bootstraps." We similarly
view the rest of our world as a collection of sharply distinct and separate
things, and ourselves as a collection of separate parts. We have sliced and
diced our world and ourselves to the point of blindness to interconnections.

MISGUIDED BELIEFS

A misperception that humans are separate from and superior to nature and
other species fuels our disastrous lifestyle as we futilely try to impose our
will on the world around us. We extend this approach to others within our
species. Our history of technological innovation, especially agriculture,
led to increased division of labor, complex hierarchical societies with large
population centers, and magnified feelings of superiority of the privileged
few over commoners.

Despite America's values of equality and freedom, revered around the
world, and despite our heroic mythology, America was built on atrocities
justified by assumptions of superiority. White people came to this country,

slaughtered its rightful owners, and forced Native Americans and Africans into slavery.[117] Women were property with no rights or property of their own. It was mostly slaves who built the White House and the US Capitol.[118]

Our current paradigm reduces citizens to "consumers" and "human resources" and puts them last in importance. Filmmaker Michael Moore, in his documentary *Sicko,* says the current regime has people where it wants them, feeling hopeless, pessimistic, frightened, and demoralized.[119] Citizens take orders and hope for the best, putting up with the top 1 percent of the world's population who enjoy 80 percent of the wealth. As former British member of Parliament Tony Benn observed, "An educated, confident, and healthy nation is harder to govern."[120]

> *An educated, confident, and healthy nation is harder to govern.*
> —*Tony Benn*

Slavery is the ultimate example (besides killing) of separation and keeping people powerless. Many people are not aware that human trafficking flourishes today. Though slavery is banned in most countries, the world currently has about forty-five million slaves in at least 167 countries, more than at any time in human history.[121]

Not all human cultures engage in arrogance. New Zealand's Kiwis believe it is the responsibility of humans to protect the natural world and that the knowledge of the ancients may hold a key to the planet's survival.[122] A little humility would lead Westerners to sign scientist David Suzuki's "Declaration of Interdependence," which affirms our intent to preserve the Earth, based on the understanding we are completely dependent on and interconnected with nature.[123]

Indigenous people—sometimes known as tribal people, first people, or native people—have historical continuity with pre-colonial societies and constitute about 5 percent of the world's human population. As indigenous societies worldwide continue to be wrecked by the juggernaut of "civilized" resource plundering, humanity is losing its ancient knowledge of plants, animals, nature, and human adaptation. Logging and mining destroy the rain forests of indigenous people who have lived in them for thousands of years.[124]

Westerners believe that "survival of the fittest" means duking it out—between or among species, with the victor surviving and the loser dying. Yet this ignores countless real-life examples in which cooperation makes species fittest, as in the case of fungi and algae living in symbiotic partnership in the form of lichen. Our hierarchical, separation-based worldview promotes a way of life based on competition rather than harmony. We think in terms of the economy versus the environment, us versus them, humans versus nature, and the mind versus the body. What an exhausting way to live.

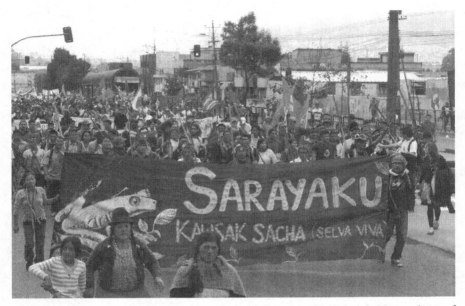

Thousands of indigenous people led by the Confederation of Indigenous Nationalities of Ecuador converged on the town of Quito, culminating a fifteen-day march demanding a new water law, land reform, and an end to open-pit mining and new oil concessions. Photo credit: ©Amazon Watch.

People on the forefront of science lament society's resistance to new information. We see this happening today with climate science denial—and even denial of evolution more than 150 years after publication of Charles Darwin's *The Origin of Species*. Of respondents to a recent poll of Americans, 45 percent agreed with this statement: "God created human beings pretty much in their present form at one time within the past 10,000 years or so."[125] Similarly, we often believe we're powerless to solve the global problems we face, even though history proves otherwise. Consider the Montreal Protocol on Substances that Deplete the Ozone Layer, an international agreement adopted in 1987 that has contributed to a significant drop in total global production and consumption of ozone-depleting substances.[126]

Author and researcher Lynne McTaggart writes that new ideas are "always considered heretical" and that "to be a revolutionary in science today is to flirt with professional suicide. Much as the field purports to encourage experimental freedom, the entire structure of science, with its highly competitive grant system, coupled with the publishing and peer review system, largely depends upon individuals conforming to the accepted scientific world view."[127]

We learn conformity at an early age. Many US schools "teach to the test," with students memorizing content asked for on standardized tests rather than learning how to question, learn, focus, listen, research, critically evaluate, and problem-solve. Author Napoleon Hill wrote that the public school system teaches children "almost everything except how to use their own minds and think independently."[128]

Knowledge is power and, according to a quote attributed to Thomas Jefferson, "Information is the currency of democracy." Democracy can't survive without free thought and a free press. The Federal Communications Commission fails to preserve competition in the citizen-owned airwaves, approving ever more media consolidation. Large absentee corporations feel freer to eliminate reporters, gut newsrooms, and replace substantive news and debate with celebrity gossip and pap.[129] Bill Moyers quotes his mentor, Paul Thompson at the University of Texas, who said, "News is what people want to keep hidden. Everything else is publicity."

We suffer from too much publicity and too little news about some of the dire issues impacting our lives. Network news typically ignores logging and mining travesties, decimation of indigenous societies, murders of environmental activists, wetlands violations, adverse health effects of synthetic chemicals, factory farming, and other health and environmental news. Network news reports those rare times when a shark bites a human, but it seldom mentions the wasteful slaughter of millions of sharks by the fishing industry that is driving some species toward extinction.[130] Climate change receives some coverage, but not with the depth the situation calls for. Luckily, alternative media provide more comprehensive reporting.

THE INDIVIDUAL HUMAN

We are designed not to "go it alone" but to live in full integration with other species and other humans. Humans and prehumans survived by cooperating and living in groups, not by living as isolated individuals.

And the individual human survives *only* by cooperating with other species. The healthy human body contains fifty trillion to one hundred trillion human cells living harmoniously.[131] Microbial cells outnumber human cells 10 to 1. More than ten thousand microbial species, mostly bacteria, occupy the human ecosystem, and microbes contribute more genes responsible for human survival than humans contribute.[132] Genes turn biological functions on and off. Beneficial microorganisms produce certain vitamins, bolster our immune response, keep harmful microorganisms in check, and more.

David Perlmutter, MD, writes that our relatively low number of human cells and genes indicates that we have "offloaded" the storage of much of our

DNA information to "the cloud" or an external hard drive that resides in gut bacteria. This microbiome, which is the genetic information contained within our gut bacteria, plays a huge role in our health outcomes. We live in a mutually beneficial relationship with these organisms whose mission is to keep us healthy, because we provide their home.[133]

Our food and lifestyle choices dictate the health and diversity of our gut microorganisms. Adverse changes in gut microorganisms have been associated with conditions such as autism, Alzheimer's disease, and inflammatory bowel disease.[134] Overuse of antibiotics may be fueling dramatic increases in many illnesses by destroying the body's beneficial bacteria.[135]

In addition, high-sugar, high-carbohydrate, and low-fiber diets; stress; steroids; birth control pills; and other pharmaceuticals may be promoting harmful yeast and fungi at the expense of beneficial bacteria.[136] Tom O'Bryan, DC, says gut dysfunction is the number one culprit in our culture today for many of the diseases we are battling.[137]

Though our body feels relatively constant and immutable, the average age of all the cells in an adult human's body may be as little as seven to ten years. Cells in our gut lining last only five days.[138] We are constantly cycling materials into and out of our bodies, including our bones.

When one considers all the other species living in us and on us, as well as all the things that go into and out of our body, we seem more like a habitat for small beings or a distribution center than a self-contained separate existence. In our delusional feeling of separateness and autonomy, we also don't notice how strongly we are shaped by external forces: our environment, family, friends, teachers, employers, religion, advertising, language, and the arts.

Our feeling of separation is not universal. In the unified worldview of the Lakota Sioux people, "each person is regarded as an intimate part of the natural world, not separate from it.... The community is the basic unit of study, not the individual.... The idea is that we are formed by relationships.... We are not individual, autonomous units."[139]

In the Western world, we identify more with our brain and mind as "ourselves" and view our body more like a machine subject to the laws of physics and chemistry. Similarly, we cut off our heart from our mind. Primatologist and conservationist Jane Goodall says science that explicitly excludes the heart is "very cold." Goodall says that "a disconnect between the human brain and the human heart ... can lead to serious problems. I truly believe that only when head and heart live in harmony can we reach our true human potential. And our potential is huge."[140]

Conventional medicine, in which most doctors specialize in one body part, system, or disease, further divides the person into a collection of disconnected parts. This may be okay for the treatment of a broken leg or another acute problem; however, this "silo" approach fails to fix many chronic illnesses. Andrew Weil, MD, writes, "Our health or lack of it is the result of biochemical interactions *and* genetics, dietary choices, exercise patterns, sleep habits, hopes, fears, families, friends, jobs, hobbies, cultures, ecosystems, and more." In addition, illnesses such as heart disease and depression are multifactorial health problems "rooted in complex interactions of biological, psychological, and social variables."[141]

> *I truly believe that only when head and heart live in harmony can we reach our true human potential. And our potential is huge. —Jane Goodall*

Within ourselves, the dueling higher self and the ego-centered "inner critic" self can destroy our peace. Furthermore, and contrary to the ideal of rugged individualism, we frequently excise and disown parts of ourselves, putting them outside of ourselves into other people. That is, instead of ultimately relying on inner guidance to direct our life choices, when we seek guidance from someone who we believe knows better—a therapist, friend, counselor, or expert—we may place greater weight on what that person says than on what our higher self says.

We fragment and compartmentalize our behaviors. A businessperson who loves his or her family and exemplifies the model citizen in the community may, at work, abuse people or the environment, rationalizing, "That's business." My grandfather remarked that when he grew up in the South, devout white people would go to church on Sunday and to a lynching on Monday.

Balancing the competing demands of our inner and outer worlds is not easy. Some tree-burning opponents I worked with focused on the need to block the biomass plants at the expense of their own health and well-being—not eating well, getting enough sleep, or sufficiently "recharging their batteries." At the other extreme, I observe people working hard to perfect their lifestyles and care for their immediate families and friends, while remaining relatively oblivious to the wider world and doing little to help it.

Striking a Good Balance. My grandfather, Paul Green, fought tenaciously for civil rights, back when it was virtually unheard of for a white person in the South to speak out for racial equality. Often, my grandfather would be the only one protesting an injustice or tirelessly traveling the state in search of a lawyer willing to represent a black defendant. A writer and teacher by profession, he kept himself strong and positive with a balance of daily physical labor (chiefly farming), eating well, engaging with his family and community, and enjoying humor and the arts. He lived a healthy life to the age of eighty-seven and accomplished so much, including the publication of a shelfful of books and plays, numerous movie scripts, and outdoor symphonic dramas, some of which are still performed regularly throughout the United States.

Insecurity plaguing many Americans and others today discourages risk-taking. With job security gone, wages flat, union power diminished, and nest eggs wrecked by Wall Street tycoons, workers—often overworked, isolated, and vulnerable—turn inward. We idle in ever worsening traffic jams, and squeeze out time for sleep, cooking, exercising, studying, discussing, citizenly duties, and pursuing our dreams and priorities. We're demoralized by all the bad news we hear from the media. With insecurity also comes the notion of scarcity. People compete more while cooperating less, asking "What can I get?" rather than "What can I give?" and "What do I really want?" It's no wonder that many of us, preoccupied by fear, distraction, and ill health, just try to get by. Meanwhile, the top 1 percent help themselves to resources while no one is looking.

THE HUMAN SPECIES

Though "developed" societies slice and dice the human species based on gender, age, ethnicity, and so on, there is no biological basis for such differentiation. The Human Genome Project shows that all human beings are 99.9 percent identical in their genetic makeup.[142] Yet fragmentation and separation extends even to the family level, and now as never before in human history. Families formerly stayed together in close geographical proximity. Now, family members increasingly live far apart geographically. Couples commonly go through divorce and separation (though, previously, many people were forced to stay together in unhappy marriages, a poor alternative). Even when families do live together, individuals increasingly fend for themselves, perhaps eating different meals at different times or watching televisions (or other devices) in their own rooms.

With the Industrial Revolution, the number of generations typically living together in close contact and cooperation shrank from three to two, with grandparents living elsewhere.[143] Once valued for their wisdom and active role in family life, elders are now sometimes seen as "over the hill," extraneous, and burdensome.

The Baby Boom that followed World War II—combined with an increase in average life expectancy—has created growing numbers of retirees. In 2011, baby boomers began reaching age 65 at the rate of 10,000 people every day in the United States alone.[144] Many elders feel cut off from the rest of Western society, which considers them to be finished contributing and tends to exclude and think negatively of them.[145] Likewise, many young people increasingly live in narrow communities—more often sharing time with their peers than with their nuclear family and only occasionally with grandparents. And young people more frequently communicate remotely over phones and the Internet.[146]

Separation allows individuals to feel freer to do their own thing. But in many ways, separation can make people feel less powerful. Solitary confinement represents the extreme condition of separation and powerlessness, and some consider it to be unconstitutional "cruel and unusual punishment."[147]

Just as an individual is most powerful when all of his or her components are working together harmoniously rather than warring against each other unproductively, peoples' power increases when they band together and cooperate in groups. Labor unions can usually negotiate higher wages and better working conditions than individuals can.

"Divide and conquer" is an ageless strategy for gaining control over others: "United we stand, divided we fall." Advertisers use the divide-and-conquer approach to make individuals feel separate and inadequate, a situation easily remedied by buying the advertisers' products.

We live in a "touch-deprived society," says Dr. Weil, observing that animal and human infants deprived of physical contact don't develop normally and can actually die.[148] Today, the connection Westerners yearn for arrives via phones and computers. Clinical psychologist Sherry Turkle says children can't resist texting in class, and "we are so vulnerable to the seduction of who wants to reach us, what sweetness is coming through the phone, that we're really at a point where we turn away from our kids." Westerners' attention is "divided between the world of the people we're with and this other reality."[149]

Separation exacts a high price. The World Health Organization reports that rates of depression are rising and predicts that by 2030, more individuals will be affected by depression than by any other health condition, representing the biggest worldwide health burden on society both economically and sociologically.[150] Dr. Weil cites modern industrial food, information overload, noise, sleep deprivation, and aggressive marketing of pharmaceuticals as factors contributing to stress. But high on his list are social isolation and "nature deficit disorder" that separate individuals from other people and from the natural world. He writes that an "astonishing" 1 in 10 people in the United States, of whom millions are children, takes one or more antidepressant drugs.[151]

By 2030, more individuals will be affected by depression than by any other health condition. —World Health Organization

---

SUPPRESSING THE FEMININE

It would take too long to cover all the varieties of discrimination among humans, though they are all critically important. Gender discrimination, which affects the most people, illustrates the general idea. More broadly, suppressing the feminine affects many aspects of our society as a whole—fostering competition and discouraging cooperation, self-control, and nurturing.

Whether from nature or nurture, Daniel Amen, MD, after examining 120,000 brain scans of people from 111 countries, concludes that female brains are dramatically more active than male brains throughout about 80 percent of the brain. He concludes that women's strengths include empathy, intuition, collaboration, self-control, and appropriate worry. On the flip side, women are more vulnerable to anxiety, depression, eating disorders, insomnia, and pain. He says it is women who will change the world and when women do better for themselves, children and men also benefit because women tend to care for them.[152]

Former US vice presidential candidate Barbara Marx Hubbard recalls when, soon after their wedding, her husband asked what kind of stove she wanted. She said she didn't want any stove; she wanted to go to Washington and get a job.[153] But instead, she capitulated, carrying out the prescribed role of wife and mother. Only much later did she enter public life, inspiring people with her writing and speaking. Deepak Chopra, MD, calls Hubbard "the voice for conscious evolution." The world could have used her genius a lot sooner, during those early years when she worked in the home.

Women's physically smaller size renders them inherently vulnerable to coercion by men. Nevertheless, cultures vary widely in how they define gender roles. Some Native American and other tribes practice gender equality. Anthropologist Margaret Mead studied cultures in New Guinea, including the Tchambuli, in which women were more dominant and men were more submissive. She concluded that "human nature is almost unbelievably malleable."[154]

Exceptions notwithstanding, males dominate females throughout most of world today.[155] In 1995, then First Lady Hillary Clinton explained: "Women comprise more than half the world's population, 70 percent of the world's poor, and two-thirds of those who are not taught to read and write ... much of the work we do is not valued—not by economists, not by historians, not by popular culture, not by government leaders.... Women also are dying from diseases that should have been prevented or treated.... They are being denied the right to go to school, by their own fathers and brothers.... They are being barred from the bank lending offices and banned from the ballot box.... Tragically, women are most often the ones whose human rights are violated.

These abuses have continued because, for too long, the history of women has been a history of silence.... As long as discrimination and inequities remain so commonplace everywhere in the world, as long as girls and women are valued less, fed less, fed last, overworked, underpaid, not schooled, subjected to violence in and outside their homes—the potential of the human family to create a peaceful, prosperous world will not be realized."[156] This horrific situation still holds today. Worldwide, 1 woman in 3 will be beaten or raped during her lifetime.[157] In the United States, nearly 1 woman in 3 has experienced domestic violence and almost 1 in 5 has been raped.[158]

> *As long as girls and women are valued less, fed less, fed last, overworked, underpaid, not schooled, subjected to violence in and outside their homes—the potential of the human family to create a peaceful, prosperous world will not be realized.*
> *—Hillary Clinton*

The World Bank "finds substantial evidence of discrimination by banks against women entrepreneurs."[159] Women also face discrimination in mortgage lending, hindering women's ability to build wealth and financial security.[160] Women are subjected to a myriad of subtler forms of discrimination. In 2011, the department store JCPenney marketed T-shirts to girls between the ages of seven and sixteen that said "I'm too pretty to do homework so my brother has to do it for me."[161] Women are the "other," the outsider (the "woman doctor").

We may have "come a long way, baby," but we still have a long way to go. Author and feminist organizer Gloria Steinem, writing that "we're not even halfway there," recently looked at unfinished goals of the feminist movement. These include equal valuing of "women's work," ending violence against women, reproductive freedom, and equality in parenthood and housework. To achieve these goals requires not only pushing ahead but also, due to "a powerful backlash to the victories won," actively holding ground women have already won.[162]

Gender Bias in My Lifetime. I was born into the first generation in human history in which many women have reproductive choice. However, vestiges of the expectation that "normal" women have children have lingered.

When my grandmothers were born, women did not even have the right to vote. Both of my grandmothers went to college, which was unusual, but after getting married, both devoted their lives to their families without pursuing careers of their own. Their daughters became highly successful in their chosen careers and did not relinquish their careers to take care of their families. They retained a residue of deference to male power, however.

I remember my mother explaining to me when I was little that the father is the "king of the castle" with the ultimate say over how things will be. I didn't buy it then, or since. I'm not sure she really bought it either.

Luckily, gender equality was much more highly valued in my family than in many others. All the boys and girls in my family did housework and yardwork chores equally.

Growing up, I was fairly sharp but often dumbed myself down in social situations to be more acceptable to males. While studying engineering in the early 1980s, I felt intimidated in the environment where men vastly outnumbered women. I worked extra hard to do well. Even on my hour-long daily walk, I'd bring a stack of index cards with notes and study them as I walked.

The glass ceiling remains. In my professional career, I still observe that men are accepted and presumed competent unless they prove themselves to be incompetent, while women are often viewed skeptically and presumed incompetent until they prove themselves to be competent. Women must prove themselves to each new person, which exacts an exhausting tax on their psyches. I still sometimes hear men call women "girls." Women are passed over for promotion, held to higher standards, and paid less.

I copresented a workshop at the Danish Technical University along with my client and my colleague, both males without PhDs. A poster at the conference listed us as presenters, with a "PhD" after each of their names but not after mine! Refusing to let that stand, I spoke with the conference organizer, who promptly corrected the error. My colleague said the conference organizers listed us that way of their own volition, likely "as a courtesy."

I feel an obligation to push for gender equality because I can, while so many cannot.

Many women are denied the human right of controlling their own bodies. Dr. Kenneth Edelin, an American crusader for legal and safe abortion and for the rights of the poor and African Americans, wrote, "For me, the struggles for reproductive rights for women and civil rights for African Americans are intertwined and at the same time parallel. The denial of these two rights is an attempt by some to control the bodies of others. Both are forms of slavery."[163]

Forty years after the landmark *Roe v. Wade* decision legalizing a woman's right to abortion, Bill Moyers said that "the forces opposed to abortion ... seem more determined than ever." More than half of all US women of reproductive age now live in a state that is hostile to abortion rights, an increase from a decade ago. Lynn Paltrow, executive director of the National Advocates for Pregnant Women, told Moyers that "women are beginning to recognize that what's at stake is more than abortion. It is their personhood—their ability to be full, equal, constitutional persons in the United States of America."[164] The "fighting for the rights of the children" ploy is unveiled when the same people who so vociferously promote the rights of the unborn also vote to slash funding for the federal Women, Infants, and Children nutritional assistance program.[165]

As bad as the gender arrangement is for women, men suffer from it too. Traditional roles that require men to be "strong" and independent, while they "bring home the bacon" and protect their families can cause isolation and pressure. Gun violence and genocide are carried out overwhelmingly by men, and the suicide rate for males is 4 times the rate for females.[166]

WAR

War, lethal fighting between groups, is like an autoimmune disease of the human species. Humans attack other humans in war the way cells attack other cells in autoimmune disease, mistakenly identifying them as enemies.

War is common but not inevitable among social animal species. Bonobos, our close relatives formerly known as pygmy chimpanzees, have not been observed making war. Similarly, though all human societies practice both violence and cooperation, a few indigenous societies do not engage in war. Peaceful human societies are typically isolated or living on marginal lands at low population densities. Victors of war benefit by capturing humans for labor; by taking possession of domesticated animals, food, land, or other valuable resources; by enhancing their prestige and reputation as "people not to be messed with"; or by keeping other people away.[167]

Nuclear stockpiles around the world represent a constant threat to everyone.[168] Ironically, nuclear weapons are so powerful that they drive us to peace—no one can afford to use them (though in a moment of weakness, someone may). Unfortunately, people can afford to, and do, use conventional weapons, though at enormous cost.

Governments have killed about 260 million people in the last hundred years.[169] The United States alone has killed more than twenty million people in thirty-seven nations since World War II.[170] The Iraq and Afghanistan conflicts together will be the most expensive wars in US history, with a total cost between $4 trillion to $6 trillion, most of which is yet to be paid.[171] Imagine what else we could do with that much money.

War is a key mode of operation and an integral part of culture in much of the world today. We practice chemical warfare on our agricultural fields. Many Americans enjoy war and violence in their free time in the form of violent movies and video games and confrontational sports. History books and media glamorize war. It seems we just can't get enough of war and violence.

CORPORATIONS VERSUS CITIZENS

The division of labor among us who live in "developed" societies makes us highly dependent on one another. A typical American relies on others for food, housing, energy, employment, and entertainment, whereas in the recent past, individual families took care of much of this on their own.

We now put the interests of corporations above the interests of citizens, supported by a framework of laws giving corporations wide latitude to harm humans and the environment. Citizens are exhorted to not ask for too much lest we harm the economy, as if the economy is some kind of god: "Safety testing of chemicals may hurt the economy!" or "Protecting that forest from clear-cutting could cost jobs!"

Our system rewards short-term greed at the expense of "the commons"— the natural and cultural resources we hold in common rather than privately, such as air, water, soil, habitable climate, and public infrastructure and buildings. Powerful individuals (via corporate entities) use their short-term gains to amass ever greater wealth and power, which they use to turn government into an enabler of corporate power. Corporations can then grab more resources and leave more damage behind.[172]

NATURE

As Westerners have increasingly exploited and subjugated nature, our misguided notion of separation from nature has become ingrained in our language. We speak of "humans" and "animals" as if they were mutually exclusive, forgetting that humans *are* animals. Our ignorance and disrespectful attitude are revealed when we use words such as "She treated him like an animal!"

Ninety percent of our human genetic code is shared with chimpanzees. Analogous percentages for some other species are: mouse, 88; cow, 85; dog, 84; zebra fish, 73; chicken, 65; fruit fly, 47; honeybee, 44; roundworm, 38; rice, 25; wine grape, 24; and baker's yeast, 18 percent.[173] Naturalist Sy Montgomery, citing "a dangerous disconnect between us and the rest of animate creation," explains that animals share a lot of the same emotions we have, because neurotransmitters in different species are similar. A clam that's being opened and thus panicking will show the same neurotransmitters in its bloodstream as a person having a heart attack.[174]

Many people in the Western world are so disconnected from nature they don't know where their food and water come from, where their waste goes, basic facts about the natural world, or even the names of common plant and animal species in their environs. Americans on average spend 90 percent of their lives indoors. In the United States, children's contact with nature and the outdoors has declined precipitously. While 96 percent of adults report the outdoors was their most important environment during childhood, in an average week, a typical child today spends less than one hour outdoors compared with fifty-two hours engaged with electronic media (television, computers, and video games).[175]

> *Today, in an average week, a typical child spends less than one hour outdoors compared with fifty-two hours engaged with electronic media.*

"Nature-deficit"–afflicted children may not become strong protectors of the environment. People who love plants, animals, water, air, and soil do not harm them without a thought or care—just as people who love other people do not harm them without a thought or care. But many of us don't get to know—or learn to care about—plants, animals, and the natural world.

Like every other organism on earth, we evolved in intimate connection with nature, and our new feeling of disconnection runs counter to our biology and psyche developed over eons. A friend of mine drove past an area near her home and saw the trees had been cut down. She started crying when she told me about it and was startled by her tears. She told me she had no idea she felt so strongly about the forest. Many people in the developed world still feel a visceral connection with nature, whether consciously or not.

The world's protected natural areas receive eight billion visits a year.[176] The National Park Service reported more than 273 million recreation visitors to US national parks in 2013.[177] Birdwatching and gardening are among the fastest growing outdoor hobbies in the United States.[178] More than sixty-five million Americans care for birds, spending many billions of dollars each year on bird food, feeders, baths, houses, and other accessories.[179]

At the same time, "eco-crime"—which includes wildlife poaching and smuggling; toxic waste dumping; and illegal fishing, logging, and mining—is the fourth-largest criminal enterprise in the world and growing fast. A lot of people have cut ties with nature.[180]

Our deadly combination of arrogance and ignorance threatens our life-support system and thus our very existence. Philosopher Kathleen Dean Moore says, "We have brought the world to the brink of ruin by acting under the delusion that humans are separate from the earth, better somehow, in control of it. We believe that humans are the only creatures of spirit in the universe otherwise made up of stones and insensate matter; that the nonhuman world was created for us alone and derives all its value from its usefulness to humanity; that we are the masters of the universe. Because of our technological prowess, we see ourselves as exceptions to the rules that govern the 'lower' forms of life. We believe we can destroy our habitat without also destroying ourselves. How could we be so tragically wrong?"

CONNECTIONS

Science—including quantum theory—increasingly shows just how interconnected everything in our world is. The individualistic story Westerners have been living, based on the work of physicist Isaac Newton, is more than three hundred years old. This story defines the world as a collection of separate and well-behaved things following fixed laws of time and space. Naturalist Charles Darwin augmented this view with the notion that individual living things compete against each other to survive in a world without enough to go around.

In her books *The Field* and *The Bond*, author and researcher Lynne McTaggart explains that new science shows there *are* no individual things, that all things are bonded, and that nature has a tendency to connect rather than to compete. She says, subatomic particles aren't "little billiard balls" vibrating independently. Rather, they are nothing more than little knots of energy that briefly emerge and disappear back into the underlying field. "According to quantum field theory, the individual entity is transient and insubstantial." The new science reveals that what's important isn't the thing but the relationship. She writes in *The Field*, "What we believe to be our stable, static universe is in fact a seething maelstrom of subatomic particles fleetingly popping in and out of existence."[181]

Further, quantum physics has demonstrated there is no such thing as a vacuum. The "Field," also called the "Zero Point Field," is the web of energy exchange in so-called "empty space" that connects everything in the universe. Frontier science indicates it's impossible to determine where one thing ends and another begins—our body and the environment, for example. McTaggart explains that we now know "genes are like the keys of a piano. They sit there silently until they are expressed. And what expresses them is a quartet of atoms called an 'epigene' that sits above the gene, which is affected by environmental influences such as food, water, and friends." Thus we are not self-contained isolated entities. Furthermore, McTaggart maintains that the science from many fields "overwhelmingly" indicates we were made to cooperate rather than compete.[182]

In the words of Albert Einstein, "A human being ... experiences himself, his thoughts and feelings as something separated from the rest, a kind of optical delusion of his consciousness. This delusion is a kind of prison for us, restricting us to our personal desires and to affection for a few persons nearest to us. Our task must be to free ourselves from this prison by widening our circle of compassion to embrace all living creatures and the whole of nature in its beauty."[183]

The Field may explain some things that prior science could not. McTaggart writes, "Some scientists went so far as to suggest that all of our high cognitive processes result from an interaction with the Zero Point Field. This kind of constant interaction might account for intuition or creativity—and how ideas come to us in bursts of insight, sometimes in fragments but often as a miraculous whole. An intuitive leap might simply be a sudden coalescence of coherence in The Field." It makes sense—something is going on when, shortly after we think of a person for the first time in years, that person calls on the telephone "out of the blue." The Field also could account for prophetic dreams, distant healing, and other phenomena conventional science can't explain.

Like everything else, our institutions and policies are extensively interconnected, feeding off and supporting each other in a complex ecosystem of their own. Consider this: the petroleum industry provides oil as raw material for the chemical industry. The chemical industry makes synthetic chemicals for big agriculture and big food, whose products cause chronic disease, thus creating markets for the pharmaceutical and health-care industries. After all, 70 percent of cancers are related to diet, and cancer is big business.[184] Keeping our petroleum supply chain going sometimes involves war (for example, in the Middle East), which creates business for the defense industry, itself a big user of oil and thus a large client of the petroleum industry.[185] And so on.

Industries give cash, often secretly, to politicians, who reward industries with subsidies and other special favors, conferring on them competitive advantages. Subsidies essentially take money from you and me in the form of taxes and gift the money to selected corporations or other institutions, sometimes ultimately as quid pro quo for campaign contributions. This extra money allows the industries to offer their goods and services to us at a lower sticker price. Competing industries not receiving subsidies must reflect all their costs in their sticker prices, resulting in prices higher than those of their subsidized counterparts. Consumers compare sticker prices and choose the subsidized alternative, thinking it's cheaper. This may be an illusion, of course, because we are—usually unwittingly—also paying above and beyond the sticker price through our taxes. Subsidies steer consumers into making choices that oftentimes are not in consumers' best interests. We pay attention to small changes in prices posted at the gas pump, oblivious to the humongous sums siphoned out of our pockets—via taxes—and delivered to the oil companies as subsidies on a regular basis. Perverse subsidies leave out the interests of citizens and their environment, essentially going behind our backs with under-the-table spending of our money.

> *Perverse subsidies leave out the interests of citizens and their environment, essentially going behind our backs with under-the-table spending of our money.*

Citizens often lose, suffering illness and death from unhealthy food and pharmaceuticals, getting wounded and killed in wars, paying for subsidies, living in a degraded environment, and foregoing advocacy by their political representatives who collude with corporate entities. This corrupt system enriches those at the top, ever widening the gap between the few haves and the multitude of have-nots. Citizens experience even more financial stress and have to work harder to put food on the table. Weak, unhealthy, worried, overworked, and frazzled citizens feel they have no time to be involved citizens, who could potentially change the parasitic industrial ecosystem. So the system perpetuates, in a downward spiral that promotes unevolved politicians and CEOs at the expense of citizens.

RECONNECTING

At the same time that Westerners feel increasingly separated, connectivity is increasing as science reveals more about reality and as humanity behaves more globally. Bruce Lipton and Steve Bhaerman write, "We are each and all cells in the body of an evolving giant super-organism we call humanity."[186] Thanks to the Internet, we now have a global brain we can tap into almost instantaneously, with abilities to both upload and download information. Telephones enable us to talk with people almost anywhere on the planet. The economy is now global, as are some environmental impacts, such as climate change. On September 21, 2014, hundreds of thousands of people in one hundred and fifty countries participated in a People's Climate March, pressing for action to address climate change. The march was reported via the Internet from all over the world.[187] When terrorists flew airplanes into the World Trade Center and other US locations on September 11, 2001, the world "stood still" and there was a worldwide outpouring of grief and support for the United States.[188]

As conventional medicine fails to address chronic illnesses, holistic medicine puts the pieces of the human back together again and also considers the person's environment. One form of holistic medicine, integrative medicine, takes account of the whole person (body, mind, and spirit) and makes use of all appropriate therapies, both conventional and alternative. Functional medicine is similar but it provides an architecture to help organize and apply medical knowledge in a systematic way to dig deeper into the origins of disease and the determinants of health.[189] These approaches strive to keep a person healthy and, barring that, to successfully treat the whole person, with his or her interrelated symptoms and systems. Dr. Hyman writes that mainstream medicine is missing synthesis and integration: "There are millions of bits of data and information, and yet for most practitioners of medicine they are strewn about the floor like a million puzzle pieces."[190] Dr. Weil writes, "Professionals are even more fed up than patients with the dead end that the drug-only approach represents."[191] Similarly, organic agriculture puts the ecological pieces back together and grows food in sustainable ecosystems rather than in industrial monocultures (single crops).

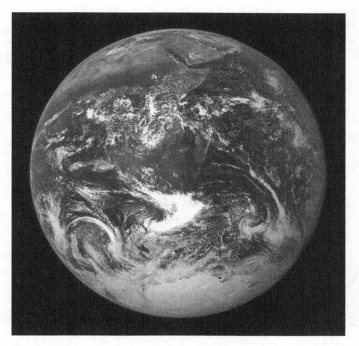

The beautiful yet sobering images of Earth from space made the concept of one unified earth and one unified human species living on a finite Earth concrete and irrefutable. Photo credit: NASA. http://www.nasa.gov/multimedia/imagegallery/image_feature_329.html.

Creating a sustainable world involves realizing we are not solitary individuals acting alone. The stakes could not be higher in our interconnected world. Pessimism and gloom can spread, easily facilitated by global communications. But so can hope and goodwill.

Humans, acting together, can create massive change. American colonists defeated England in the 1700s by joining together. Adolph Hitler was defeated in the 1940s when countries of the world joined together in common purpose in World War II. American citizens banded together to stop the Vietnam War in the 1970s. Today, hundreds of nongovernmental environmental organizations are driving change.[192]

LEARNING FROM INDIGENOUS SOCIETIES

It seems as if Western society is on the verge of leaving its adolescent phase and entering adulthood. This involves transitioning from awkwardness, impulsiveness, rudimentary skills, and, perhaps, illusions of invincibility to a state in which we have greater awareness, skills, command of ourselves, sense of purpose and responsibility, and recognition of our mortality.

Many Westerners now feel the urge to break out of our unsustainable and combative way of life. As spiritual teacher Eckhart Tolle writes, "Humanity is under great pressure to evolve because it is our only chance of survival as a race."[193]

We can learn from other societies. Humans have come up with a range of solutions to universal problems in learning how to live almost anywhere on Earth. Civilizations and writing arose only 5400 years ago. Therefore, people living in civilizations are a tiny and unrepresentative slice of humanity. Indigenous societies, which are far more representative of the totality of humanity, can teach us about what is "typical" for humans—and also what is possible.

There are 370 million indigenous people—a population larger than that of the United States—living in ninety countries in all regions of the world.[194] Many indigenous societies have lived in harmony with their environments for thousands of years. Indigenous people spend much more of their time outdoors than Westerners, and they often feel deeply and spiritually rooted to the land, in contrast to Westerners' sense of disconnection with nature.

Similarly, social bonds in indigenous societies are stronger than in Western societies. Loneliness is relatively uncommon, in contrast to the 1 in 5 Americans who experience persistent loneliness.[195] Because their members typically do not travel far, indigenous groups of people end up living together for their entire lives and sharing with each other, even when they have very little. Evolution did not prepare us for the American way of living in relative isolation and frequently relocating to new homes. People who have moved from indigenous societies to Western ones report that they miss the lifelong social bonds of their former community.

Habits of indigenous societies indicate the wide range of diets humans evolved to eat—including, in the Arctic region, diets comprised exclusively of meat. And they show humans did not evolve to eat the "standard American diet," which is high in animal fats, unhealthy fats, and processed foods and low in fiber, complex carbohydrates, and plant-based foods. People living in indigenous societies typically do not die from chronic diseases that kill Westerners—stroke, diabetes, and heart attacks. But if they adopt the standard American diet, they begin contracting chronic diseases.[196]

CHAPTER 4
EXAMPLES OF INTERCONNECTIVITY

Man is a part of nature, and his war against nature
is inevitably a war against himself.

—*Rachel Carson*

WESTERNERS ARE PRONE TO FRAGMENTING our world and attending to its individual parts, not seeing how the pieces fit together. Consequently, our chosen solutions to problems often don't consider potential side effects in other areas and may end up creating additional, and sometimes worse, problems. Because of the extensive interconnections between humans, the environment, and the economy, an action in one area will often have ramifications in other areas, benefiting or damaging all together.

Biologist David Suzuki explains how migrating salmon bring nitrogen within their bodies from oceans to rivers to land. When bears catch salmon, they typically carry the fish away from the river before eating them and discarding their carcasses, providing forests with nitrogen, which is in limited supply because it is easily washed from the soil. This nitrogen supply helps huge trees flourish in forests along the West coast of North America.[197]

Wolves were reintroduced to Yellowstone National Park in 1995, after an absence of 70 years. The reintroduced wolves not only killed some of the numerous deer but also changed the behavior of the deer. Deer steered clear of dangerous areas such as valleys and gorges, and once denuded areas revegetated. Valley sides became forested, attracting songbirds, migratory birds, and beavers. Beavers engineered dams and habitats that attracted otters, muskrats, ducks, fish, reptiles, and amphibians. Wolves killed coyotes, causing populations of mice and rabbits to increase. This attracted hawks, weasels, foxes, and badgers. Carrion left by the wolves attracted ravens, bald eagles, and bears. Bears also killed some of the calves of the deer. The revegetated valley sides reduced erosion. Rivers meandered less and channels became narrower and more fixed. New habitats were created as more pools and riffle sections formed. All this, from reintroducing wolves.[198]

This chapter examines four examples of how human actions can simultaneously help or harm diverse aspects of life. The examples show that beneficial and practical alternatives are available to replace destructive practices. The first example explains how wood-burning power plants generate a stunning array of damaging impacts. The second example explores how the Green Belt Movement, based in Kenya, nurtures rather than destroys trees and in so doing propagates beneficial impacts into many areas of life. The third and fourth examples describe the widespread impacts of industrial and organic food production.

These examples are particularly useful to examine because they concern practices central to our adaptation on Earth. Forest cover is essential to the Earth's biosphere, and food is the most basic way we humans fit into the web of life, as the Earth's top predator. Furthermore, agriculture, logging, and other land use generate about one-quarter of the global greenhouse gas emissions wrecking our climate.[199] The UN Food and Agriculture Organization estimates agriculture alone causes one-third of global greenhouse gas emissions.[200] However, forests and agricultural fields offer potentially vast repositories for the carbon damaging our climate, if we take better care of them. These topics are not well publicized. Consequently, I cover them in some depth.

> *Forests and agricultural fields offer potentially vast repositories for the carbon damaging our climate.*

WOOD-BURNING ELECTRICAL POWER PLANTS

This example shows how one action can generate an array of intertwined negative impacts on our environment, health, economy, and democracy. Wood-burning electrical power plants, often euphemistically called "biomass plants" supplying "bioenergy," are touted by their developers as providers of clean, green, and renewable energy. However, biomass plants supply no such thing. Citizens seem to sense this: according to a 2012 survey, 81 percent of Americans think that other energy-producing options should be explored before biomass energy production is explored.[201] However, many governments are pushing damaging bioenergy projects in lockstep with project developers—and rewarding the developers with generous subsidies funded by citizens.

Biomass plants devour many resources of great value: trees, wildlife habitats, soil fertility, water, petroleum, and money. They produce a multitude of damaging byproducts—among others, greenhouse gases, other air pollutants, water pollution, ash, adverse health impacts, and economic damage. It would be a challenge to design a more damaging industry if one tried. Recognition of the devastating effects has been slow to take hold, perhaps partly because the term "biomass plants" sounds cozy, nice, "green," and maybe even organic, and also because of our obsessive desire for more energy, especially energy that is homegrown and does not involve fossil fuels.

Biomass plants can be fueled by trees, contaminated wood ("construction and demolition wood" can contain hazardous chemicals), tires, or just about anything that can burn. Many biomass plants combust whole trees, which biomass plant owners often refer to as "forest debris" or "waste wood." Hundreds of biomass plants operate in the United States, with more proposed. Meanwhile, a number of existing biomass plants sit idle, often due to financial difficulties.[202]

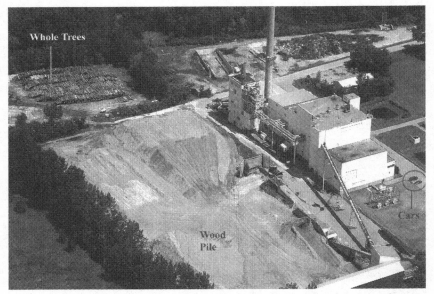

The Joseph C. McNeil Generating Station, a 50-megawatt biomass plant in Burlington, Vermont. https://www.burlingtonelectric.com/about-us/what-we-do/joseph-c-mcneil-generating-station. Photo credit: Chris Matera.

Of all the available combustion-based electricity generation technologies, biomass plants are the least efficient, converting only 20 percent to 25 percent of the energy in the wood to electricity and wasting the rest as heat. Like other types of power plants, biomass plants need cooling, and river water is often used for that purpose. A typical 50-megawatt plant requires 800,000 gallons of water per day, vaporizing 85 percent and returning only

15 percent—heated and contaminated—to the river.[203] (A 50-megawatt plant can power thousands of homes.[204])

Due to inefficiency—wasting three or four trees for every tree that is converted to electricity— biomass plants require gargantuan quantities of fuel. That's one reason the technology is so expensive. If all the trees in the United States were burned for bioenergy, our national energy needs would be met for only one year.[205] A 50-megawatt biomass plant burns 1.2 tons of wood each minute. Supplying this fuel devastates forests and the wildlife that depend on them for food and habitat. It also permanently removes nutrients from the forest ecosystem rather than recycling them, thereby degrading soil quality and rendering the process unsustainable.[206]

Despite unrealistic industry-funded fuel supply studies to the contrary, the supply of nearby trees is quickly exhausted. Shipping wood chips from distant sources is expensive (but even so, some biomass plants in Europe turn to the United States and elsewhere for wood chips). A common strategy is for biomass plants to switch to burning contaminated wood for fuel. This can be lucrative because, rather than having to purchase a resource (wood chips), biomass plant owners are paid to take a waste product (contaminated wood) off other peoples' hands. Once the expensive biomass incinerators have been built, regulatory agencies find it hard to say no to fuel-switching requests.

Due to their inefficiency, biomass plants emit more carbon dioxide per unit of electricity generated than any other energy source—about 1.5 times that of coal. Many proponents claim that burning wood is "carbon neutral," that the carbon emitted during combustion is reabsorbed by growing trees. However, they egregiously neglect the mismatch in rates—while it takes a minute to burn a tree in a biomass plant, it takes decades to grow a tree back.

Regulators generally ignore scientific research demonstrating bioenergy's damaging climate impacts.[207] While they consider the burning of tropical rain forests to be environmentally damaging, they paradoxically regard bioenergy as not only acceptable but even worthy of economic incentives, even though the carbon dioxide goes right out the smokestack. Bioenergy likely emits *more* carbon dioxide than tropical forest burning does, due to the emissions associated with the burning of fossil fuels to cut the trees, chip them into small pieces, and transport them. What's more, oil is often sprayed on the green wood chips to get them to ignite. Add to that the environmental toll for biomass plant construction (including production and transport of huge amounts of cement and steel used to build the incinerators, which typically cost several hundred million dollars).

Biomass plants not only emit more carbon dioxide than any other energy technology per unit of electricity generated, but they also destroy the very trees that remove carbon dioxide from the atmosphere. The world's forests are much more important in the carbon cycle than previously thought, soaking up as much as one-third of the planet's fossil fuel emissions.[208] If developed countries burn their own forests for electricity, it shatters their credibility when they ask developing countries to preserve their forests in order to mop up carbon dioxide emissions emanating primarily from developed countries.

As yet another consequence of their bottom-of-the-barrel efficiency, biomass plants (despite air-pollution control equipment) release copious amounts of air contaminants besides carbon dioxide: fine particles (soot), carbon monoxide, sulfur oxides, nitrogen oxides, heavy metals, volatile organic compounds, radionuclides, and dioxins. Emissions of pollutants from biomass plants are similar to those from coal plants.[209] Biomass plant developers estimate, during their permitting process, the amounts of air pollutants they expect their project will routinely emit. Those estimates don't include emissions from fuel pile fires, a common occurrence when fuel is stored uncovered outdoors, as is invariably the case because of the mammoth fuel quantities required. Such fires can burn for weeks, with zero emissions controls.[210]

Like emissions from coal-burning plants, air pollutants emitted from biomass plants hurt and kill people by causing or exacerbating asthma and other respiratory diseases, heart disease, and cancer. The Massachusetts Medical Society, among other medical societies, has spoken out vehemently against biomass plants.[211] Increased illness from biomass plant emissions costs not only lives, pain, and suffering, but money and jobs as well. Yet biomass plant owners bear none of the costs of these impacts.

Asthma Attack. One of the most moving public comments I heard during biomass controversies occurred at a hearing for a biomass plant developer seeking a permit to discharge air pollutants in a low-income urban neighborhood. A woman simply held a small tape player up to the microphone and hit the "Play" button. We all heard the disturbing sound of a child wheezing and coughing, having an asthma attack. It brought tears to my eyes. The moderator made the woman stop the tape even though her time (three minutes, if I recall correctly) was not up.

When it was my turn to speak, I was unexpectedly overtaken by anger as I wrapped up my comments at the microphone. I was angry the regulators had for years consistently ignored solid and compelling public comments—even from professionals such as medical doctors—instead unquestioningly accepting the developers' junk science and approving their permits. I was angry the burden of exposing developers' misleading information fell on unpaid citizens rather than on the regulators the citizens were paying to do this job. Above all, I was angry at the greedy developers who were proposing these horrible projects in the first place, and always proposing them in low-income communities with thin resources for fighting back.

As I concluded my comments, I turned from the audience to the chief regulator, glared, pointed right at him, and said, "People will die if you approve this air permit." I afterward thought to myself, "Ooh, maybe I've gone a little too far here." However, I felt vindicated when, a few speakers later, a medical doctor said pretty much what I had, though without the drama.

Despite overwhelming evidence that human health and the environment would be harmed, the regulatory agency conditionally approved the discharge of almost a ton a day of pollutants into the air, not counting the massive carbon dioxide emissions, which (absurdly) were not a part of the permitting process. The permitted emissions included carbon monoxide; fine particles; and Hazardous Air Pollutants, a list of 187 chemicals that includes dioxin and arsenic.[212]

Before the biomass wars, I thought we were doing reasonably well with environmental issues, changing course, albeit gradually, to a more healthy one. Now I see I was naïve. The primary concern evidently is not about whether children can breathe. It's about corporate power and profits.

Another dangerous product that comes out bioenergy's back end is ash. A typical 50-megawatt biomass plant produces 1.5 tons of ash per hour.[213] Ash from burned wood, even trees taken directly from the forest, contains dioxin and heavy metals, including arsenic.[214] Radionuclides, such as cesium-137—originally released from nuclear testing and nuclear accidents and taken up by trees—end up in the ash (and/or in air emissions).[215] Regulators turn a blind eye to radionuclides, however, and typically do not require testing for them. They likewise often do not require testing for dioxin, a known human carcinogen.[216] Regulators usually allow the ash to be spread on farmers' fields, thereby allowing contaminants to enter the food supply and, subsequently, our bodies. Up to 80 percent of wood ash generated in the Northeast is spread on agricultural soils.[217]

The primary concern evidently is not about whether children can breathe. It's about corporate power and profits.

Largely owing to their insatiable demand for wood and their clunky inefficiency, biomass plants require massive infusions of cash in order to be financially viable (unless they are allowed to burn contaminated wood), in the form of taxpayer and ratepayer subsidies.[218] These subsidies are not insignificant—amounting to hundreds of millions of dollars over thirty years in the case of just one plant proposed in Massachusetts—and they divert funds that could instead be used for cleaner energy.[219]

Supporters argue that biomass plants create jobs. However, the jobs created are few and costly. The investment required to create each permanent full-time job typically exceeds $3 million.[220] Biomass also damages the economy by hurting tourism (often a much larger job creator), driving down nearby property values, and driving up the price of wood needed for other purposes.

Biomass plant developers argue that biomass plants should be "part of the energy mix." That's as absurd as saying Westerners should keep using slide rules in modern computing, bloodletting in modern medicine, or horses and buggies in modern transportation. With increasing atmospheric carbon dioxide concentrations, we need our trees more than ever before. It's time to close the chapter on combustion energy and ramp up and carefully deploy readily available, cleaner technologies. It's time to further develop our expertise in the areas of conservation, efficiency, solar, geothermal, wind, hydropower, and fuel cells.

THE GREEN BELT MOVEMENT

The Green Belt Movement illustrates a positive response to the environmental impacts of deforestation—a response that snowballed to create positive effects in many areas of life. The Green Belt Movement is an example of observing and honoring life and interconnections. It grew into a nationwide campaign to safeguard the environment, defend human rights, and fight government injustice.[221]

Wangari Maathai (1940–2011), the first African woman and the first environmentalist to receive the Nobel Peace Prize (in 2004), appreciated the value of trees. By the early 1970s, Kenya's forests had shrunk to less than 5 percent of their former area in just one century, and Kenya's entire ecosystem was threatened.[222] British colonials cut down native forests, believing the forests should be replaced with eucalyptus and pine plantations for timber (largely to be used for railway construction and industrial tea drying). Maathai recollected, "I grew up in a beautiful part of the countryside, full of trees, full of food, a lot of happiness, a lot of water, a lot of firewood, a lot of building material. Everything that I am now trying to replenish, there was plenty of when I was a child." Educated in the United States, she returned home to a drying and devastated landscape.[223] Topsoil erosion had made farming difficult, and children were suffering from malnutrition. Families were in need of firewood, food, clean drinking water, and income.

Maathai earned a doctorate in veterinary anatomy from the University of Nairobi and became a university professor.[224] She studied the brown ear tick in an effort to combat a fatal East African cattle fever. She came to realize the real threat to cattle in Kenya was not the brown ear tick, but the deteriorating environment. There was little grass and other fodder, and the animals were suffering from hunger. Rivers were low. Maathai further realized the deteriorating environment threatened not only the livestock industry but also her, her children, her students, and the entire country. The deteriorating environment was related to deforestation, soil loss, pollution, and unsustainable land practices.

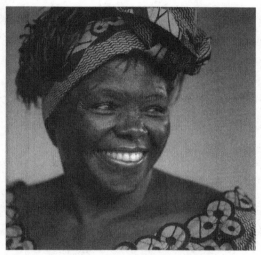

Wangari Maathai. Image ©Brigitte Lacombe.

The Green Belt Movement began with a simple act, when Maathai planted seven trees on Earth Day in 1977.[225] She realized that a positive step was needed to break the cycle of disempowerment and lack of hope and planting a tree is a simple and easy positive step almost anybody can take. The Green Belt Movement has since planted more than fifty million trees across Africa, reducing soil erosion and reforesting and protecting thousands of acres of forest. The Green Belt Movement encouraged rural Kenyan women to work together to grow seedlings and plant trees to bind the soil, store rainwater, provide food and firewood, and receive, in return, a small monetary token for their work.[226]

Thousands of community tree nurseries are the heart of the Green Belt Movement. Each begins when an interested person in a community contacts a Green Belt representative, who advises the person to invite everyone in the community to a meeting in a school or church. A Green Belt staff member attends the meeting, helps the community choose leaders, and teaches them how to collect tree seeds and select a good site for a nursery. The Green Belt Movement provides materials to the new local chapter. The community members plant the seedlings at homes, at schools, and in forests, and tend them for three months. At that point, the Green Belt Movement pays the local chapter about 7 cents per seedling.

The Green Belt Movement expanded in scope and became a vehicle for empowering women to become champions for sustainable resource management, equitable economic development, good governance, and peace. "I started planting trees and found myself in the forefront of fighting for the restoration of democracy in my country," Maathai said.[227] The Green Belt Movement recognizes a healthy, natural world is at the heart of an equitable and peaceful society, and vice versa.

Maathai inspired women to work hard at planting trees, which involved routinely hauling heavy loads of water and seedlings in wet soil. At first, the political establishment was unfazed by the actions of a bunch of second-class citizens (women). However, as the movement grew, the political establishment felt threatened. Nevertheless, Maathai remained unwavering in her determination and outspokenness, risking death and enduring beatings and imprisonment. When the then-president of Kenya was selling off pieces of the Karura National Forest, Maathai said "[it is] on my dead body that Karura will ever be subdivided by individuals" and went to retake Karura symbolically by planting a tree. There, she and her supporters faced a police blockade armed with daggers, whips, and machetes. Despite the misgivings of some of her supporters, she insisted on going forward, carrying a seedling in one hand and a crucifix in the other, saying, "This is the day that we are going to plant this tree. We must do it today." As she was digging a hole in which to plant the seedling, Maathai was attacked and was subsequently hospitalized with head injuries. Protests grew, the names of some of the people involved in the real estate transactions were published, and the destructive project was halted.[228]

As the Green Belt Movement grew, the focus moved from largely local concerns to overarching ones. Maathai began addressing the connections between Kenya's degraded land and its political leadership. Life was easier for political leaders if the people remained poor and disempowered. Things came to a head when Maathai campaigned against plans to construct a sixty-story building and a four-story statue of Kenya's president in Nairobi's Uhuru Park. Later, she helped a group of mothers of young men who were being held as political prisoners. The mothers built a camp in the public park and held all-night candlelight vigils. For three days, security personnel surrounded the women, and on the third day, with the help of guns and soldiers, they uprooted the women from the camp. Maathai was clubbed unconscious. The protestors were given protection in a church basement for months, until nearly all their sons were freed. "What began as a three-day hunger strike became a year-long struggle to open up Kenya's political system."[229]

Maathai entered the political system in 2002, having won a seat in the Kenyan Parliament by a landslide. Soon thereafter, she was named deputy minister of the environment. In 2004, she won the Nobel Peace Prize.

The Green Belt Movement solves community problems of all kinds, empowering and improving the status of women in the process. Part of the effort to raise the status of women involves teaching about proper nutrition, traditional foods, and family planning.[230] Wangari Maathai risked her life trying to benefit everything and everyone around her.

INDUSTRIAL FOOD

The problems described below are avoidable and solvable. I promise much more positivity after this discussion.

Industrial agriculture provides an extreme example of ignoring interconnections. I use the word "industrial" rather than "conventional," because industrial agriculture is totally unlike agricultural methods humans used for thousands of years. Also, the word "food" in this discussion refers to all plant, animal, and synthetic materials consumed.

Today, the United States focuses on large-scale, short-term exploitation of soil, water, energy, plants, and animals. Small farmers don't do well under the current system.[231] Many family farms have been bankrupted, cutting in half the number of US farmers in the last forty years, with the largest 2 percent of farms now producing 50 percent of the US food supply. Industrial producers grow varieties not primarily for their nutrition and taste but for their high yield and ability to withstand long-distance travel, distribution, and storage. One example of such a variety is bland, tough, and pale supermarket tomatoes.[232] Long-distance transport favors highly processed food ingredients such as white flour and preservatives. Long-distance transport also contributes to the transmission of food-borne pathogens.

Empty Shelves. In October 2011, a devastating "nor'easter" storm in my region brought down many trees and power lines. Shortly after the weather cleared and roads reopened, I drove to a large health food store for supplies. It's amazing the store had opened at all, given the circumstances. All the conventional grocery stores in the area were closed. I was unnerved by the small selection of food and the rows of empty shelf space, having taken for granted the availability of unlimited food supplies at all times. I was shocked that a severe weather event could cut off my food supply so suddenly.

A handful of gigantic companies control most of the world's seed sales.[233] Big producers grow large swaths of monocultures rather than resilient mixed communities of organisms. They apply broad-spectrum pesticides, chemicals that kill good and bad organisms indiscriminately and contaminate soil, water, and air (not to mention food and farm workers). Among the casualties of pesticides are pollinators—birds, bats, bees, and butterflies—upon which 90 percent of all plant species, including most crop plants, depend. By disrupting nitrogen-fixing bacteria that fertilize the soil, pesticides decrease crop yields.[234]

Rachel Carson warned the public about pesticides in the 1960s, writing of a future in which birds and fish would die and humans would fall victim to mysterious illnesses due to the use of the pesticide DDT. "As crude a weapon as the cave man's club, the chemical barrage has been hurled against the fabric of life—a fabric on the one hand delicate and destructible, on the other miraculously tough and resilient, and capable of striking back in unexpected ways," Carson wrote. "These extraordinary capacities of life have been ignored by the practitioners of chemical control who have brought to their task no 'high-minded orientation,' no humility before the vast forces with which they tamper."[235]

Pesticide use continues, however. Annually, more than 1 billion pounds of pesticides are used in the United States and 5.6 billion pounds are used worldwide, with twenty-five million agricultural workers worldwide experiencing unintentional pesticide poisonings.[236]

We are exposed to pesticides through food, water, home and garden use, termite control, spray drift, and residues in household dust. Americans on average each consume approximately one gallon of neurotoxic pesticides each year.[237] The US Department of Agriculture has estimated that fifty million people in the United States obtain their drinking water from groundwater that is potentially contaminated by pesticides and other agricultural chemicals. Various pesticides have been implicated in chronic diseases ranging from cancer to diabetes; neurodegenerative disorders including Parkinson's and Alzheimer's diseases; birth defects; reproductive disorders; respiratory diseases such as asthma; cardiovascular diseases; kidney diseases; and autoimmune diseases including lupus erythematous and rheumatoid arthritis.[238]

We grow fewer crop varieties than before, threatening the resiliency of our food supply to withstand challenges such as climate disruption and drought. Since the 1900s, approximately 75 percent of plant genetic diversity has been lost worldwide as farmers have given up growing multiple local varieties and turned instead to genetically uniform, high-yielding varieties. In addition, 30 percent of livestock breeds are at risk of extinction. Today, 75 percent of the world's food is generated from only twelve plants and five animal species.[239]

Industrial farms grow food as intensively as possible, packing as many plants or animals into as small a space as possible to get the maximum yield. When inputs such as organic matter are not adequately replenished, as is often the case for industrially farmed fields, the soil becomes depleted of organic carbon and micronutrients, and the soil's capacity to retain water is diminished.

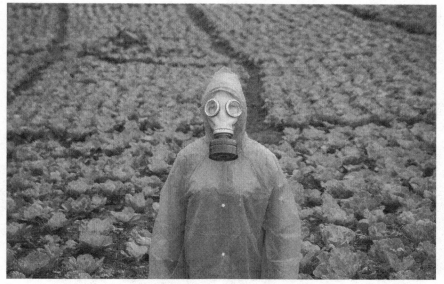

Farmer in a field of industrially grown lettuce. Photo credit: ©Istockphoto.com/Bubbers13.

Other agricultural practices deplete finite water resources. Up to half of the water used in irrigation is lost or unaccounted for in developing countries, and up to 30 percent of irrigation water is wasted in developed countries.[240] That's a big deal, because about 70 percent of all the world's freshwater withdrawals are for irrigation.[241] Overpumping of aquifers for irrigation is a particular concern in America, India, and China, and the Middle East is seeing "the first collision between population growth and water supply at the regional level."[242]

Falling Water Table. In my work, I am used to seeing data showing groundwater elevations at a given site fluctuating seasonally, with water table elevations typically several feet higher in the spring than in the fall. I'll never forget looking at a ten-year record of groundwater elevation data for a site in Kansas atop the Ogallala Aquifer, where the water table elevations went down about a foot per year, year after year. This drove home for me the frightening unsustainability of our industrial agricultural system.

Industrial agriculture uses a lot of petroleum—emitting copious amounts of carbon dioxide—to produce and apply petroleum-derived chemical fertilizers and pesticides, plow and irrigate fields, and process, store, and ship food. Our industrial food production system uses much more energy than it produces. David Suzuki writes, "For every unit of energy recovered from plants, industrial agriculture expends 6 to 10 units in fossil fuels."[243]

Industrial farmers often apply excess nutrients (fertilizer) that are highly soluble. Nutrients, along with pesticides, run off into surface water or percolate through soil and into groundwater, contaminating them. Nutrient-caused oxygen depletion has created more than 400 dead zones in the world's oceans, some as large as New Jersey.[244]

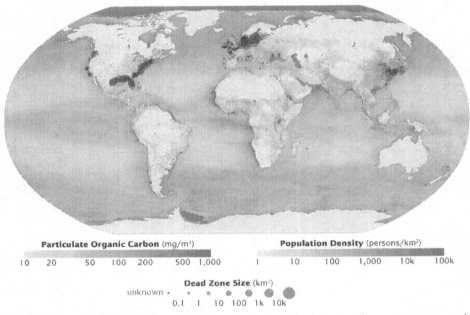

Dead zones, areas where the deep water is so low in dissolved oxygen that sea creatures can't survive. Note the dark areas along the coasts. Credit: NASA. http://earthobservatory.nasa.gov/IOTD/view.php?id=44677.

Industrial agriculture often involves tilling the soil and then failing to prevent soil from running off when it rains. Our food supply—our very survival—depends on topsoil we are losing at an astonishing rate, one that far exceeds the soil replenishment rate.[245]

Industry claims industrial methods are the only way to produce enough food to feed everyone. However, studies show efficient organic agriculture can achieve yields comparable to those produced by intensive industrial agriculture.[246]

More than a third of the world's ice-free land is dedicated to raising crops and livestock, and clearing grasslands and forests for agriculture is a major driver of wildlife extinction and rain forest destruction.[247] Meanwhile, as much as half of all the food produced in the world ends up being thrown away.[248]

Similarly, we overfish many target species and kill ecologically valuable nontarget animals in the process. Nontarget sea animals injured or killed but not harvested ("bycatch") are estimated at 40 percent of the world's catch, totaling sixty-three billion pounds each year.[249] Farm-raising salmon and other seafood not only damages habitat, but it also transmits parasites to the salmon's wild cousins swimming nearby. We also kill seafood nurseries by creating ocean dead zones and damaging coastal wetlands, driving up the costs of seafood.

LIVESTOCK

Only 55 percent of world crop calories feeds people; 36 percent feeds livestock, and 9 percent is used for biofuels and industrial products.[250]

Livestock production requires vastly more water, land, and energy than do plant foods and is a major cause of some of the world's most pressing environmental problems: climate change, land degradation, water pollution, biodiversity loss, and more.[251] Raising farm animals uses three-quarters of the world's agricultural land and accounts for one-third of our global fresh water consumption.[252]

> *Raising farm animals uses three-quarters of the world's agricultural land and accounts for one-third of our global fresh water consumption.*

Meat consumption may be the leading cause of species extinction, destroying habitat and overwhelming ecosystems with wastes from meat production that are wiping out freshwater life throughout the world.[253] Animal waste is less of a problem with grass-fed and pasture-raised animals, which roam over large areas of land rather than being confined in small areas. Their manure is dispersed over fields and becomes incorporated into the soil. However, in the western United States, grazing has negatively impacted 80 percent of stream and riparian habitats (the banks of rivers, streams, and other water bodies).[254]

The meat industry is estimated to generate 18 percent of global greenhouse gas emissions.[255] Greenhouse gas emissions per unit of beef protein are 150 times that of soy protein. Chicken protein generates 20 times as much greenhouse gas emissions as soy protein.

According to the UN Food and Agriculture Organization, "Livestock's contribution to environmental problems is on a massive scale and its potential contribution to their solution is equally large. The impact is so significant that it needs to be addressed with urgency. Major reductions in impact could be achieved at reasonable cost."[256]

Farm animals raised outdoors on family farms are a minority.[257] Huge numbers of animals crammed indoors or in outdoor feedlots are fed foods they weren't designed to eat (for example, corn fed to cows). This practice can not only make them sick, but it also disrupts the carbon cycle by essentially exporting the rich soils of mid-America, developed over eons, via animal feed to distant factory farms. Crowding means manure is concentrated in one location, becoming a water pollution and odor problem instead of a beneficial soil amendment. Many regulations exempt factory farms that would otherwise require pollution control.[258]

Author–activist Michael Pollan writes: "The industrial animal factory offers a nightmarish glimpse of what capitalism is capable of in the absence of any moral or regulatory constraint whatsoever.... Here in these wretched places life itself is redefined—as 'protein production'—and with it 'suffering.' That venerable word has become 'stress'.... It all sounds very much like our worst nightmares of confinement and torture, and it is that, but it is also real life for the billions of animals unlucky enough to have been born beneath those grim sheet-metal roofs into the brief, pitiless life of a production unit." Pollan suggests if factory farms had windows and we could see in, it would revolutionize the food system because the average person could not abide it.[259]

We sustain the tormented lives of farm animals in unsanitary, crowded conditions, using antibiotics and hiding this inhumane treatment using "ag gag" laws that criminalize taking photographs of "concentrated animal feeding operations."[260] Our inhumanity came back to bite us when Mad Cow Disease (bovine spongiform encephalopathy) arose after producers put cow byproducts into cow feed, turning herbivores into cannibals.[261]

It would be difficult to devise a more pathogen-friendly food system if we tried. "Beyond organic" farmer Joel Salatin describes how pathogens thrive when animals live close together, indoors, with no sanitizing sunlight or fresh air. Indoor air pollution abrades their respiratory pathways, providing entry points for the pathogens. The animals are fed "Frankenfood" and dosed with antibiotics, hormones, and other chemicals (which make their way onto our dinner plates).[262] Antibiotics, which are administered to kill pathogens and promote faster animal growth, can lead to the development of antibiotic-resistant "superbugs." Superbugs could kill more people than cancer by 2050.[263]

GENETICALLY MODIFIED ORGANISMS

Some industrial agriculture produces GMOs, in which the DNA from two species is combined, something that would not occur in nature or in selective breeding.[264] In most cases, a primary goal is to make the GMO plant crops resistant to herbicides, which threaten human and environmental health. The approach is to blitz everything with herbicides, including the herbicide-tolerant GMO crop plants, in the hopes the GMO crop will be the only plants left standing. Other GMOs are designed to produce their own pesticides, such as the Bt toxin.

The US Food and Drug Administration approved the first genetically modified crops in 1994, and GMO crops were first planted in the United States in 1996. In the United States, more than 90 percent of corn, soybeans, and cotton are GMOs.[265] More than 75 percent of processed foods on US supermarket shelves contain GMOs.[266] A coalition of environmental, consumer, and commercial and recreational fishing organizations is challenging the US Food and Drug Administration's approval of the first-ever genetically engineered food animal, an Atlantic salmon engineered to grow quickly. If accidentally released to the environment, these salmon could threaten wild populations by mating with them, by outcompeting them for scarce resources and habitat, and/or by transmitting diseases.[267]

GMO crops—grown in 28 countries—include corn, soy, sugar beets, canola, cotton, alfalfa, papaya, zucchini, and summer squash. GMO crop cultivation is banned in 38 countries.[268] Sixty-four countries—with more than 40 percent of the world's population—require foods containing GMOs be labeled as such.[269] Thirty of the United States have introduced legislation to require GMO labeling and several states passed such laws.[270] But the food industry has fought back hard. President Obama signed into law a sham federal GMO labeling law that negates the state laws.[271] The food industry might be afraid that if American consumers know GMOs are in a food product, they won't buy it.

Agriculture via a chemical arms race is not working. Genetically engineered Bt insecticide corn has created resistant superbugs, and one study found Bt toxins in 93 percent of maternal blood samples and 80 percent of fetal blood samples.[272] Roundup™ herbicide, used on "Roundup Ready" GMO corn and soybeans, has been linked to crop disease, livestock infertility, and herbicide-resistant superweeds.[273] In 2015, the World Health Organization determined the primary active ingredient in Roundup, glyphosate, is "probably carcinogenic to humans."[274] (Roundup is widely used on both GMO and non-GMO crops.) Evidently, you and I are not "Roundup Ready."

INDIA

Government policies favor large growers and dependence on agrochemical companies for seeds, pesticides, and fertilizers. One example of how this system ravages smaller farmers, the environment, and the economy can be witnessed in India, where more than a quarter million indebted farmers have committed suicide, about one every half-hour—many by drinking pesticides.

In an agricultural experiment known as the "Green Revolution" undertaken in the Punjab state of India in the 1960s, high-yielding varieties of rice and wheat seeds were introduced in an effort to radically increase food production. The seeds were used, in conjunction with new chemical fertilizers and pesticides, to grow monoculture crops. Irrigation costs increased with time as water tables dropped due to unsustainable water usage.

Negative impacts of the Green Revolution proliferated throughout many aspects of Punjabi life. Soils are now "weak and in many ways dead," depleted of micronutrients and beneficial microorganisms, and contaminated with pesticides. Other problems include breakouts of new and devastating pests and diseases, pesticide poisoning, drinking-water contamination, and increased incidence of cancer. The Green Revolution also increased levels of debt and social inequality for small farmers.

Traditional farming methods before the Green Revolution incorporated crop diversity, sustainable water use, low input costs, recycling of soil nutrients, farmer self-sufficiency, and mutual cooperation. Hunger problems were not caused by farming methods, but rather by large-scale exportation of food out of the countryside beginning after 1860 with the advent of British rule.[275]

This example from India highlights the connections between people, food, water, soil, synthetic chemicals, corporations, governments, and the economy, and all the damage done by misguided agricultural policies and methods. The "Green Revolution" might be one of the earliest instances of "green-washing" (that is, claiming something is environmentally friendly when it isn't).

HEALTH AND ECONOMIC IMPACTS

Food quality is foundational to our health. Diet is a significant factor in three of the major causes of death in the United States—heart disease, cancer, and stroke, which account for more than half of all deaths—as well as diabetes, hypertension, obesity, osteoporosis, and nonalcoholic fatty liver disease.[276] Food allergies can lead to a whole host of psychological symptoms: fatigue, "brain fog," slowed thought processes, irritability, agitation, aggressive behavior, anxiety, depression, schizophrenia, hyperactivity, autism, learning disabilities, and dementia.[277]

Dr. Fuhrman estimates about 90 percent of what US doctors do wouldn't be necessary if people took care of themselves, including by eating a better diet containing more plants.[278] Dr. Hyman writes that our "human capital" is being lost due to poor diets, and our federal budget deficit is driven mainly by "diabesity," a range of health problems that is almost 100 percent preventable.[279] Consider that 27 percent of young Americans are too overweight to join the military and another 32 percent have another disqualifying health problem.[280] Politicians ignore a major cost of skyrocketing health-care costs—our disastrous diet.

The problem is global. The World Health Organization reports that noncommunicable diseases (NCDs)—principally, cardiovascular diseases, cancers, diabetes, and chronic lung diseases—are the leading global causes of death, causing more fatalities than all other causes combined. NCDs are due primarily to tobacco, inactivity, diet, and alcohol and have reached "epidemic proportions." Almost two-thirds of the deaths that occurred globally in 2008 were caused by NCDs.[281] NCDs are often long-term; they elevate health-care costs and push one hundred million people worldwide into poverty each year.[282]

Big Agriculture means big money, which buys government influence, cushy subsidies, and a system rigged to reward the food industry for feeding us unhealthy food full of sugar, harmful fats, refined carbohydrates, GMOs, pesticides, antibiotics, artificial hormones, and chemical additives.[283] It buys food safety regulations that squeeze out local producers. As Joel Salatin observes, "our culture now considers it perfectly safe to feed your kids Coke, Twinkies, and Cocoa Puffs, but raw milk, compost-grown tomatoes, and Aunt Matilda's pickles are hazardous substances."[284] To make you buy and eat ever more, the food industry adds addictive substances (salt, sugar, and fat) to their products and promotes them with slick advertising.[285]

The US government kowtows to the food industry and allows industry representatives to make policy in government agencies such as the US Food and Drug Administration and the US Department of Agriculture.[286] Leading experts say lobbying skewed the 2015 US Dietary Guidelines.[287]

The government paid out $332 billion in farm subsidies from 1995 through 2014.[288] Support is highly skewed toward the largest and most financially secure producers growing corn, soybeans, wheat, cotton, and rice. Corn and soy are used mainly for junk food and meat production. Fruit and vegetable producers receive little support. "We subsidize large agribusiness and the wealthy at the expense of the family farmer and the taxpayer," says US Congressman Paul Ryan, who describes the practice as "an egregious example of cronyism."[289]

While the US government feeds large companies this corporate pork, sixteen million children in the United States on food stamps know what it's like to go hungry, and the United States has one of the highest relative child poverty rates in the developed world.[290]

Our food system ignores the financial benefits of ecosystem services. We put a financial value on pesticides but not on birds that eat pests. When coffee is grown under tall forest trees, birds eat insects that would otherwise damage the crop. Researchers quantified the effect of birds on coffee crops in Jamaica by using nets to experimentally exclude birds from certain areas. The research concluded birds provided $310 worth of value per hectare (or $125 per acre). Other research in East Africa, for tea cultivation, showed trees not only provide habitat for hundreds of species of birds, but they also keep the atmosphere moister, provide wood for drying tea, conserve soils, help ensure rivers continue to flow during droughts, and act as corridors for the movement of birds and other wildlife.[291]

ORGANIC AND LOCAL FOOD

Well, that was depressing.

Fortunately, the problems described above are unnecessary and largely reversible, using solutions that already exist. Organic corn and soy yields outperformed industrial yields in thirty-year, side-by-side trials while emitting less greenhouse gases, using less energy and water, decreasing erosion and groundwater pollution, and enhancing soil quality and biological resources.[292] Organic growing is the only way to feed the world sustainably, according to a UN report aptly titled *Trade and Environment Review 2013: Wake Up Before It's Too Late.*[293]

Organic farming emits less greenhouse gases than industrial farming.[294] Furthermore, Frances Moore Lappé, author of books about world hunger, democracy, and the environment, writes that by shifting to organic farming practices, agriculture could become carbon neutral.[295] According to Rattan Lal, a professor of soil science at Ohio State University, the world's cultivated soils have lost 50 percent to 70 percent of their natural carbon since people began farming. This number is even higher in some parts of the world. Agricultural fields offer a potentially vast repository for the carbon that is warming the atmosphere. Restoring lost carbon to the soil also increases its ability to support crops and withstand drought.[296] Nadia Scialabbe of the UN Food and Agriculture Organization asserts currently available knowledge and technologies, including ecological and organic agriculture, "would be sufficient to counter greenhouse gas emissions of the entire agricultural and forestry sectors combined."[297]

Organic growing is the only way to feed the world sustainably.

Currently, less than 1 percent of US farmland is dedicated to organic agriculture, while organic sales account for more than 4 percent of total US food sales.[298] What are we waiting for? And why are we exporting the environmental benefits of organic growing?

Organic farming often raises different species and varieties of plants together in communities and relies on enhancing interconnections among plants, animals, soil, water, air, the sun, and people. It creates harmonious ecosystems in which all elements benefit and no pest is allowed to rage out of control.

Writer and garden designer Jeff Cox elegantly describes the connections inherent to organic farming:

> The organic grower works within the natural system to strengthen and intensify it for the betterment of the crops. This leads to ecological diversity, among other benefits. The more participants in the growing system, the healthier the system becomes. One reason that organic growers can do without chemical pesticides is that a naturally occurring mix of insects will include beneficial insects and other animals that feed on the pests. Surviving pests target weak and sick plants first, just as a pack of wolves will target a weak or sick animal. This has the effect of culling the crop so that the strong and healthy plants survive and reproduce. The surviving healthy, organically grown plants tend to resist pests and diseases, just as healthy human beings resist diseases…. Without pests, what would the beneficial insects eat? Without beneficials, who would pollinate the crops? Without compost plowed into the soil, what would the earthworms eat? Without earthworms, what would nourish the plants? Without the plants, what would the pests eat? And so the interwoven web of life forms circles within circles, great and small, that add up to health and—in the case of organic food—good eating.[299]

Many of the bacteria, fungi, and other organisms in healthy soil decompose organic matter, such as plant stems and roots remaining after harvest, to humus and, eventually, to nitrogen, phosphorus, potassium, and other elements necessary for plant growth. Humus also promotes beneficial soil texture that allows air exchange and appropriate water retention and drainage. Well-managed organic soil becomes richer and healthier with time, unlike industrial agricultural soil.[300]

Soil health translates to the health of the plants and animals the soil supports. Healthy plants produce phytochemicals to defend themselves against pests. Many of these phytochemicals turn out to be very beneficial to the health of the humans who consume them.[301]

Organic farming is also better for air and water quality. Water supplies remain cleaner in the absence of applied pesticides, hormones, and antibiotics and from the use of slower-releasing forms of nutrients. Because approximately 41 percent of US land is farmland, the potential environmental benefits of switching to organic methods are immense.[302]

> *Because approximately 41 percent of US land is farmland, the potential environmental benefits of switching to organic methods are immense.*

Will Harris, a beef producer in Georgia, switched from industrial to grass-fed methods. Before he made the switch, his eight hundred cows were confined, fed corn and soy, and treated with antibiotics and artificial growth hormones. "Here I was fighting nature every step of the way," he said. When he learned of consumers who want grass-fed beef, he discarded the drugs, hormones, corn, soy, pesticides, and chemical fertilizers and switched to pasture feed. He says he has only one metric for humane livestock husbandry: "Can you pour yourself a glass of wine, sit back, and enjoy watching your animals?"[303]

Food grown not only organically but locally piles on even more benefits. Local food growing can take many forms, including household gardens, school gardens, and community gardens. Community-supported agriculture involves consumers buying shares of a farmer's crop for the growing season in advance, thus assisting with cash flow and sharing in the risks inherent in growing food (for example, weather and pest problems). Consumers share in the bounty of the growing season, receiving a variety of fresh, local produce every week. Many farmers sell food at roadside stands, pick-your-own fields, farmers' markets, local food cooperatives, or nearby supermarkets. Farmers' markets, becoming more numerous, increasingly serve as social nuclei for local communities.

Community partnerships include local farmers selling (or donating) produce to food pantries, helping to provide fresh, nutritious produce to the 1 in 4 American children without enough food to eat.[304] In a recent invention called "crop mobbing," farmers put the word out over the Internet requesting assistance with a labor-intensive activity such as harvesting. Interested citizens pitch in and enjoy the chance to get dirt under their fingernails and connect with nature, the source of their food, and fellow humans in the process.

Local food production decreases energy use and greenhouse gas emissions associated with transportation, while delivering fresher food to the consumer faster. Nutrients and flavor and fragrance molecules typically begin to break down as soon as produce is harvested, so fresher produce is often particularly nutritious and delicious. Local food can be harvested ripe, unlike food that is harvested hard and unripe for long-distance transport to the supermarket.[305]

Local food keeps money in the local economy and supports local jobs and land preservation. Consumers connect with producers, strengthening the community and reducing dependency on large corporations. Local farmers can be held accountable for their practices—for example, if their dairy contaminates a local stream—in ways that industrial producers are not. Small farmers working their own land tend to take better care of it and its inhabitants.

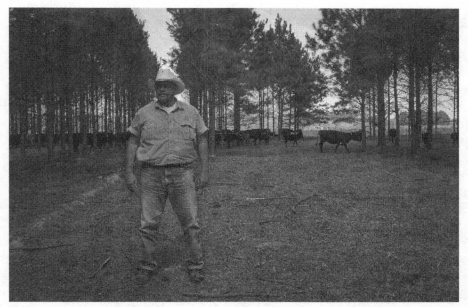

Will Harris, owner of White Oak Pastures, and grass-fed cows. Photo credit: White Oak Pastures.

UPWARD OR DOWNWARD SPIRALS

As evolutionary thinker and author Barbara Marx Hubbard points out, our problems are "dys-synergistic," meaning one problem creates another, which creates another, which creates another. Environmental pollution leads to health problems, which lead to financial problems, which lead to depression, which lead to vocation problems.[306] But the synergistic flipside also holds—

one solution creates another, which creates another, which creates another. Just as we can have downward spirals, so can we have upward ones.

A downward spiral often begins with a misguided notion. In the biomass burning and industrialized food examples discussed earlier, foundational misguided notions include "burning trees will produce clean, green, and renewable energy" and "industrial food production will solve hunger problems." These conceptual errors lead to a slew of ill environmental, health, social, and economic effects.

An upward spiral begins with a "right" idea. The right ideas in the Green Belt Movement and organic farming examples include "planting trees can begin to restore our world" and "nurturing the entire ecosystem is the most effective way to grow food." Because of the way problems and solutions are connected, we do not need to solve each and every problem directly. If we begin tackling a few key problems, such as deforestation and unhealthy industrial food, with a few key solutions, such as preserving and expanding forests and producing food organically, other positive effects will automatically follow.

We tend to focus on economic, health, and other immediate problems that grab our attention, and put concerns about the environment aside. Meanwhile, our house may be flooded or perhaps we're battling chronic illness. We may not realize that environmental problems—climate change or hazardous synthetic chemicals—are the cause of our ills, or at least making them worse.

By making a manageable number of important changes, we can create an exponentially increasing spiral of solutions that address many connected problems. Wonderful and doable alternatives are available now.

The pervasive problem of climate change connects with many aspects of our lives, causing ecological disaster, increased poverty, resource scarcity, mass migration, violence, and conflict, as people compete for resources.[307] Fixing the climate will help solve these other dire problems.

Climate change serves as a single barometer for measuring how we're doing in diverse areas—harnessing energy, producing goods, growing food, creating the built environment (buildings and infrastructure), and more. Climate change is feedback from the universe saying "whoa, whoa, whoa—stop burning things, killing life, and tearing up the land." It is measurable by concrete criteria—temperature, sea level rise, carbon dioxide concentrations, and ice, glacier, and snowpack areas and volumes.

Climate change connects generations of humans because it unfolds over long time frames and requires long-term solutions that work for multiple generations. This is, by definition, sustainability.

Because human and environmental health are one, actions individuals take to improve their health—such as eating organically grown food or bicycling instead of driving—help the climate at the same time. Conversely, actions we take to help the climate—such as stopping burning fossil fuels for energy—simultaneously help human health.

Environmentalist Gus Speth writes that the failure of the United States to lead the world on the climate issue over the past three decades is "probably the greatest dereliction of civic responsibility in the history of the Republic."[308] We have also exported our toxic chemicals, unhealthy agriculture, and deadly diet to the rest of the world. We have stirred up violence in other parts of the world, such as Iraq. Since in many ways, Americans have led the world into its current mess, out of basic fairness, we should lead the way out. But success will require global action.

The rest of *Our Earth* discusses and illustrates how humans can create the upward spirals necessary to survive and thrive, both as individuals and as a species. We can work on both fronts simultaneously, and we can begin right now.

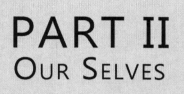

PART II
OUR SELVES

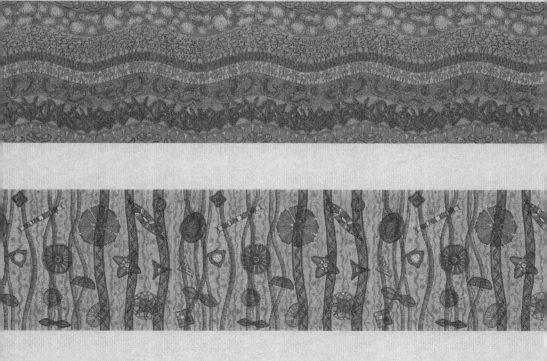

CHAPTER 5
POTENTIAL

When you have exhausted all possibilities, remember this: you haven't.

—*Thomas Edison*

EACH OF US IS BORN with vast and unique potential. In addition, people in the developed world today are blessed with extra years with which to use and express this potential. These years are added to our active adulthood rather than tacked on at the end of life when capacities may be diminished.

We design our lives on multiple levels, from life goals to our daily practices. Changing our life design can be easier than we may think. Author and philosopher Wayne Dyer wrote, "Never underestimate your power to change yourself. And never overestimate your power to change others."[309]

THINK YOU'RE NOT AMAZING? THINK AGAIN.

We are far more gifted than we realize. The Olympic Games every few years showcase human physical (and mental) potential from around the world. By the time Wolfgang Amadeus Mozart was five years old, he was playing keyboard instruments and violin and composing music, and he wrote his first symphony at the age of eight. Leonardo da Vinci's genius manifested in architecture, painting, sculpture, mathematics, engineering, geology, botany, cartography, writing, and music. In 1977, Shakuntala Devi, known as "the human computer," could correctly multiply two 13-digit numbers and recite the answer in twenty-eight seconds.[310] My father described the amazing memorization abilities of Joseph Romel, a blind Haitian violinist, who heard a musician play the violin part for the first movement of Beethoven's Symphony no. 1, one time. The next day, Romel played back the first movement, true to the original, note for note.

You may be thinking, "Come on, these are unusual humans." Yet other species of animals, supposedly less advanced, are also amazing. Dogs rescue humans against incredible odds or find their way home over long distances months after getting lost. Dogs and dolphins perform complex wartime tasks, including finding bombs. Lipizzaner horses perform complex choreographed maneuvers. Octopuses use remarkable intelligence to create camouflage or figure out how to unscrew the lid on a glass jar to access a tasty shrimp.[311]

In light of the amazing capabilities of "ordinary" animals, humans must have at least equally amazing capabilities. Each person is unique, and propensities often show up early in life.

Having a Path and Not Knowing It. At an early age, I was crazy about plants and animals. I would cry out to flocks of blackbirds flying overhead. Working in the vegetable garden felt special and meaningful to me, especially handling the soil. Among various pets, I kept tropical fish. I took pains to arrange rocks and abundant plants in the aquarium and filtered and frequently replaced the water to create a healthy, lush environment.

My best friend and I played with small plastic dinosaurs, dozens of them, and also trolls, small plastic figures with wild, bright-colored hair. We made clothes for the trolls out of felt and sewed our own colorful clothes, wearing matching outfits to school.

I collected rocks and was fascinated by geology, archaeology, and different cultures from around the world. I devoured books. Living in a family of musicians, I was immersed in music from day one. I always loved art and over the years explored many media—oil and watercolor painting, drawing, pastels, sculpture, pottery, silk painting, silversmithing, photography, pen and ink, and fabric design.

Some of my seemingly trivial childhood events turned out to be prescient. One time, I was designing houses with my cousin—drawing plan views with paper and pencil—and I designed a house with a circular fish pond at its center. This foretold my interest in green buildings that incorporate plants, animals, and water. As a very small child, about five years old, I made up a silly song called "Please May I Have a Pink of Water?" (yes, "Pink") that may have pointed to my future career in the field of water resources.

My interests as a kid were all over the place and consistent with exactly the way I turned out: I am a generalist, anthropologist, environmental engineer, writer, and artist, with strong interests in music and health.

After finishing a bachelor's degree in anthropology, I was at loose ends and working at restaurant and secretarial jobs. I took extensive aptitude tests to help me decide my next path. Recommendations based on test results were that I pursue medicine or environmental engineering.

At first, I was not excited about these recommendations, but after some months I decided to go to graduate school to study environmental engineering. I've been at it happily ever since.

Writing this book, I get to be a true generalist again, which feels so right. Earlier in my life, I mistook being a generalist as not having direction. But now I see that it all fits together as well as if it had been painstakingly planned. A person can have a life direction and only realize it retrospectively, and early interests may point the way.

Helpers can make a huge difference. Napoleon Hill, author of the best-selling book *Think and Grow Rich*, grew up in poverty and ignorance in a log cabin in the Appalachian Mountains of West Virginia. His mother died when he was ten, and his behavior became increasingly rebellious. His father remarried, and the boy's stepmother nurtured him and inspired him. She interested him in writing and talked him into trading his six-shooter for a typewriter. He went on to become a wildly successful researcher and writer.[312]

My Grandfather's Helpers. My paternal grandfather, David Moyer, launched his music career at an early age partly because of an intense and determined woman—Mary Walsh—who mentored, managed, and promoted him.

One day when my grandfather was about five years old, a woman knocked on the door and said to his mother, "Through the window ... while I was walking by, I saw a nice piano in your living room." She explained her intention to start a music studio in the neighborhood and said she was looking for a place to live, a piano, and children who might be interested in taking music lessons. At that moment, my grandfather's life was launched on an amazing trajectory. Under the tutelage of the resourceful but strange Mary Walsh (not her real name), he went from a conventional happy, active kid to a child prodigy. Before David was six, his parents allowed Mary to take him from Philadelphia to live in New York City for intense piano studies that included piano lessons nearly every day and two hours of practicing every day. She legally adopted two younger boys, teaching them violin and cello, to form a trio. David, so young and small that he stood rather than sat at the piano, began performing recitals in public when he was eight. At the age of ten, he performed at the White House for President Theodore Roosevelt. Soon thereafter, Mary Walsh (then going by the name "Madame Marie Berlino") began touring the trio all around the United States and then Europe.

David lived in Europe for eight years, meeting, studying with, and performing with and for the famous musicians of that era. He returned to the United States and began teaching piano at Bucknell University. After military service in Europe in World War I, he became a professor of piano at Oberlin Conservatory in Ohio, where he spent the remainder of his career.

My father carried on the musical tradition as a trombonist and later as personnel manager of the Boston Symphony Orchestra. And Bill's son (my brother) mirrored David's life as a child prodigy and concert pianist.

Though musical success might seem to be due to innate genius, David quoted Mary Walsh as saying "it's 90 percent hard work and 10 percent talent." My grandfather had the gift, and he also had amazing teachers to help him develop and express his gift of music.[313] And the mentorship of Mary Walsh influenced not only my grandfather, but his son and grandson too.

LIMITATION

To train a baby elephant, the handler tethers the baby elephant's leg to something sturdy (such as a tree), using a rope. The elephant tugs and tugs, trying futilely to get free. It eventually gives up and internalizes the thought that whenever the rope is around its leg, it can't get away. It grows up to be a gigantic animal that could easily snap a rope with the tiniest effort. But it does not try because it is held captive by its own belief.[314] We learn the same way.

As babies we cry and laugh and do whatever we want, in the now. We have no control, are extremely limited, and depend on others for all our basic needs. As our capabilities and our awareness of them gradually develop, we become less dependent on others. When young kids are asked what they want to do when they grow up, they might reply "be the President," "be an astronaut," or "be a rock 'n' roll star." Never is the answer to "endure a stultifying and thankless job until I can retire," which is where many eventually end up.

This boundlessness of preschool years ends when society tells us to rein in our behavior to conform to societal norms—no more running around screaming in restaurants, for example. We repeatedly hear "no," "stop," "be quiet," and "do what I say." In school, we are instructed to quietly sit in rows unless we are given permission to move or speak. Soon "no," "stop," and "be quiet" becomes internalized, and we think of this voice as our own as we police and disapprove of ourselves on behalf of society.

In addition, advertising increasingly bombards us with messages that we are inadequate. Only 8 percent of an ad's message is received by the conscious mind. The rest is worked and reworked deep within the brain.[315]

Some people endure an additional helping of disapproval piled on by religious dogma, which calls them "sinners." And corporations often view their employees as liabilities—with profits and stock valuations improving when employees are fired. This creates immense pressure for employees to go along and not make waves.

We conclude others know better than we do, so we disconnect our inner guidance system and discount our intuition. We learn to avoid negative feedback from the outside world by conforming, dimming ourselves down, and shrinking from life as we avoid challenging tasks at which we might fail.

> *We learn to avoid negative feedback from the outside world by conforming, dimming ourselves down, and shrinking from life.*

Of course, exceptions abound. At the same time that we dim down, some teachers and other mentors encourage us to excel. And rebelliousness and spunk prompt many of us to take risks. Still, even rebels struggle with the inner voice that says "be careful," "watch out," "don't get hurt," "be good," "keep low." These are limiting beliefs.

Self-development author and motivational speaker Wayne Dyer identified eighteen of our most popular excuses, which he also called "mind viruses" because of the way they duplicate, infiltrate, and spread:

1. Change is difficult.
2. Change is risky.
3. It will take a long time.
4. There would be family drama.
5. I don't deserve it.
6. It's not in my nature (for example, "I'm shy").
7. I can't afford it.
8. No one will help me.
9. It has never happened before.
10. I'm not strong enough.
11. I'm not smart enough.
12. I'm too old (or not old enough).
13. The rules won't let me.
14. It's too big.
15. I don't have the energy.
16. Personal family history makes it tough (for example, "my parents divorced when I was four").
17. I'm too busy.
18. I'm scared.[316]

Striking the right balance between fearlessness and caution will allow us to accomplish big things yet stay safe and viable.

Limiting beliefs not only diminish us—they erode our happiness. We punish ourselves for mistakes and misdeeds, vividly reliving them for decades. Eckhart Tolle writes about the "pain-body," which is an accumulation of our old painful experiences in our energy field.[317] The pain-body feeds on more pain and attracts more painful experiences. We may try something and fail and then be told (either by ourselves or by others) "you're not good enough." We internalize that belief and are less confident when we try again. We're more likely to fail due to lack of confidence. When we fail again, it reinforces the belief.

Guilt With No End. I had a pen pal in India with whom I corresponded when I was a kid. We wrote letters back and forth, and then one day I received from her a package of beautiful gifts, including small painted wooden containers and dolls. I wanted to return the gesture and mail her some quintessential American gifts. I wracked my brains as to what those would be. A tricornered hat? No, that was not current and would cause confusion. A toy that makes colorful red, white, and blue sparks? No, that was made in China. Native American arrowheads or pottery? No, that could be confusing. I just could not figure out what was American. I never sent her anything, not even another letter. I still feel bad about it, decades later.

All this limitation depletes our self-esteem, and as a result we may not take good care of our health, well-being, relationships, finances, and spiritual or personal development. We adopt a "can't do" attitude. Frances Moore Lappé writes that spreading disillusionment and feelings of powerlessness among citizens underlies deepening poverty, global warming, and other massive problems we face today.[318]

CONSCIOUS UN-LIMITATION

We tend to think barriers holding us back are outside of us—that we don't have enough money, education, time, connections, opportunity, or luck to be able to do what we are called to do. But barriers are usually an inside job, though individuals face a wide range of external hardships. Except in extreme circumstances, the only person powerful enough to stop us is ourself, and the only person powerful enough to free us is ourself.

Daniel Siegel, MD, teaches that we literally shape our brains: "One of the key practical lessons of modern neuroscience is that the power to direct our attention has within it the power to shape our brain's firing patterns, as well as the power to shape the architecture of the brain itself."[319] Research shows regularly playing the violin, as Albert Einstein did, causes a specific area of the brain to physically grow larger, and regularly playing the piano causes a different specific area of the brain to grow larger.[320]

If we are to bravely actualize our potential, fear and failure will never be far away. When we attempt something beyond our current level of proficiency, we have a good chance of failing. If we're feeling confident about everything and not failing or feeling fear, then we're aiming too low. We can learn from failures, make corrections, and charge onward without waiting until we "feel ready." We may never feel ready.

We can't suppress or destroy fears—of failing, disapproval, hurting someone, or being wrong—so a better approach is to "feel the fear and do it anyway."[321] Another tactic is to stop and pay attention to what we are sensing—what are we seeing, hearing, touching, smelling, and tasting? Paying attention to sensation puts us back in the present moment and shifts our focus away from the fear. Another strategy for fear management is to get oneself out into nature. The vastness of the night sky dwarfs our fears to manageable levels. We can also remind ourselves of our past successes and remember we're as smart as everyone else out there.

We can defuse fears by repeatedly asking "what if" to identify the worst-case scenario. For example, *If I don't finish this assignment on time, my boss will be mad; if my boss is mad, I may lose my job; if I lose my job....* Chances are, if we review our past fears, we'll realize most things we worried about never did, in fact, happen.

Personal transformation leader T. Harv Eker advises us to not believe everything we think. If a negative thought comes in, say, "Cancel!" "Next!" or "Thank you for sharing."[322]

Nelson Mandela endured twenty-seven years in prison before becoming South Africa's first black president and receiving a Nobel Peace Prize. During eighteen of those years, he was confined to a small cell, given horrific "food," and forced to do hard labor in a quarry. Each year, he was limited to having one visitor for thirty minutes, receiving two letters, and sending two letters. He controlled his mind and refrained from expressing bitterness over his harsh treatment. "Through his intelligence, charm, and dignified defiance, he eventually bent even the most brutal prison officials to his will, assumed leadership over his jailed comrades, and became the master of his own prison."[323]

Ask "How Can I?" Rather Than "Can I?" Many times, my parents decide what they want and then figure out how to get it—often by innovative, unconventional means.

- My parents wanted a compact Japanese-style house on a large parcel of land, but they realized they could afford this only if they achieved it gradually. They first purchased the land, on which we lived in a tent all summer long, for years. Eventually, they built a tiny building with running water and electricity. Many years later, they could finally afford to build a house on the site.

- My mother wanted a harpsichord but didn't have enough money for it. She had one custom-made by master harpsichord maker Frank Hubbard, paying for it partly by typing the manuscript for his book *Three Centuries of Harpsichord Making*.[324] Her father provided the wood for this instrument by cutting down one of his black walnut trees.

- My father, personnel manager of the Boston Symphony Orchestra, wanted to eliminate any possibility of bias in the auditioning process. He persuaded management to conduct all rounds of auditions with applicants playing behind a curtain, with no talking, so only their music-making could be judged. The practice of "blind" auditions became common in major orchestras.

- Despite blind auditions, my father was troubled by the lack of applicants of color. So he began a nonprofit organization called Project STEP (String Training and Education Program) to provide intensive training for minority students. Now more than thirty years old, Project STEP trains children starting as young as five years old until they are of college age. Every Project STEP graduate has gone on to college, and many have pursued professional music careers.

The current times call us to live more conscious and empowered lives so we can get to work quickly to help create a sustainable world. The rest of Part II describes how we can develop and grow ourselves, both to have more fulfilling lives and to more effectively participate in change-making.

CHALLENGE

We can learn how to keep limiting beliefs from stopping us, to live life from the "higher self" or "true self" rather than as dictated by the "inner critic" that tries to keep us safe. This learning can happen gradually or suddenly. There is nothing like a catastrophe to call forth unlimited behavior, which teacher and philosopher Jean Houston calls "emergence through emergency."[325] Women of ordinary strength have single-handedly lifted cars to free children trapped underneath ("hysterical strength").[326] To respond to an emergency, we may react with uncharacteristic intelligence, consciousness, speed, and physical ability.

There is nothing like a catastrophe to call forth unlimited behavior.

Many leaders in history grew themselves to greatness in response to crises: Martin Luther King Jr. struggling against racism, Harriet Tubman rescuing slaves via the Underground Railroad, Rachel Carson exposing the devastating impacts of pesticides, Mahatma Gandhi struggling against British domination, and Susan B. Anthony fighting oppression of women and slavery, to name a few.

Survivors of serious illness may realize what is really most important to them and that their way of life had not been supporting those values. They may switch to a healthy lifestyle, quit comfortable and predictable jobs to pursue lifelong dreams, or forgive decades-long resentments towards others. Some feel grateful to their illness for prompting their monumental life changes.

Barbara Marx Hubbard met a man who, after twenty-seven years in solitary confinement, now works for prison reform but said if he had it to do over again, he wouldn't change anything.[327] Veteran Reg Twigg, one of the longest-surviving prisoners of the Japanese during World War II, endured three years of hell on the River Kwai, building the infamous Burma railway and dealing with deadly jungle diseases. He said, "If I could have my life over again I wouldn't change a single thing." [328]

Learning

Humans possess an amazing capacity to learn and to consciously change their own way of thinking. Success coach Michael Neill says, "You're one thought away from changing your life."[329]

So much information is available now we are at risk of information overload. Google CEO Eric Schmidt said, "We create as much information in two days now as we did from the dawn of man through 2003."[330] One edition of the *New York Times* contains more information than the average person living in the seventeenth century would come in contact with during his or her entire lifetime.[331]

Information uptake can come with a cost. We may become discouraged from knowing about so many problems all over the world. And information can crowd out attention to art, wisdom, intuition, spirituality, nature, other people, and our life's purpose.

Still, knowledge is power. Plantation owners in the United States deprived slaves of education and prohibited them from learning to read to keep them powerless. More recently, the Taliban in Pakistan's Swat Valley region banned girls from attending school. In 2009, preteen Malala Yousafzai began speaking out for girls' education. In 2012, when she was fifteen years old, Taliban gunmen shot her in the head and neck in an assassination attempt as she returned home from school one day. She eventually recovered, and the UN Special Envoy for Global Education launched a petition in her name. The petition called for Pakistan to educate every child, for all countries to outlaw discrimination against girls, and for international organizations to ensure the world's sixty-one million out-of-school children would be in school by the end of 2015. On her sixteenth birthday, Yousafzai spoke at the United Nations "for the right of education for every child." She cited the ideas and human rights struggles of Mahatma Gandhi, Martin Luther King Jr., Nelson Mandela, and Mother Teresa. She concluded her address by saying, "Let us pick up our books and our pens. They are our most powerful weapons. One child, one teacher, one book, and one pen can change the world. Education is the only solution. Education first."[332]

Education expands our world, bringing us ideas and information from others with whom we have no direct contact. Education saves us the trouble of "reinventing the wheel," and it inspires us by showing us what people are capable of.

PERSISTENCE AND REPEATED SMALL ACTIONS

Having and knowing one's "burning desire" is not enough to succeed.[333] Persistence and hard work, often in incremental daily efforts, are necessary. Many wait for opportunities to take a few large steps toward their goals rather than taking many small steps. People may wait until they have a big chunk of money to begin saving for retirement, or wait until they have a big chunk of time to start writing a book. This kind of thinking can lead to procrastination and failure.

Persistence means doggedly continuing despite obstacles, which invariably show up. That's why the desire has to be a burning one. Otherwise, it's easy to give up.

Inventor Thomas Edison perceived as progress his attempts that didn't pan out. Of his efforts to develop a commercially viable light bulb, he is reported to have said, "I have not failed 10,000 times. I have succeeded in proving that those 10,000 ways will not work. When I have eliminated the ways that will not work, I will find the way that will work." Success and fulfillment guru Jack Canfield endured one hundred and forty-four rejections of his manuscript for *Chicken Soup for the Soul,* but he kept submitting his book to publishers until one said yes. To date, his *Chicken Soup* series has sold more than half a billion copies.[334]

The power of daily incremental actions can move mountains, just as increments of wasted time really add up. Plus, daily practice cultivates focus and discipline, increasing the practitioner's power and effectiveness. To create the lives we want, we can weed our garden to get rid of counterproductive practices while cultivating practices that strengthen us. This puts us in a better position to do the same on a collective level, so we can create the world we want.

CHAPTER 6
HEALTH AND HAPPINESS

Your health is your greatest wealth.

—Joel Fuhrman, MD

Happiness is when what you think, what you
say, and what you do are in harmony.

—Mahatma Gandhi

NO BRIGHT LINES DIVIDE PHYSICAL, financial, mental, spiritual, and emotional health and happiness. They are interconnected. A quote attributed to the classical Greek philosopher Socrates states, "There is no illness of the body apart from the mind."

BASIC HEALTH

Body and mind tend to heal themselves, given the opportunity.[335] Progressive-thinking doctors help their patients optimize diet, exercise, rest, and state of mind in order to maintain health and promote self-healing when problems do crop up. Mainstream medicine is beginning to embrace this strategy. Note that no well-funded advocates promote broccoli, whereas well-funded advocates push pharmaceuticals.

It's up to each of us to manage and advocate for our own health rather than rely on the mainstream medical system to do it. For example, no one keeps all our health-related information organized in one place for us (as much as it may seem otherwise). And each of us decides when to get a doctor involved.

Dr. Fuhrman writes, "Almost every person eating the standard, toxic, American diet develops strong physical addictions" to sweeteners, white flour, salt, and artificial flavors. Robert Lustig, MD, observes that our "sugar glut" is generating obesity, hypertension, diabetes, and heart disease and may be driving cancers and cognitive decline.[336]

Heart disease, now the leading cause of death in the United States, hardly existed in 1900.[337] We eat too much junk, or "edible food-like substances," and not enough plants, but stress and our sedentary and toxic lifestyle also fuel health problems.[338] Mainstream medicine falls short in addressing these drivers, though they are becoming harder to ignore. Paraphrasing Dr. Fuhrman, we don't want to have people falling off a cliff and have ambulances waiting at the bottom to pick them up—we want to keep people from falling off the cliff in the first place.

Yet mainstream medicine (also known as "conventional" or "Western" medicine) typically waits for things to go wrong and then identifies the best drugs or surgery to address symptoms. This disease-management approach, focusing on one body part or ailment at a time, neglects to identify the root causes of health problems. It is common to prescribe antidepressants for depression without even determining whether the cause of depression is physical. Our health-care system originally focused on battlefield injuries and infectious diseases. Dealing with chronic disease is not its forte. Mainstream medicine is particularly ignorant of environmental toxins and nutrition.

DIET

You are what you eat. Food becomes your physical manifestation and fuels your actions. It is easy to be confused by the constantly changing advice regarding diet. We can cut through this by focusing on guiding principles on which knowledgeable experts agree.

Journalist and author Michael Pollan sums them up by advising us to "Eat food. Not too much. Mostly plants."[339] By "food" he means whole, organically grown plants and animals, not processed foods, synthetic additives, pesticides, antibiotics, hormones, or other substances not originally present.

Eat food. Not too much. Mostly plants. —Michael Pollan

It can be a challenge to remove synthetic food-like substances from our diet. "We make our food very similar to cocaine now," says Gene-Jack Wang, MD. "We purify our food…. Our ancestors ate whole grains, but we're eating white bread. American Indians ate corn; we eat corn syrup." Many processed food ingredients cause people to eat unconsciously and unnecessarily, and will also prompt an animal to eat like a drug abuser uses drugs.[340]

High-fructose corn syrup and hydrogenated fats are relatively new substances, in widespread use, that our bodies were not designed to deal with.

Dr. Hyman says, "[These] are toxic foods that everyone should eliminate from their diet today, *immediately*. In fact, go right now to your cupboard and throw out everything with these two ingredients, because they damage your brain (and the rest of your body as well). But be prepared. There may be nothing left in your cupboard."[341]

One area receiving more attention lately is food allergies and sensitivities. Wheat and dairy have undergone so much selective breeding (the regular, non-GMO kind) that some people who were not sensitive to these foods in the past now react badly to them. Dr. Hyman reports the new modern wheat strains contain a starch that is super-fattening, a form of gluten that is super-inflammatory, and wheat polypeptides that are super-addictive and make you crave and eat more.[342]

Another concept experts agree on is that we should drink a lot of (clean) water. We hear conflicting advice about vitamin, mineral, and herb supplements. It makes sense that certain supplements could help optimize our health, in light of our degraded agricultural soils, our increased exposure to environmental toxins, our high stress levels, and the low availability of some nutrients in food. For example, most North Americans are deficient in vitamin D, an essential nutrient. Because supplements undergo little regulatory control, it's essential to buy high-quality supplements.

Dietary Changes Can Be Easy. About five years ago, I stopped eating wheat, dairy, and eggs. My diet was fairly healthy (mainly whole, real, organic foods), and I wasn't experiencing symptoms. But I had read about food sensitivities and was curious to see if I'd feel better without these substances. My plan was to go without them for two weeks and then gradually reintroduce them back into my diet, paying attention to how I felt, in an effort to identify sensitivities. I thought it would be tough, but endurable for a couple of weeks.

It was far easier than I anticipated. Within days I experienced greater vitality, sharper thinking, and improved mood. Furthermore, I simply lost all interest in these foods and I've continued to avoid them since. I also avoid large fish (due to mercury contamination), all flours, and refined sugar. I feel great!

PHYSICAL EXERCISE

Lack of exercise kills us slowly, and it doesn't take much exercise to satisfy minimum requirements. Exercise is not just good for our bodies, but also for our minds, enhancing overall brain health, learning, and memory. Exercise reduces risks for diabetes, hypertension, and cardiovascular disease, which converge to cause brain dysfunction and neurodegeneration.[343] Exercise decreases inflammation and works better than Prozac in treating depression.[344] Ideally, exercise should increase heart rate and aerobic activity and enhance strength, flexibility, and balance. It may be good to engage in different kinds of exercise to accomplish all these objectives, though some—such as yoga— can potentially do it all. But any kind of exercise that works for you is great. Just move!

Excessive sitting turns out to be one of the most dangerous things we could possibly do. The average American sits for eight or more—sometimes a lot more—hours per day. Sitting causes muscle activity, calorie burning, fat burning, blood flow, artery dilation, insulin sensitivity, and brain function to decrease. Sitting also increases bad cholesterol levels and blood pressure. Consequently, chronic sitting can cause a huge array of diseases and ailments, including the major killers cancer and diabetes.[345]

To cut back on sitting, use a standing desk or a workstation with a treadmill at work, if possible. If you must sit, get up and walk around often. The Mayo Clinic says: "No exaggeration: sitting is the new smoking."[346]

> *Sitting is the new smoking. —The Mayo Clinic*

TOXINS

Toxins may be natural (such as cyanide, radon, asbestos, heavy metals, and toxic mold) or synthetic (such as pesticides, PCBs, chlorinated solvents, and flame retardants). Our bodies have not had the opportunity to adapt to the tens of thousands of synthetic chemicals that we encounter in our food, water, air, soil, and built environment.

Toxins can be hard to eliminate once they enter our bodies. Creating optimal health includes minimizing exposure to toxins and promoting detoxification. A healthy diet not only can reduce new exposure but help eliminate toxins. Foods that enhance detoxification include cruciferous vegetables (which include broccoli, kale, Brussels sprouts, cauliflower, and cabbage), cilantro, green tea, watercress, dandelion greens, and garlic.[347] Clean water similarly is key—for reducing new exposures and eliminating toxins. Sweating from exercise and heat (from taking saunas, steam baths, or hot baths) helps our bodies get rid of toxins.[348] We take in toxins through our skin, so try to avoid touching objects containing toxic chemicals—such as receipts (which often contain BPA), glues, and conventional cleaning products—and wash immediately if you do.

Exposure to air pollutants is particularly difficult to avoid because we have no choice about whether to breathe. The typical built environment contains toxic chemicals that off-gas, such as paints, glues, and furniture.

Green buildings typically strive to minimize toxic chemicals in building materials and furnishings and provide adequate ventilation. Indoor air quality can also be degraded by things you bring into your home, such as dry-cleaned clothing, cleaning products, personal care products, and art supplies. If something emits a chemical odor, there's a good chance it's releasing toxic chemicals into the air. Houseplants can help clean the air.[349]

Avoiding toxins is hardest for those of limited means, partly due to the widespread practice of "environmental injustice," whereby we site polluting facilities such as hazardous waste handling facilities in disadvantaged communities where people are ill-equipped to fight back. People in disadvantaged communities also are less able to afford to buy cleaner food and filter their water and indoor air, and their access to cleaner food is limited. The solution, for all of us, is to insist that our government should protect us from toxic chemicals.

SLEEP

Many of us try to cope with over-busy lives by cutting back on sleep. Since the time of the Industrial Revolution, our workaholic society has devalued sleep, admonishing us to work, work, work. Arianna Huffington, editor-in-chief of *The Huffington Post* and author, calls sleep deprivation "the new smoking" because it is linked to heart attacks, strokes, diabetes, obesity, Alzheimer's disease, and a weakened immune system.[350]

Sleep deprivation is the new smoking. —Arianna Huffington

In our increasingly light-polluted world, we let electric lights and electronic devices interfere with sleep and disrupt our circadian (daily) rhythms, which are based on natural cycles of light and dark.[351] Throw in unhealthy diet, lack of exercise, and too much stress, and it's a wonder we can sleep at all.

The main function of sleep may be to "take out our neural trash," cleaning out wastes that accumulate in our brains from our daily thinking.[352] Sleep deprivation makes people irritable and moody and curtails their creativity and problem-solving abilities, Huffington reports, robbing them of joy and the ability to be fully present.

The Centers for Disease Control and Prevention estimate that more than 1 in 3 American adults don't get enough sleep, which the agency describes as seven hours per night.[353] American adolescents—who need about nine hours of sleep per night—fare even worse, with more than half suffering "severe sleep deprivation," sleeping six hours or less on most school nights.

STRESS

Many factors contribute to our stress: information overload, advertising, isolation, bureaucracy, transportation delays, discrimination, overcrowding, job insecurity, poverty, overcommitment, poor diet, lack of exercise, and noise. The US Department of Labor says the workplace is the greatest single source of stress, no matter what one does or how much one earns.[354]

> *The workplace is the greatest single source of stress. —US Department of Labor*

Stress is not only unpleasant, it also leads to a fight-or-flight reaction that shuts down growth and the immune system. When stressed, we resort to reflexive behavior rather than thinking behavior and essentially become less intelligent.[355]

Taking care of oneself in the areas of diet, exercise, toxins, and sleep helps reduce stress. A full menu of de-stressing methods is available for us to choose from—meditation, exercise, massage, heat, and journaling, to name just a few.

FINANCIAL HEALTH

Officially coined or stamped metal currency was invented within the past several thousand years. Other items not directly utilitarian in themselves, including shells and beads, were used as a means of exchange for the sharing of goods and resources long before that, and livestock and grain were used in barter or gift economies.

Money in itself is neither good nor bad. People doing bad things can do more bad things with more money, and people doing good things can do more good things with more money.

> *People doing good things can do more good things if they have more money.*

Winning the money game is an inside job. T. Harv Eker says that to be financially successful, we must be a success ourselves—in character, habits, attitude, fortitude, body, and spirit. Success with money can inspire us to reach for success in other areas of life as well.[356]

Financial health is having the money we need and want to help us fulfill our life's purpose and develop to our full potential. The amount of money individuals need and want varies tremendously. The amount of money is secondary to how the person uses it. A billionaire who hoards money and hides in a cocoon of fear and isolation may not have financial health.

Money enables us to have and do more, experience less stress, and feel more confident and secure. If we have an "emergency fund" that could tide us over during times of no income, we can afford to take more risks in our careers. We can become "financially free" when our passive income—that is, income that does not require us to put in time working, such as income from investments—exceeds our living expenses. Then our time is our own, and we work only if we want to.

Personal finance expert Suze Orman says, "If you are strong, you have the ability to lift up everybody.... Put the financial oxygen mask on yourself first so you can save your children.... When I say 'people first, then money, then things,' you have to care about people more than you care about money."[357] In our society, we have made money paramount—more important than our health and happiness, environment, other people, and so on.[358]

In the United States, fifty million people live in poverty, and another hundred million are on the brink of it.[359] That totals about half the population. Both external and internal reasons account for this situation.

The American Dream once promised a decent life for those who work hard and follow the rules. For many, the American Dream has become just getting by and surviving.[360]

Limiting beliefs—among them, "money is the root of all evil," "it's hard to make money," "if you have more money, it means that I have less money," and "rich people are greedy cheaters"—erode our financial health from within. Such beliefs may cause a person to unconsciously repel money to avoid becoming a "greedy cheater."

Many limiting beliefs are predicated on the "I win/you lose" orientation of Western society. However, when money circulates around and around—like water—profits can increase for the many parties the money touches.

Our first step toward financial health is to identify our limiting beliefs about money, examine and realize how fraudulent they are, and replace them with empowering beliefs. We can replace a "poverty mentality"—a belief that there is not enough money, time, or [fill in the blank]—with an "abundance mentality" and gratitude for all we have. Many of us have much more than we appreciate and vastly more than many people on Earth have—especially if we enjoy clean water, adequate food, and electricity.

A poverty mentality keeps us preoccupied with the mechanics of survival, distracting us from deeper subjects. It can allow us to be victims to whom "unlucky" things happen, justifying our "staying small" and avoiding more challenging pursuits.

Abundance is more about the way we feel than about what we have. Expect the universe to provide, because it is a friendly and abundant place, and maybe it will. Expectation of deprivation—whether due to a smallness of self or universe—invites it. If I want something but don't feel confident I'll get it, I may not even try for it, pretty much guaranteeing I won't get it and also reinforcing my "can't do, can't have" attitude. This makes it less likely I will give something a try next time, and the situation will spiral down from there. Whereas if I feel confident, I'll try and maybe succeed, which will reinforce my "can do, can have" attitude, leading to greater confidence and increased willingness to try next time, and so on, in an upward spiral.

Tiny actions can help foster an abundance mentality. Instead of searching for a quarter to feed a parking meter every time we need one, keep a roll of quarters in the car. Similarly, stock extra consumables, perhaps for the kitchen or bath, to promote the sense that we have plenty of everything.

T. Harv Eker talks about "raising your money setpoint," which is the point above which you feel uncomfortable earning or receiving money. If your income exceeds your money setpoint, you will somehow lose the excess money, just as when casino winners blow through their winnings, ending right back where they started. If your current income is below your money setpoint, you may take actions, perhaps working more hours, to bring in more money and return to your money setpoint. Much like setting a thermostat, you can consciously raise your money setpoint by establishing financial goals that exceed your current status.[361]

How can you reach your financial goals? Learn about money. Many people receive scant training in personal finance. Though the prospect may seem daunting, it really is not that hard to learn the basics from a book or a community college course. Do what you love in your work life. If you do, you'll probably be good at it and more enthused to put in time and effort, leading to higher rewards. If what you do helps people, they will want to pay for your service or product. It usually doesn't work well to chase money as the goal. If you are in a service mindset and fulfilling your life purpose, rather than pursuing money as an end in itself, money may come in more easily. Invest time and money in yourself through education and personal development. Your education can't be taken away.

Save money to provide for your future. Savings grow, thanks to the power of compound interest. As you save, track how you're doing over time, such as by calculating your net worth, maybe every six months or so. Add up your cash, savings, and the value of what you own, plus what's owed to you that you expect will be paid, estimating where necessary. Then add up your debts. The difference is your net worth.

Give more. The universe seems to fill the vacuum created by giving you more money. Deepak Chopra, MD, writes about the Law of Giving and

Receiving: "The universe operates through dynamic exchange—giving and receiving are different aspects of the flow of energy in the universe. And in our willingness to give that which we seek, we keep the abundance of the universe circulating in our lives." Gifts can be in the form of material or money, but the most precious gifts are "caring, affection, appreciation, and love."[362]

When you feel abundant, you are more inclined to share. Sharing increases your happiness, gratitude, and feeling of abundance. In addition, the people you have shared with feel more happiness, gratitude, and abundance. Giving is contagious. Lynne McTaggart describes the power of generosity, explaining how a woman who worked in a "typical dog-eat-dog" office, wanting to change the culture, left change in the soda machine one day and put up a small sign that said, "Your soda has been bought for you. Keep the spirit alive and pay it forward." This small action ultimately catalyzed a complete culture change of that company.[363]

People sometimes "pay it forward"—respond to a person's kindness by being kind to someone else—at tollbooths. A driver who pays his or her toll plus the toll for the car following behind potentially sets off a chain of forward payments if subsequent drivers choose to follow suit. Drivers feel good that someone paid their toll, and they feel good when they pay the toll for the next person.

Paying It Forward. One day recently, I was at a university for a meeting. My colleagues and I took a break and went to a campus cafe for lunch. I ran into an old friend who happened to be standing in line behind me. She said, "Let me buy your lunch for you." I said, "Great, what's the occasion?" She said someone had bought lunch for her the other day and she was just passing the gesture along. A few days later, I in turn bought lunch for a friend. She likely paid for lunch for a friend of hers, and who knows how far this went before someone stopped the chain. Or maybe the chain continues.

Finally, use some money to have a little fun. While it's great to be disciplined and allocate money for living expenses, savings, education, and giving, money for fun allows us to be full human beings and not deadly serious. We are more than scientific, disciplined, materialistic, and responsible beings. We didn't come here just to work.

HAPPINESS

By *fun*, I mean a lighthearted good time delighting in the present moment, while *happiness* refers to a broader, deeper, and more long-term satisfaction—feeling vital, living your values and your purpose, making a difference, and feeling connected with the world. Happiness adds more meaning to the equation, allowing us to thrive. People yearn to transcend just satisfying their basic needs.[364]

Preconceptions that it is selfish to want happiness often spring from puritanical modes of thinking that say we should deplete ourselves for others and follow orders. When we're happy, we're more motivated, effective, productive, self-sufficient, caring, and giving—helping us and everything and everyone around us. When people are unhappy, they tend to cocoon, neglecting themselves and others, and maybe even bringing them down. So it's helpful—not selfish—to be happy.

We can deliberately raise our setpoints for happiness and its relatives such as love, gratitude, and forgiveness.[365] Your happiness setpoint determines how naturally happy you are, and you tend to return to the setpoint from a relative deficit or surplus of happiness. Some people tend to see "the glass half full," whereas others tend to see "the glass half empty," depending on their happiness setpoint.

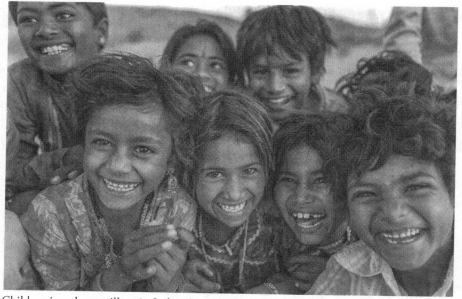

Children in a desert village in India. ©Istockphoto.com/Bartosz Hadyniak.

Happiness is related to fulfilling our life purpose rather than just satisfying our ego. Jack Canfield says we know we're fulfilling our life purpose when we feel joy. Joy is a compass.[366]

Living things have the urge and tendency to grow and express at a higher level of complexity and beauty over time. An acorn becomes an oak tree. A flower bud becomes a flower. A caterpillar becomes a butterfly. A person does good art and then does great art.

A lion lying in a cage is not the full expression of a lion. The full expression of a lion is out in nature, moving freely. It is hard to imagine a lion could be happy in a cage. Similarly, the full expression of a human is not someone in a self-created cage feeling afraid and isolated. At the end of life, old folks usually don't regret the risks they took and failed at, but they sometimes regret not taking certain risks. They may regret not allowing themselves to be happier, not going after their dreams, worrying too much about scary scenarios that never came to pass, or not having better relationships.[367]

STEERING THE SHIP

Happiness is a choice, whether conscious or not. Motivational speaker and author Marci Shimoff advises how we can be "happy for no reason … from the inside out," by practicing happiness habits that take us beyond barriers to happiness such as fear and anxiety.[368] She deconstructs a common misconception—that success will bring us happiness—saying it's actually the other way around.

To run our lives proactively and happily, we must discern what makes us happy, which may be different from what society says *should* make us happy. Transformational leaders Janet Bray Attwood and Chris Attwood write that passions are like pipelines to your soul and when you do what you're passionate about, you are doing what's meaningful.[369] This applies not only to one's vocation, though vocation is a big part of the picture because we spend so much time at it. Vocation connects us with others we serve by delivering a product or service, and our vocation feels like a vacation when it's aligned with our aptitudes, passions, values, and intention to give to the world.

Advice from many camps urges us to identify what we truly want and consciously set and work toward big goals, even if it takes many small increments of progress to get there. Billionaire Bill Bartmann uses the example of the game Pin the Tail on the Donkey, in which a blindfolded player tries randomly, and generally unsuccessfully, to pin a paper tail on a paper donkey. "If you can't see the goal, you have very little chance of success."[370]

One of educator and author Stephen Covey's "7 habits of highly effective people" is "beginning with the end in mind," discerning what is deeply important to us and managing ourselves each day to be and do what really matters most. He advises developing a personal mission statement. A sense of mission gives you the vision and values that direct your life and the basis for setting your long- and short-term goals. "People often find themselves achieving victories that are empty, successes that have come at the expense of things they suddenly realize were far more valuable to them."[371] Life is too short for a Pin-the-Tail-on-the-Donkey approach.

We typically have multiple goals, therefore, taking charge of our lives requires organizing our lives around the goals we value most. T. Harv Eker recommends "big rocks planning." Imagine you have a collection of rocks (representing goals) of all sizes and you want to fit them all into a jar (representing your life). If you fill the jar by putting in the little rocks first, the big ones won't fit in the jar. Fitting all the rocks into the jar requires prioritizing, putting the big rocks in early and fitting the little rocks in secondarily, around the big rocks. This means entering priority actions on your calendar first and then working other things in around them, realizing that some things may not fit on your calendar at all.[372]

Do your top-priority activities first thing in the morning so they can't be crowded out by other demands of the day. Many people do the opposite, first checking e-mail or otherwise attending to other peoples' wants.

Figuring out what we really want and letting our goals be as big as they want to be requires us to override the fears, inner and outer critics, and limiting beliefs that try to keep us small and safe. Belief in success is an absolutely essential characteristic of successful people and the driving force and power behind all great books, plays, scientific discoveries, and other human creations.[373]

Err on the side of being outrageous, and ask for what you want—all of it—for yourself and others. This includes asking people around you for help. They are often surprisingly happy to assist you.

A Small Ask, Leading to a Large Ask. When I was a kid, I had a feisty Welsh pony named Hurricane. Every summer, my family would move ourselves and Hurricane to western Massachusetts. Hurricane was ornery when it came to the horse trailer. Before we got under way, he didn't want to get in, and then at the end of the line, he didn't want to get out. He had to be coaxed out, with oats. One summer, we forgot to bring oats, and Hurricane would not budge from the trailer. So my parents drove to some nearby stables, with Hurricane in tow and an empty coffee can at the ready, to ask for oats. At several stables, stable hands refused us, saying, "I'm not authorized to ... [blah, blah, blah]." (We're talking about five cents worth of oats here!) Then my parents tried a residence less than a mile from our summer place, a house they had never noticed before. "Of course! I'll call down to the stable and have someone bring up some oats." My parents stayed for about half an hour and became acquainted with the Right Reverend Anson Phelps Stokes and his wife, Hopie.

Though my parents didn't know this until later, at around this time, the Stokes visited a mission of the Sisters of St. Margaret in Haiti. They were enthused about the work being done at the orphanage there, which included a fledgling youth orchestra. Having met my parents from the oats incident, the Stokes recommended the Sisters get in touch with my father.

That fall, back at Symphony Hall in Boston, Dad received a phone call in his office. "Mr. Moyer, there's a nun down here and she wants to come up and see you." He replied, "Well, I've never been visited by a nun before. Send her up." In flowed a nun in her long black robe and a starched white wimple that quivered whenever she spoke, which was often. She explained, "We have a mission in Haiti and a small but growing orchestra, and I have come to find out what you and the Boston Symphony Orchestra can do for us." She had targeted the right person. My father is an open-minded, creative, compassionate, and unlimited thinker. He said, after pondering this a bit, "There's probably quite a bit we can do for you—providing music, instruments perhaps, reeds and strings for instruments, perhaps even musical instruction." After a pause he continued, leaning forward, "But what can you do for us?" Sister Anne Marie, never at a loss for ideas or words, replied, "We have beautiful weather there in February and perhaps we could provide a week of respite for some of your players in exchange for a few hours of instruction for our musicians."

My parents attended a concert of the youth orchestra in Boston and were smitten by the children's enthusiasm, though their sound was pretty raw and their instruments were not very good. Dad became determined to help grow the Orchestre Philharmonique Sainte Trinité (OPST). On his first trip to Haiti (of many), he coached the brass section and helped organize the music library. My mother coached some piano students. My brother Fred performed on piano with the orchestra in the first of many such collaborations. My sister Annie played violin in the orchestra. On later trips to Haiti, Dad sometimes brought along instruments for the players. I remember seeing a stockpile of thirty or so instruments, including adorable quarter-size violins and cellos, in my parents' guest room before a trip.

Numerous BSO musicians visited Haiti during their orchestra time off and taught students, always returning refreshed and excited about the students they had worked with. Things skyrocketed from there. With Dad's encouragement, the BSO invited OPST to be their guests at Tanglewood for a month, where they received free private lessons and sectional coaching from BSO members and attended BSO rehearsals and concerts for free. Then the BSO invited OPST to perform in a festival of orchestras. Several years later, Dad arranged a second one-month residency for OPST at Tanglewood, and several of the top string players returned on scholarship as BSO Berkshire Music Center students.

When Sister Anne Marie needed an architect to design a concert hall for Holy Trinity School, Dad brought in his best friend, Frederik Christiansen, who designed the hall and traveled to Haiti to supervise its construction, gratis.

Today, the school building lies in rubble due to the earthquake of 2010. Underneath the rubble are the many instruments donated by BSO musicians, including the trombone Dad had played in the BSO. But the spirit of the group is undaunted, and the school has relocated within Haiti.

The moral of the story is this: know what you truly want and ask for it. You may be shocked at the overflowing abundance that comes back. Limiting beliefs could have kept Sister Anne Marie from asking one of the best orchestras on Earth to help a ragtag orchestra of destitute orphans. But she asked.

Personal growth pioneer Shakti Gawain recommends "creative visualization," consciously using the power of your imagination to create what you have decided you want in your life. She points out that when we create something, we always create it first in thought. We think about preparing a meal before we make dinner; a house design precedes house construction.[374]

Motivational speaker Debra Poneman used creative visualization for her very first presentation on creating prosperity at the Santa Monica, California, Public Library. She was financially strapped at the time. But she held strong convictions about how people can create abundance in their lives. She chose the library as a venue because it was free, and she put up posters all around town announcing her talk. Before the event, she visualized not only attendees packing the room, but also their joyful faces as they were transformed by the knowledge she would be delivering. She visualized the scene as being real in the present moment. As it turned out, the room was indeed full of happy listeners. This talk led to a long-running series of *Yes to Success* seminars, some graduates of which went on to develop their own personal development programs and become best-selling authors.[375]

People can use autosuggestion to influence their own minds by repeating affirmations to themselves. Affirmations are statements declared to be true, such as "My mind and body are in perfect balance. I am a harmonious being."[376] Consciously repeating affirmations can eventually make them more unconscious and automatic, like riding a bicycle.

Dr. Chopra says since most of our thoughts are not our own, it's wise to evaluate thoughts that come up and decide whether we want them to guide us. Meditation and journaling can help us increase awareness and control over our thoughts.

LOVE, FORGIVENESS, AND GRATITUDE

All wrapped up with happiness are love, forgiveness, and gratitude, which in turn are wrapped up with our physical being. The HeartMath Institute researches these connections and has found that when you feel positive emotions such as love, forgiveness, and appreciation, your heart rhythm pattern consists of synchronized, coherent waves. By contrast, when you feel negative emotions that create stress—such as anger and impatience—your heart rhythm pattern is jagged, irregular, and disordered. The heart, with its electric and magnetic fields, acts like a radio transmitter and receiver, transmitting our emotional state and receiving the emotional states of others. When you walk into a room after two people have argued, you can feel the emotion hanging in the atmosphere.[377]

Love is absolutely required for the survival of our species because our young depend on intensive care, attention, and protection in their early years, and their caretakers must be protected too. Babies thrive on love and wither without it. Love can apply to everything—oneself, family, generations long gone and yet to come, friends, other humans, humanity as a whole, plants, animals, the natural world, the universe, the Creator, the arts, technology, activities, and just being in the present moment. Love leads to responsibility, the taking care of what is loved.

Love reduces stress, and stress reduces love. Love seems in short supply in our modern world. We are stressed to the max by exploding e-mail inboxes, work and interpersonal conflicts and commitments, financial challenges, bureaucratic rigmarole, traffic, noise, advertising, and unhealthy lifestyles and environments.

Marci Shimoff teaches us ways to "love for no reason"—regardless of external events. When we give love, love comes back to us. Shimoff maintains we all have a love setpoint, "an invisible ceiling limiting your ability to experience love."[378] Love triggers more happiness, so raising our love setpoint is desirable.

Human survival requires that we once again love the natural world. Writer and environmental activist Wendell Berry told Bill Moyers that "the world and our life in it are conditional gifts. We have the world to live in and the use of it to live from on the condition that we will take good care of it. And to take good care of it, we have to know it, and we have to know how to take care of it. And to know it and to be willing to take care of it, we have to love it. And we've ignored all that all these years."[379]

Human survival requires that we once again love the natural world.

Similarly, human survival depends on once again loving future human generations. Our current course involves sticking them with a big environmental mess, in a case of what David Suzuki calls "intergenerational crime."[380] We even lack love for people living today, such as people in island nations and polar regions that are being devastated by climate change.

Love for other living things motivates us to protect habitats, shut down cruel farm animal "concentration camps," preserve forests, and stop slaughtering elephants for their ivory.[381] If we don't love and take care of the natural world, each succeeding generation will be left with less of Earth's bounty and more challenges. Environmental activist Derrick Jenson writes that our inaction "reveals nothing more or less than an incapacity to love." He fights for the environment, he writes, "because I'm in love. With salmon, with trees outside my window, with baby lampreys living in sandy stream bottoms, with slender salamanders crawling through the duff. And if you love, you act to defend your beloved. Of course results matter to you, but they don't determine whether or not you make the effort. You don't simply hope your beloved survives. You do what it takes. If my love doesn't cause me to protect those that I love, it's not love."[382]

We are taught that it's selfish to love yourself, just as we're taught that it's selfish to be happy. But loving oneself is good for the world because it increases our vitality, positivity, capability, and motivation. Loving ourselves and being our own best friend means overriding our inner critic, who can be downright mean. Treating a friend this way would end the friendship.

If we have gratitude for our challenges, we're less attached to outcomes. We resist less what life throws at us, believing "it's all good." Appreciation expands and opens us, and the universe reciprocates by filling the space created by gratitude. Human behavior specialist John Demartini writes, "To those who are grateful, more is given."[383]

We can be grateful for being alive during this most important and exciting point in human history. We can be grateful for our parents, grandparents, and ancestors going back hundreds, thousands, millions of years who struggled and sacrificed for their children, enabling the human story to go on and for us to be here. We can be grateful for our gifts, which allow us to contribute to the saga, and for the wondrous natural world.

Forgiveness recognizes the fallibility of us all and expresses love and compassion for all, including ourselves. We often are faced with a choice of either feeling right or feeling happy. Feeling right can feel bad in several ways: separate ("I am this right person here, and you are that wrong person over there"), anxious about the potential repercussions of being judgmental (will the person retaliate?), and worried that I am uncooperative and unlovable. And if I harshly judge others, there is a good chance I'll harshly judge myself, making myself miserable.

Using Our Lives to the Max

Maximizing our personal efficiency, in alignment with "big rocks" planning, allows us to use our limited time and energy to get more done, have more fun, and provide the most service to the world.

It's easy to waste time. The average employee in the United States admits to wasting two to three hours per workday.[384] Successful people can focus like a laser beam and shut everything else out. A great musician or sports star does not check e-mail or answer phone calls while practicing his or her craft.

Clutter-clearing—on many levels—increases efficiency. We can clear mental clutter: negative self-talk, judgment, resentment, worry, and mundane details. Methods for clearing might include reconnecting with our sense of purpose, practicing compassion, or making lists or calendars.

Author Denise Linn says physical clutter clogs your life. If you hang onto something you haven't used in fifteen years, you're telling yourself, "I have been okay for fifteen years, but someday I may not be okay; someday I might need this." This affirms future lack. Instead, clear out the object, confident that the universe will bring you whatever you need. Also clear out things that are damaged or that you don't love.[385]

Fun

Regularly having fun means we are enjoying the journey as well as our achievements. For many animals, fun, joy, and playfulness are part of growing up. Play and laughter existed in other animals long before humans came along, and circuits for laughter exist in very ancient regions of the human brain.[386]

Fun has taken a back seat in American society. The average worker fails to take almost five vacation days per year, and 61 percent work while they are on vacation.[387]

What qualifies as fun is unique to each individual. For one person, attending a football game is lots of fun, whereas for another person this would be anything but fun. Fun ranges from memorable major travel vacations to enjoying simple tasks, even mundane chores. In one sense, fun is a state of mind. Dr. Chopra says, "Have some fun. If you do that, life will be much better. I ask myself three questions. Is it fun? Is it with people who are fun? Does it help people to have more fun?"[388]

Journey Versus Destination

There is an apparent paradox between working toward big goals and being fully alive in the present moment. We want to have goals, but simultaneously release them and live in the present—not clutching our goals desperately.

Right here, right now, we have the power to change our lives. Yet many of us alternately dwell on the past and the future. We regret things we've done (or not done), which cannot be changed. We worry about what might happen, often engaging in debilitating exaggerated fantasies, or feel overwhelmed, fretting about all the things we "should" be doing. Dr. Chopra advises, "The most important time in your life is now. The most important person in your life is the one you are with now. The most important work that you're doing in your life is the work you're doing right now. And if you just remember that, that's the life you want to live."[389] Eckhart Tolle writes, "It is not uncommon for people to spend their whole life waiting to start living."[390]

Living in the now can save us from being "achievement junkies" who think *I'll be happy when I ... lose ten pounds* or *find my soul-mate* or *land my dream job*—and on arriving, immediately start on a next *I'll be happy when....* We can maximize our happiness by enjoying the long journeys as well as the fleeting moments of arrival at milestones, especially if we can even find enjoyment in chores, errands, dealing with challenges, and just being alive.

Journey Versus Destination: My Struggle. I have long struggled to overcome a fundamental focus on achievements and view of the journey as a nuisance.

For me, moments of achievement are thrilling but disappointingly fleeting. Each time I finished an academic degree after years of study, the sense of satisfaction lasted maybe a day before I'd think, Okay, what's next?

As a potter, another thrill for me is lifting the lid of a kiln. This moment comes after weeks of shaping, drying, bisque-firing, and glazing pottery, a day of firing, and an excruciating waiting period overnight to allow the kiln and its contents to cool. It's so exciting to see all the finished pieces, once drab and now colorful, shiny, and ready to be put into service. I can't honestly say I much enjoyed the time-consuming shaping, drying, bisque-firing, and glazing processes, but I loved the finished products.

CHAPTER 7
How We Can Each Help

Unless someone like you cares a whole awful lot,
Nothing is going to get better. It's not.

—*Dr. Seuss*, The Lorax

WE EACH MAKE A SIGNIFICANT positive or negative difference in the world—whether we try to or not, whether we know it or not, and whether we like it or not. And if we put our hearts and minds to it, we can make a massive difference by our individual actions. Actions tend to snowball—motivation leads to action, which leads to success, which leads to satisfaction and increased motivation, which leads to larger action, and so on.

We each make a significant positive or negative difference in the world.

We sometimes assume that deliberately changing our lifestyle would be a form of sacrifice. However, philosopher Kathleen Dean Moore points out that sacrifice is what we are doing now. We're "sacrificing what is big and permanent to prolong what is small, temporary, and harmful. We're sacrificing animals, peace, and children to retain wastefulness, while enriching those who disdain us."[391] Addressing climate change does not require most citizens to sacrifice. We can still live well—using smarter, greener practices that get more done with less and prevent damage. However, a tiny minority of people—those amassing huge financial wealth by plundering the commons—*will* be called upon to sacrifice or pursue different work.

This chapter focuses on actions individuals can take on their own—without depending on anyone else for anything—to help create a sustainable world. Part III will focus on collective actions, which are likewise critically important.

It's important to avoid being a perfectionist or overwhelmed, but to do what feels right and doable and perhaps work additional actions into your life over time. If a lot of us did a bit more than we're doing now, it could make a big difference.

Climate change especially calls on Westerners to help create a sustainable world. South African social rights activist Desmond Tutu highlights the grave injustice that people in Africa are being forced to pay the price for the West's consumption of oil—in the form of droughts and crop shortages—when they don't reap the benefits. Moore says climate change is "poised to become the most massive human-rights violation the world has ever seen."

Intergenerational issues are likewise important, as many people unwittingly destroy the world on which their children's lives depend. Moore says retired people feel like the world owes them a rest since they've worked all their lives. "Old age is precisely when we need to pay the world back. Yes, we have worked hard, but our successes depended on a stable climate, temperate weather, abundant food, cheap fuel, and a sturdy government—all advantages that our children and grandchildren will not have if we don't act…. We've got to remember that the next generation will have to live in whatever is left of the world after we get done with it."[392]

AWARENESS

Awareness of the current dangers comes first. Otherwise, we'd continue on our current path, like lemmings blithely running off a cliff. Whether humans will skillfully turn away from the cliff and onto a path of survival, growth, and happiness largely depends on how we who are alive today choose to act.

The transition time, while old ways unravel and we change course, can feel painful, scary, and unfair. Feeling outraged or sad is understandable—and possibly even necessary.

French diplomat, ambassador, and Holocaust survivor Stepháne Hessel at the age of 93 wrote in *Time for Outrage,* "The reasons to get angry may seem less clear today, and the world may seem more complex. Who is in charge, who are the decision makers? It's not always easy to discern. We're not dealing with a small elite anymore, whose action we can clearly identify. We are dealing with a vast, interdependent world that is interconnected in unprecedented ways. But there are unbearable things all around us…. The worst attitude is indifference. 'There's nothing I can do; I get by'—adopting this mindset will deprive you of one of the fundamental qualities of being human: outrage. Our capacity for protest is indispensable, as is our freedom to engage."[393]

BELIEVE AND ACT

Keeping human success going will entail a combination of many "ordinary" people taking many small actions—individually and collectively—along with some of us stepping up further to take larger actions. One person can catalyze monumental change when followers join in. In 1955, Rosa Parks—a forty-two-year-old African American woman on her way home from work as a seamstress—quietly refused to give up her seat on the bus for a white passenger. Her act of defiance led to the Montgomery Bus Boycott, followed by a Supreme Court decision declaring segregated buses unconstitutional, and ultimately helped end racial segregation in America.

Mahatma Gandhi began the Indian independence movement in 1930 with a 241-mile march to the sea with 278 followers to protest the British monopoly on salt. Along the way, he addressed large crowds and ever more people joined the march. At the end of the march, with tens of thousands of followers, he reached down and picked up a clump of natural salt out of the mud, thereby defying British law. Thousands followed his lead, and the independence movement snowballed from there.

Each year, the Goldman Prize recognizes grassroots environmental heroes from around the globe who acted to protect the natural world, often at great personal risk. The prize seeks to inspire people to take extraordinary actions to protect the natural world.[394] People in the developed world—who largely drive and benefit from resource extraction and environmental destruction and generally face less risk speaking truth to power—need to speak out and act more simply because we can. As antinuclear advocate Helen Caldicott, MD, said with regard to the United States and nuclear proliferation, "Rise up. It's this country that has to save the earth. You have no right not to do anything."[395] Because change requires both courageous leaders and courageous followers, we can each make an important difference, either leading or following.

Jim Kouzes and Barry Posner, authors of *The Leadership Challenge,* write, "Leadership is not about personality; it's about behavior—an observable set of skills and abilities." From studying and teaching leadership for more than 30 years, they offer Five Practices of Exemplary Leadership that "liberate the leader in everyone" and enable ordinary individuals and groups of people to achieve extraordinary results, often in a series of small steps:

1. Model the way—find your values and voice, and set an example in how you do things and what you do.

2. Inspire a shared vision—envision the future and enlist others, appealing to common ideals.

3. Challenge the process—search for opportunities to change the status quo, seize the initiative, experiment and take risks, and learn from mistakes.

4. Enable others to act—foster collaboration and strengthen others.

5. Encourage the heart—recognize contributions and celebrate values and victories.[396]

MINIMIZE OUR ENVIRONMENTAL FOOTPRINT

The impacts of our small, day-to-day actions add up significantly. We vote with our wallets every time we buy something, and consumer spending comprises more than two-thirds of the US economy.[397] Ideas for minimizing our individual environmental footprint are suggested below. Choose those that work for you. Some likely will not be appropriate for your situation.

FOOD

- Get rid of junk masquerading as food in your kitchen. Increasingly choose organically grown food—preferably, locally grown and predominantly plants.[398]

- Cook at home more often—using food ingredients you understand. Read labels and avoid the 10,000 or so chemicals the food industry adds to food to improve their bottom line, including dyes, preservatives, and "natural flavorings."

- Grow your own food, or start a community garden.

- Eat less meat.

- Reduce food waste and compost the plant-based foods you do discard.

ELECTRICITY

- Replace incandescent light bulbs with energy-efficient ones.

- Get into the habit of automatically turning off lights, appliances, computers, printers, and other equipment when they are not in use and unplug chargers (such as for phones and toothbrushes) when charging is complete.

- Reduce standby power consumption (also called "Dracula," "vampire," or "phantom" load), the electricity used by devices when turned off that can account for up to 10 percent of household electricity.[399] One way is to plug devices with standby power—such as televisions, DVD players, stereos, computers, printers, copiers, and cordless phones—into an appropriate power strip, which you turn on and off.[400]

- Maintain your appliances—for example, vacuum your refrigerator coils.

- Avoid using electricity at times of peak demand and avoid running multiple appliances at the same time. Peak demand typically draws power from the least efficient and dirtiest power plants and it drives the construction of new power infrastructure. Peak demand varies with location and season. You can call your electric company to find out when peak demand occurs in your location.

- Consider installing a solar electric system, if appropriate.

HEATING AND COOLING

- Avoid going overboard on heating in the winter months and cooling in the summer months.

- Use programmable thermostats that vary room temperature settings throughout the day, reducing energy demand when it won't be noticed (such as when people are asleep).

- Tighten up the building—caulk cracks and improve insulation. Some states have programs offering free home energy audits. However, ensure that the caulk is safe and that ventilation is adequate to avoid accumulation of indoor air contaminants.

- Service your heating, ventilating, and air conditioning (HVAC) equipment periodically.

- Consider installing a solar heat and/or hot water system or geothermal heating and cooling system, if appropriate.

- Let trees help—deciduous trees situated on the south side can shade the house in the summer and let sunlight through in the winter, while evergreen trees on the north side may shield the house from winter winds.

TRANSPORTATION

- Do shopping, banking, and other errands on efficient "milk run" circuits.

- Have the car tire pressures checked and optimized every time the oil is changed, to maximize fuel efficiency.

- Consider fuel efficiency when shopping for vehicles.

- Keep the car clear of unnecessary stuff to avoid hauling weight around needlessly.

- Use alternative transportation when possible—walk, bike, carpool, or take public transportation.

- If possible, live near your work or work from home on some or all days.

WATER (INCLUDING HEATING ENERGY)

- Use water-conserving appliances and fixtures such as low-flow showerheads.

- Run the dishwasher and clothes washer only when they are full, and air-dry dishes and clothes.

- Wash clothes in cold or warm rather than hot water when appropriate.

- Harvest rainwater for landscape watering; for example, funnel water from the roof into a fifty-five-gallon drum.

- Landscape with plants, especially native plants, with low water requirements. Avoid automatic sprinklers.

- Reuse water when you can.

- Fix leaks and don't leave the faucet running.

FORESTS AND WILDLIFE

- Print documents double-sided, print out less, or don't print at all.

- Use the back sides of paper and reuse gift-wrapping paper.

- Avoid the use and purchase of excess packaging.

- Cut down on junk mail. If a return envelope is provided, send the junk back with a note to remove you from the mailing list. Otherwise, call the company and ask to have your name removed. Call the phone company to stop them from sending unwanted phone books. Go online to Catalog Choice or other services, or call the phone numbers on catalogs to unsubscribe.[401]

- Stay off mailing lists in the first place. When giving your contact information to stores, companies, associations, or charitable organizations, tell them to keep your name off mailing lists and to not share your information with other organizations.

- Recycle paper and opt to buy things made from recycled paper. Buy copy paper with recycled content, even though—perversely—it may be more expensive.

- Opt for less lawn and more woods, and plant native trees.

- Leave natural areas, such as wetlands, wild.

- Pick up litter, to prevent ingestion by wildlife.

- Grow native plants that provide food and habitat for pollinators (bees, butterflies, birds, and bats) and other wildlife.[402]

MATERIALS

- Buy quality items that you love, are made to last, and won't go out of style.

- Reuse bags and packaging.

- Cut back on gifts—consider having a "Yankee Swap" or some other system whereby each person brings only one gift to a gathering.

- Strive for a clutter-free home and workplace.

- Opt for things made of organic and recyclable materials that are themselves recyclable. Avoid buying things made of synthetic materials such as plastic or high-environmental-impact metals such as aluminum or rare earth metals—even if they can be recycled.

- Buy nontoxic household cleaners, personal care products, paints, and other items.[403]

- Steer clear of items that emit chemical odors or fragrances.

INVESTING

- Consider socially responsible investing, which encourages corporate behavior in the direction of the investor's choosing. This can include the promotion of human health, environmental health, human rights, peace, consumer protection, and/or animal welfare.

- Grow the next generation to care for the environment—by taking kids outdoors and decreasing their screen time. Teach them about the natural world, food, gardening, and environmental challenges we face.

> **Special Trees.** My family planted a special tree in our yard for each of the four kids—moraine locust for me, maple and pine for my brothers, and weeping willow for my sister. We watched our trees grow over the years. Even after we moved away, we occasionally went by the old house and loved to see how our trees were doing.

MAXIMIZE OUR HANDPRINT

In addition to minimizing our environmental footprint, we can each maximize our individual contribution to the world by becoming more actualized in general and by taking specific actions.

Jack Canfield writes, "If you want to be successful, you have to take 100 percent responsibility for everything that you experience in life."[404] We each have the opportunity to develop ourselves, pursue our goals fearlessly, and stay healthy, balanced, relaxed, and happy. This increases our courage and power to do, say, and demand things. We can develop and empower ourselves by following the advice outlined in Part II of this book—by replacing limiting beliefs with unlimited thinking, identifying what we truly want, getting organized, learning, persisting in actions toward our goals, optimizing our personal and financial health, loving, and enjoying our journey. While no one can do our personal development for us, a lot of help is available given the recent explosion of personal development books and programs—identifiable through word of mouth or Internet search—that began with The Esalen Institute retreat center in California in the 1960s.

Here are a few examples of things we can do immediately, on our own, to increase consciousness, relaxation, enjoyment, and happiness:

- Smile.
- Take five deep breaths.
- Write down five successes you had today or yesterday.
- Write a list of things you are grateful for.
- Give a book to a friend who would enjoy it.
- Make a contribution to a nonprofit organization.
- Meditate for five minutes.
- Walk outside for ten minutes.
- Forgive someone (possibly yourself) for something.

Personal Development Workshops Helped Me Increase My Handprint. Until about ten years ago, I went about my life relatively quietly. One exception was the writing and speaking I did as part of my consulting work. Though the subjects I touched on were controversial, this work felt safe and fulfilling because I was presenting technical and impersonal information, not my opinions, and the information would help people clean up environmental contamination.

Outside my work, I tended to shrink from expressing myself publicly. For example, I created lots of art but didn't show or sell much of it. Growing up, my siblings and I were required to study music and perform publicly from time to time, which made me uncomfortable unless I was in a big group, playing in an orchestra or singing in a chorus. I looked at public self-expression as anything but enjoyable.

I experienced a major breakthrough during a five-day personal development workshop that, among other things, helped participants identify limiting beliefs and declare who we really are.[405] In a key exercise, I showed my art to the other attendees. Wearing around my neck silk scarves of my own design, I showed them paintings, pottery, photos, jewelry, and other items I had created. I declared that I was heartbroken about all the environmental destruction going on and committed to doing more about it. That workshop experience galvanized my resolve. The seminar inspired me to create the cosmology graphic on this book cover; the humans depicted in it are the workshop attendees. I began showing and selling more of my art.

I still regarded speaking out on many environmental issues as scary, but when the biomass issue exploded in western Massachusetts, to have any influence, I felt that I had little choice but to speak out and write about it. Despite risks to my career, I became a leading critic and endured attacks from the other side. To a large extent, I credit my willingness to speak out to personal development workshops. As a stronger person, I can make a bigger difference.

Specific things we can do, on our own, to help the world include:

- Voting. Staying informed and voting in elections matters, even if one vote seems insignificant. Almost half of those eligible to vote in the United States do not participate in presidential elections, and even fewer vote in other elections. It would astound people who fought and died for our right to vote to learn of America's abysmal voter participation rate.[406]

- Supporting organizations. We can vote with our dollars not only as consumers but as citizens, supporting people and organizations doing work that aligns with our values. We can provide nonfinancial support by volunteering our time. Carefully research the organization before you donate.

- Choosing work that aligns with our values. We can insist on taking our heart and soul to work with us, transitioning out of jobs that require us to check our heart or soul at the company door. Life is too short to live it half-way.

- Letting our concerns and opinions be known—by calling or writing our representatives and senators, sharing on social media, in conversations and writings, and perhaps with bumper stickers and lawn signs. Our viewpoint is just as valid as anyone else's, and we may inspire others to speak and act.

- Protecting our backyard. The phrase "Think globally, act locally" advises well, and there is nothing wrong with a "not in my backyard" approach.

If we each protected our local environment, the Earth would be in better shape. "Not in anyone's backyard" is even bolder. Local action can have wider impacts than one might imagine—often setting precedents and sparking actions that snowball, as when Wangari Maathai planted a few tree seedlings or Mahatma Gandhi picked up a handful of salt.

- Signing petitions. With the Internet, it's easier than ever to weigh in on important issues. Some debate the efficacy of petitions, but successes are real. Vani Hari ("Food Babe") launched a petition pushing for Subway to remove azodicarbonamide—a substance used in shoe soles and yoga mats to add elasticity—from its breads. Soon after 67,000 people signed the petition, the company removed this ingredient.[407]

Sign Petitions. I sign a lot of online health and environmental petitions. One day my brother Fred told me he gets inundated with e-mails asking him to sign petitions and doesn't have the time to evaluate them to determine which he should sign. He asked me to forward to him the petitions I recommend he sign. He'd sign only those and mark others as "junk." Several other people expressed interest in the idea, and it became clear that my vetting of petitions helped people. Fred created a system for streamlining the process, which he called "Ellen's List." Each week, I e-mail subscribers a link that lists my recommended petitions of the week. The subscriber selects the ones he or she wants to sign, and Ellen's List fills in the subscriber's signing information. In a minute or two, subscribers can make their voices heard on a dozen or so worthy campaigns. It's a fantastic way to quickly keep up to date on the critical environmental issues of the day while simultaneously taking action to help. I invite you to subscribe at www.ellenslist.org.

JOIN HANDS WITH OTHERS

Creating a sustainable and less violent world involves reaching out to others, including people not like ourselves. This takes effort, because the people nearest at hand tend to be generally like us, and reaching out to people not like ourselves can involve language barriers and differences in customs and opinions.

The idea that one can "go it alone" is a fallacy. We humans stand on the shoulders of those who came before us. Even activities that seem solitary—such as writing a book—actually are performed by large groups of people.

This Book Was Created by Countless People. When I started this project, I looked forward to a solo activity and not having to deal with a lot of people.

Wrong on both counts! Dealing with a lot of people ended up being both necessary and fun.

This book incorporates and builds on the knowledge of others cited, who in turn built on the work of others before them. Others' knowledge was made available through books, magazines, courses, seminars, interviews, TV, radio, and the Internet, which in turn were created by other legions of people.

Dozens of teachers taught me about the subjects in this book and how to write. Publishers, editors, literary agents, and allies provided valuable feedback, contacts, information, and other assistance. I'm bowled over by the generosity of other authors who provided significant help along the way.

Specialists helped with book production, distribution, and marketing. Still others provided speaking opportunities and spread the word about the book.

Yet you are the most important of all. Without you, the book has no reason to exist.

Although people acting individually can contribute significantly, massive change is usually created by large groups; this is discussed in Chapter 12. Groups are typically started by one or a few individuals. Recall Margaret Mead's famous words, "Never doubt that a small group of thoughtful, committed citizens can change the world. Indeed, it is the only thing that ever has."[408]

In her book *Jump Time*, Jean Houston advises individuals to "join or start a teaching–learning community that keeps you growing along with like-minded friends and allies committed to discovering and nurturing each other's hidden talents. Then together, move out in the community, see what needs vision and renewal and, using your new capacities, go out and do it."[409]

The nonprofit environmental organization Center for Biological Diversity began when three men surveying owls for the US Forest Service opposed a massive timber sale that would destroy rare owls and old-growth trees.[410] People joined to help. Since its founding in 1989, the organization has used existing environmental laws within the existing system with astounding success. Through passion and persistence, they have protected more than 550 species on more than 472 million acres of federally protected habitat preserves for endangered animals and plants. This acreage of lands and waters is larger than that of all the national parks and national forests combined, and more than the combined area of California, Texas, and Florida.[411] A million members and online activists support the Center for Biological Diversity's efforts.[412]

The Power of Ordinary Citizens. One day, blue markings appeared on trees in some areas of Robinson State Park in western Massachusetts. Wondering what was up, local residents contacted the Massachusetts Department of

Conservation and Recreation (DCR) and were informed of plans to log 133 acres. At the citizens' request, DCR representatives met with them. The DCR claimed that logging was needed to improve the long-term health of the forest; reduce threats from windstorms, insects, and wildfire; and enhance public safety and natural resources.

For two years, with the help of scientists, the citizens refuted a total of 22 excuses the DCR put forth to justify forest "treatment," "harvesting," and "management," all euphemisms for clear-cutting. (In truth, the best course for a forest is usually to leave it alone.)[413] After none of their excuses held up and the DCR ran out of new ones, the DCR canceled the logging contract.[414]

The local resistance effort had been led by a core group of about five people, and a dozen people regularly attended meetings. An e-mail list of about 350 and well over 2000 petition signers provided additional support.

Ripple effects spread out far from Robinson State Park. The citizens who blocked the logging at Robinson can largely be credited with inspiring the state to undertake a "Forest Futures Visioning Process" to evaluate a wide range of ecosystem services that public lands provide. This resulted in the state's designating some forests and parks as off-limits to commercial logging. Unfortunately, the state still allows commercial logging on other public lands, despite public comments that overwhelmingly opposed it.

Though this is just a start, it's an improvement that protects some forests. And it shows how ordinary citizens can change the game.

In 2014, I interviewed Marion Stoddart, an environmental hero who rescued the polluted Nashua River. What she told me highlights many of the concepts in Part II and can be applied to other environmental problems. Summarizing her wisdom seems like a fitting way to end this section.

In the 1960s, the Nashua River was starved of oxygen, biologically dead, and one of the ten most polluted rivers in the United States.[415] The sludge-filled river, which flows through New Hampshire and Massachusetts, was a different color every day, depending on what chemicals had been discharged. People could smell its stench from a mile away. At that time in the United States, it was legal to dump sewage and industrial waste into rivers.

In 1962, Marion Stoddart moved to the area with her family. Stoddart made it her life mission to restore the river to its preindustrial condition—running clean and clear, teeming with fish and wildlife. She mobilized industry leaders, government officials, and concerned citizens and ultimately accomplished her goal.[416]

One of Stoddart's initial tasks was to push hard for federal and state legislation that made the cleanup of the river possible and set the stage for other states to follow suit. She then persuaded municipalities to appropriate their share of funds for wastewater treatment. Wastewater treatment plants were constructed and put into service in the 1970s.

In 1969, Stoddart founded the Nashua River Watershed Association (NRWA) to protect the river and educate the public.[417] A key objective was to permanently protect the land adjacent to the river—continuous "greenways" extending at least three hundred feet back from the river and major tributaries. These buffer zones protect the river from storm water runoff—which often contains lawn-care and agricultural chemicals, petroleum from vehicles, and other contaminants. Greenways also provide wildlife habitat and corridors, protect the floodplain and wetlands, and enable people to enjoy the river. With its goal about half completed and approximately two hundred miles of shoreline protected, continuing efforts are funded by contributions to the Marion Stoddart Greenway Fund, which was created in 2013 on her eighty-fifth birthday.[418]

Fish, turtles, mink, otters, ospreys, and bald eagles returned to the river. People now flock there to fish, boat, hike, and bicycle. The clean river boosted the economy of cities along its route, increasing property values and attracting new businesses. Ordinary citizens learned that they have the power to create change.

Today, segments of the river are candidates for "wild and scenic" designation. The designation would provide federal funds to preserve the river and bordering land in its natural state due to outstanding scenic, recreational, ecological, and historical values.[419]

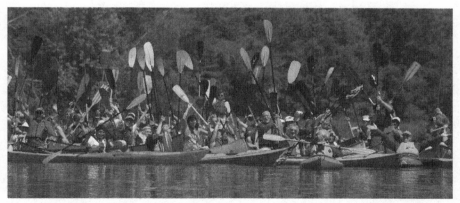

Marion Stoddart and friends celebrating the Nashua River with a paddle wave. Photo credit: Hugh F. Stoddart.

Stoddart received a UN Environment Programme Global 500 Award, was profiled by *National Geographic* magazine, and was the main character in Lynne Cherry's best-selling children's book *A River Ran Wild*.[420] The National Women's History Project honored her as a "woman taking the lead to save our planet."[421]

Stoddart attributes her success to the following factors:

Longing for a larger purpose—Shortly after moving to the area, Stoddart asked herself, "Why am I here?" She wanted to do more than simply make her family happy.

Inspiration—Stoddart was inspired by a radio program she heard. It asserted that with vision and commitment, one person can do the work of a thousand people. Through her work in the League of Women Voters, she knew the environmental advocate Allen Morgan and admired his commitment, drive, and collaborative approach. Rachel Carson's *Silent Spring* further ignited her.

Vision—One day, standing in her backyard, looking out over the fields and woods toward the reeking Nashua River a mile away, Stoddart created a vivid picture in her mind of the river and adjacent land restored to its original beauty, abundant with wildlife and attracting people as in times past. The vision came easily and never left her mind.

Commitment—Stoddart thought to herself, "I will never know what it is I am supposed to be doing, but I will take on the greatest challenge I believe I can accomplish in my lifetime and commit to that." She made a lifetime commitment to herself to restore the river—certain she would find a way—without initially discussing the idea with anyone or knowing how she was going to do it.

Homework—She informed herself on the issues, players, politics, existing laws, and process for creating new laws. She studied ways to change the laws to stop the polluting.

Collaboration—Stoddart's work required helpers. She contacted the leaders of every local industry; service, social, fraternal, recreational, and conservation organizations; and city and town mayors and boards of selectmen, planning boards, conservation commissions, boards of health, and recreation commissions. She met with state and local leaders, stakeholders, and citizens, becoming their friend, and listening, educating, and successfully enlisting them in her vision. When the NRWA was formed, the largest paper company joined. Its chief executive, Don Crocker, sent a letter to the executives of other local industries to convince them that they all would benefit from clean water. Crocker and the mayor of Fitchburg, Massachusetts, Bill Flynn, joined NRWA's board of directors. Stoddart's team amassed 6287 citizen signatures protesting the condition of the river and presented them to Massachusetts Governor John Volpe, along with a bottle of the revolting river water—with mayors and selectmen from all the riverside cities and towns, as well as legislators, photographers, and reporters, in attendance. The bowled-over governor vowed to keep the bottle of water on his desk as a reminder of what needed to be done.

Asking for what you want—Many thought Stoddart's goal of a clean Nashua River not only preposterous but threatening to the local economy as well. One riverside industry asked its employees, "Which would you rather have—clean water or your jobs?" (This false choice was later dispelled.) Stoddart received death threats. In 1966, US Senator Ted Kennedy toured polluted rivers in the northeast with Secretary of the Interior Stewart Udall. At the airport, Stoddart and her entourage of hundreds of citizens greeted Kennedy and Udall with a bottle of putrid Nashua River water. State officials, including the governor, also attended. As she prepared notes for a brief speech, Stoddart listed ways in which the public desired to use the Nashua River. She wrote "fishing, boating, irrigation, swimming." Then she crossed off "swimming," thinking the idea would strain credibility, given the horrific state of the river and because making the water clean enough for swimming would greatly escalate wastewater treatment costs. As she pondered whether to add "swimming" back in, Lieutenant Governor Elliot Richardson leaned over and whispered, "Ask for swimming. If you don't, you'll never get it." So Stoddart asked for swimming, and she got it. On returning to Boston that same day, Governor Volpe signed into law the Massachusetts Clean Water Act.

Surrounding yourself with positive-thinking people—Stoddart avoids spending time with negative-thinking people, noting "you'll never change their minds and they'll only pull you down." When you work with positive-thinking people, she says, things move quickly and become synergistic and fun, magnetizing more positive-thinking people to the effort.

Seeing challenges as opportunities—Stoddart treats obstacles as exciting challenges. When blocked, she simply looks for another way—devoid of anger, frustration, or discouragement.

Involving the media—Doing so creates pressure for change and informs citizens their voices are being heard, supported, and acted on.

Welcoming help—Stoddart says support sometimes arrives unexpectedly. In 1968, she received a call from Commanding Officer Jack Cushman of Fort Devens, a nearby military installation. Eight miles of the river flow through the army base. Cushman offered to help. Stoddart met with him, and he gave her everything she asked for, plus more—a two-story building with heat, lights, and a telephone, as well as the services of engineers, draftspeople, and other staff with specialized training. Fort Devens designated the land beside the river as a greenway. The army provided approximately thirteen Green Berets with dump trucks to transport and supervise approximately four hundred high-school dropouts sponsored by the US Department of Labor to clean up riverbanks and build trails along the river.

Persistence—Mayor Flynn remarked that in the 1960s, activists visited polluted rivers to protest and make headlines, and then they left. Stoddart was different—she was "in it for the long haul" with her relentless, collaborative approach.

Knowing the work will never be completed—Today, Stoddart continues advocating for greenways and ensuring laws are implemented and kept strong to prevent backsliding.

Stoddart provides a powerful example of collaboration, passion, and persistence. She says, "You don't have to be super-smart or super-anything, only committed." [422]

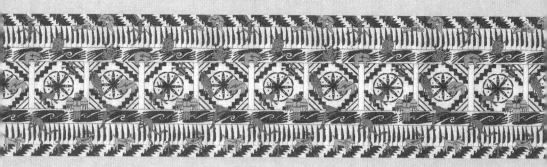

PART III
OUR SPECIES

CHAPTER 8
CRISIS IS OPPORTUNITY

We don't succeed in spite of our obstacles and challenges.
We succeed precisely because of them.

—Janet Bray Attwood and Chris Attwood

WHEN LIFE IS EASY, WE may choose the path of least resistance that requires only light use of our capabilities. When things are really bad, big change is possible. Garden-variety stress may prompt a caterpillar to become a better caterpillar, but only extreme crisis signals that it's time for the butterfly.

Crisis either does us in or kicks us into overdrive, making us do things we never thought possible. A disastrous tornado changed the world from black-and-white to color and precipitated the epic journey and transformation of Dorothy and her friends in *The Wizard of Oz*.[423]

We don't need a crisis to get something done, but it sure helps. Marion Stoddart remarked, "Most action, unfortunately, takes place only when things reach a critical stage; the Nashua River was in its death throes.... It was the right time."[424]

Sometimes, the pace of the response is similar to the pace of the crisis. A sudden crisis such as an explosion will be met with a fast response, whereas a slowly developing crisis such as climate change, weight gain, or chronic disease may be met with a slower response. However, crises can build gradually and then culminate in a rapid change. The "Arab Spring" that swept the Arab world in 2010 followed decades of trouble involving dictatorships, human rights violations, corruption, unemployment, poverty, and climate change.[425]

Life force tries to counteract entropy (the tendency of things to gradually decline into disorder) and strives for more order, healing, and growth. The current state of social and environmental disorder calls people to respond, as evidenced by global attention on climate change. At the same time, many people feel overwhelmed by the number and enormity of our problems. We now face a high-stakes choice: we can sink into despair and incompetence, or we can roll up our sleeves and get to work—and even welcome a grand opportunity for global collaboration and uplift.

We can respond to crises by creating large goals and committing the necessary resources. Often these responses come with unexpected ancillary benefits. During World War II, women filled positions in the workforce left vacant by men who went to war, becoming skilled at these jobs and gaining confidence that they could perform well in the professional work arena. Though women lost their jobs when men returned from war, according to US Representative Tim Ryan, women "forever changed the American workforce and broadened and enhanced the role of women in our society. Women in America turned a crisis into an opportunity."[426]

> *We can respond to crises by creating large goals and committing the necessary resources.*

During the Cold War, the state of political and military tension following World War II, the Russian launch of the first satellite (Sputnik) prompted President John Kennedy to resolve to put a man on the moon before Russia did. Though many thought this impossible, our government poured on the resources to develop the necessary new technology, and succeeded. The research program gave us solar technology, and the photographs of Earth from space, showing it as a small and vulnerable planet, profoundly affected viewers. "We went to explore the moon, and in fact discovered the Earth," said Apollo 17 astronaut Eugene Cernan.[427]

In 1964, with the nation reeling from the assassination of President Kennedy, President Lyndon Johnson launched the Great Society and the War on Poverty, a bold and almost utopian set of domestic programs to address problems in such areas as education, medical care, civil rights, environment, poverty, labor, transportation, and cities. Medicare, Medicaid, the National Endowment for the Arts, the National Endowment for the Humanities, and the Corporation for Public Broadcasting are still with us. A short time later, environmental crises prompted President Richard Nixon to institute visionary environmental institutions and policies.

The above examples involved strong presidential leadership. Grassroots movements—such as the Occupy Wall Street movement that began in 2011—did not have such strong leaders. Yet one month after the beginning of Occupy Wall Street in New York City, protests were taking place in eighty countries.[428]

Humanity has even responded globally to global crises. In 1987, the Montreal Protocol was the first universally ratified treaty, signed by 197 countries, in UN history. This global response phased out certain chemicals responsible for depleting the Earth's ozone shield in the upper atmosphere. According to *USA Today,* "the world came together and averted a catastrophe," and the Montreal Protocol "is proof positive that the Earth's nearly 200 countries can cooperate to save their citizens from a planetary pollution catastrophe."[429] Hopefully, the UN Intergovernmental Panel on Climate Change established in 1988 to deal with climate change will be equally successful.

The existence of the United States owes itself to crises. Religious and ethnic persecution and economic calamity led (and still lead) migrants to take frightful and often lethal journeys to what is now the United States.

FILTHY CITIES

The British Broadcasting Corporation explored examples of health and environmental crises driving massive positive change from the ground up in a series titled *Filthy Cities.* The episodes describe the histories of medieval London, revolutionary Paris, and industrial New York. The parallels between then and now are striking.

In medieval London, people routinely threw all kinds of waste into unpaved streets, open gutters, rivers, and streams—including excrement, tannery waste, and animal guts and blood. Platform overshoes were invented to lift people above the squalor when they walked. Many complained. The "Assize of Nuisance" documents grievances Londoners brought to the attention of the government from 1301 to 1431, such as pipes discharging waste from one dwelling into the basement of another.[430] As the city population exploded, the situation became intolerable. The average life expectancy was thirty-five years. The filth created a paradise for rats, fleas, and pathogens such as bubonic plague bacteria, which arrived from Central Asia by boat in 1348. By 1349, this "black death" had killed off more than half the population.

Death, disease, dirt, and squalor sparked a revolution in which Londoners came together to declare a "war on filth." New jobs were created: "muckrakers" to gather filth and take it beyond the city walls; "surveyors of the pavement" to remove waste from the streets, and "dung farmers" to clean out cesspools and privies. Fines for dumping waste were greatly escalated. The number of civil servants tripled. To address the selling of putrid and disease-ridden meat, butchers were ordered to sell meat only by the light of day, not by candlelight.

The ability to cooperate and take collective effort—even in the face of a catastrophe such as the plague—proved vital for the expansion of urban life. London, once a filthy city, ultimately became the center of the richest and most powerful empire in history.[431]

Two hundred years ago, Paris was one of the foulest and smelliest cities in Europe. City dwellers lived with grotesque filth, poverty, sickness, and starvation. The Seine River was an open sewer for human, animal, and industrial wastes, as the Thames had been in England. The average life expectancy of a poor laborer was only twenty-three years.

After generations of injustice, filth became a catalyst for political change and drove Parisians to revolt. Some Parisians surveyed the city to evaluate the link between filth and disease. As the world's first modern city to look at the science of waste, scientists and intellectuals offered an alternative to the putrid life in Paris. "The Enlightenment" included a vision for a healthier and cleaner future. An educated and literate middle class emerged. In response to mounting unrest, the king commissioned a survey of his subjects' concerns. The resulting written complaints were documented in "Books of Grievances," kept in the National Archives. Issues included odors, polluted water, and worries about potentially poisonous dyes. The idea of a right of access to clean water and decent living conditions emerged, and it was linked to political rights.

The king ignored the survey, and the people revolted, demanding a cleaner city and an end to tyranny. In 1789, the Declaration of the Rights of Man and of the Citizen spread like wildfire throughout Europe and became a cornerstone of Western democracy and a model for the UN Declaration of Human Rights in 1948. In less than one hundred years, Paris was transformed into a model city, the blueprint for every modern metropolis. However, the transformation was a bloody and violent revolution.[432]

In the nineteenth century, New York City was undergoing transformation by the Industrial Revolution and waves of immigrants from Europe. In many ways, New York City was worse than the places the immigrants had fled, with residents crammed into slums, along with farm animals, that were ravaged by epidemics of cholera, typhus, and typhoid. While poor New Yorkers were decimated, the rich didn't much care because a steady stream of fresh immigrants kept coming. The poor had privies that spilled into the streets. Sewers were built only in affluent areas.

Corruption and injustice afflicted the poor along with disease. The infamous Tammany Hall political machine stole massive sums of money from the city, including monies paid for rubbish removal, which were pocketed while waste accumulated. In the mid-1860s, Stephen Smith, MD, campaigned unsuccessfully to get rich slumlords to improve conditions. In 1865, with another wave of cholera on its way from Europe, Dr. Smith and other reformers released a detailed study, the "Citizen's Association's Report on the Sanitary Conditions of the City."

The authorities could no longer ignore the horrific conditions—horse carcasses rotting in the street and sewage in drinking water. They established the first independent Board of Health, through which Dr. Smith mobilized an army of cleaners. In just the first six months of 1866, the following were removed: 160,000 tons of manure, 38,000 cartloads of "night soil" (human excrement), 103 dead horses, and 3800 dead cats and dogs. The cleanup successfully dampened the impact of the cholera wave, with one-tenth the number of fatalities as in the previous outbreak seventeen years earlier.

By the 1880s, half of New York City's population lived in slums, to which the city's rich and powerful turned a blind eye. Flash photography exposed the horrors and had a seismic effect across America. The rich and powerful finally tackled corruption, including Tammany Hall, and cleaned up the city's streets and its politics. New York City soon overtook London to become the world's wealthiest city.

In 1882, a groundbreaking paper proved that bacteria cause disease, and the new science of microbiology was born. Attention turned to the scandalous practices of the sausage industry, which turned rotten pigs' head, hearts, lungs, and other leftovers into "food." In 1898, with only ten food inspectors for New York City's more than 25,000 food establishments, backyard butchers could do as they pleased. After journalist Upton Sinclair exposed "the horrors of the American food industry" in his 1906 book, *The Jungle,* New York City got serious about food hygiene.[433]

Do the stories about these three filthy cities sound familiar? They bring to light common themes, many of which resonate with us today and bode well for our ability to turn things around:

- Filth caused disease and death, leading to strong action to clean up the environment and the government. *The new filth—chiefly, greenhouse gases and synthetic chemicals—causes disease and death but has yet to spur strong action.*

- Income inequality, injustice, and greed drove health impacts and environmental devastation. *As explained in Part I of this book, this is the case today.*

- Secret food practices caused illness and death. *Today's secret foods include factory-farmed animals and undisclosed food ingredients such as GMOs.*

- Without enough inspectors and controls, greed ruled and people suffered. *Contemporary examples include eco-crimes and inadequate food inspections that lead to foodborne illness.*[434]

- Those in power refused to act until pushed hard by ordinary citizens. *The US government is fiddling rather than acting decisively to solve the problems summarized in Part I—because ordinary citizens have not yet pushed hard enough.*

- Documentation of the horrific conditions powerfully catalyzed bold action. *We're documenting the sobering impacts of climate change and other problems. People are beginning to wake up, but bold action is yet to come.*

- Solving the health and environmental problem created jobs and economic prosperity. *We are developing profitable green technologies in response to the problems.*

- The cooperative efforts to solve the problems elevated the societies to a higher level of effectiveness and functionality. *We are working on this.*

- Bottom line: Addressing health and environmental problems made life a *lot* better and caused the cities to flourish. *We too could have this. Are we on the cusp of transformation?*

To be fair, several noteworthy differences exist between our situation and those of the three cities. Some of our problems today are global and will be resolved over longer timeframes. And we can't simply take filth outside the city gates. Some of the damage we have done is irreversible—for example, species extinctions and the release of persistent pollutants into the biosphere. However, we have much more powerful tools with which to solve problems.

A NEW STORY, WITH BIG GOALS

While threats to humanity call for emergency response, our species lacks clear goals. The late writer and social critic Kurt Vonnegut observed, "One thing that no Cabinet has ever had is a Secretary of the Future, and there are no plans at all for my grandchildren and my great grandchildren."[435]

We can't even strongly rally behind the notion of preserving our life-support system, though the international climate agreement reached in Paris in 2015 represents a start. However, the US government keeps allowing fossil fuel extraction on public lands, and many US entities, including my home state of Massachusetts, make grand long-term plans to cut greenhouse gas emissions and then don't execute them.[436] Actions continue to be driven by two-, four-, or six-year election cycles and quarterly or fiscal-year business cycles.

The "Occupy Wall Street" movement brought income inequality and excessive corporate influence prominently into the national conversation. But who knows how much more could have been accomplished if the movement had developed clear goals?

Humanity seems plagued with low self-esteem and hopelessness based on limiting beliefs—that corporations rule, humans lack power, and problems are bigger than we are. Economist and corporate globalization critic David Korten wrote: "According to conventional wisdom, hierarchies of dominance are required to bring order to human societies because we humans are by nature an inherently unruly and self-centered species prone to violence and lawlessness."[437] Beliefs that keep societies stuck look a lot like beliefs that keep individuals stuck—"it will be too hard to change," and so forth (see page 93). We may be the Earth's first species with the option to consciously choose its story, its goals, and its path forward.

We need a new story because the old one is killing us. The old story maintains war solves problems; pollutants are unavoidable; exploitation and unbridled growth create economic health; and if citizens win, corporations lose. The current lack of support for the space program in the United States illustrates how we play small, in contrast to the grand vision of the 1960s of putting a man on the moon.[438] We pour our resources into military campaigns and the top 1 percent.

The current story provides short-term relief to both corporations and citizens. Profiteers get to continue exploiting humans and the Earth for short-term gain, and citizens are let off the hook—as if "there's no point in doing anything to help because it's hopeless." However, the "it's hopeless" story diminishes our quality of life to a fraction of what's possible.

Social psychologist Erich Fromm wrote, "I feel that the only thing that will save civilization ... is a renaissance of the spirit—a rebirth of the belief in man himself, in his essential creativeness."[439] We need a new story that says we have purpose and magnificent capacities to live creative, courageous, and loving lives.

In David Korten's view, "The human species is entering a period of dramatic and potentially devastating change as the result of forces of our own creation that are now largely beyond our control. It is within our means, however, to shape a positive outcome if we choose to embrace the resulting crisis as an opportunity to lift ourselves to a new level of species maturity and potential. The outcome will depend in large measure on the prevailing stories that shape our understanding of the traumatic time at hand—its causes and possibilities. Perhaps the most difficult and yet essential aspect of this work is to change our stories."

> *We need a new story that says we have purpose and magnificent capacities to live creative, courageous, and loving lives.*

Korten explains that the old story holds that prosperity comes from worshipping money and material acquisition and security comes from strong coercive police and military forces. A new story can hold that prosperity is measured by the quality of our lives and realization of creative potential, predicated on a "life-serving" economy; security is the outcome of strong relationships of mutual trust and caring; and everything in the cosmos is an "integral, interconnected whole." The new story can be "grounded in a love of life rather than a love of money," with humans capable of solving problems of pollution, war, resource depletion, and injustice to create a happier way of life on Earth, and with corporations thriving by serving rather than exploiting.

People can be inspired by large collective goals that set aside limiting concerns. Goals could include creating a sustainable way of life that restores and enhances life on Earth and provides a decent life for people, promoting the full expression of human potential and creativity, and exploring the universe.

REACH HIGHER

Individuals create standards or practices to live by in order to achieve their goals—such as daily requirements for exercise, sleep, and diet. Similarly, societies create laws, regulations, and standards to help them achieve collective societal goals. For example, to protect human and environmental health, our society limits the amount of carbon monoxide vehicles may emit.

Many areas of life require governments rather than individuals to set and enforce standards. Expecting each citizen to evaluate the 85,000 synthetic chemicals in commercial use and determine which chemicals they should avoid and how to go about avoiding them would be unrealistic. (Yet that's what we do, and it's not working.) Expecting corporations to voluntarily rein in their use of harmful chemicals at the expense of their short-term profits, in the absence of standards, similarly would be unrealistic.

Common sense and the Golden Rule, "do unto others as you would have them do unto you," provide a starting point for standards. Many of our societal standards fail to meet this minimum threshold. Inadequate restraints on the speculative practices of big banks led to the economic collapse of 2008, hurting societies and individuals worldwide. Yet, due to lax standards, big banks are right back at it with their reckless behavior. As Bill Moyers explains it, they are "making risky bets with our deposits and sticking us taxpayers with the bill if the gambles fail."[440]

Corporations invariably fight higher standards, often making exaggerated claims that their businesses will be ruined if they try to meet them. Former BP (British Petroleum) CEO John Browne told *Fortune* magazine "Every time there's a new piece of regulation, we say it's the end of our industry.... The oil industry has an appalling track record in this regard."[441] However, the new standards quickly become the new business-as-usual, without the world ending, and often drive innovation and job creation. Despite pitiful yet predictable corporate whining, President Barack Obama's doubling of fuel efficiency standards provided a "win-win-win" for consumers, manufacturers, and the environment.[442]

According to green business expert Andrew Winston, choosing weaker environmental regulations actually makes the United States less competitive and "saying that stricter pollution standards will cost enormous sums of money shows a staggering disregard for our capacity to innovate." He cites a battle over Clean Air Act Amendments of 1990 provisions to reduce emissions of acid rain–causing sulfur dioxide. Industry claimed compliance would cost up to $1500 per ton of sulfur dioxide reduced. For the next decade, the industry never spent more than $200 per ton, and usually far less.[443]

Cleaner Air Standards Boost the Economy. In 2012, I wrote to then US Senator John Kerry urging strengthening of the Clean Air Act. He replied back: "The Clean Air Act has been a remarkable success for our environment and our economy. For example, from 1990 through 2008, emissions of six common pollutants dropped by 41 percent while our economy grew by 64 percent. In addition, the air in our nation's cities is substantially cleaner than in 1990.... The experience with the Clean Air Act has shown that cutting pollution and building a strong economy can go hand in hand. The Act has also spurred investments in pollution control equipment, developed cleaner facilities, and helped build new industries here in America. Today, clean air technology generates approximately $300 billion in revenues for American business and supports more than 1.7 million jobs."

Many of our standards, too weak in regulating greenhouse gas emissions and other harms, result in tragic consequences. We are like someone who limits himself to one pack of cigarettes, three alcoholic drinks, and one junk food meal per day. Yes, this is better than no control at all, but meeting these standards won't create health.

Creating health and sustainability involves upping our game with higher standards—while avoiding useless, frustrating red tape—in areas such as food quality, environmental quality, chemical safety, health care, education, economic fairness, equality, and justice. It doesn't have to hurt, and everyone can win.

Companies can find they (not just their customers) benefit by voluntarily adopting standards higher than those of their competitors. Whole Foods Market has profitably led the way in food quality and labeling, food waste minimization, green building standards for their stores, treatment of their employees (the company regularly makes *Fortune* magazine's list of the "100 Best Companies to Work For"), sustainable fishery standards, animal welfare standards, and customer satisfaction (they offer a 100 percent satisfaction guarantee for their products).

Adequate enforcement of standards is as important as the standards themselves. However, lax enforcement is rampant. According to *The Wall Street Journal* in 2012, wood-burning biomass plants nationwide had received at least $700 million in federal and state green-energy subsidies since 2009. Yet of 107 US biomass plants that the *Journal* could confirm were operating at the beginning of 2012, some 85 had been cited by state or federal regulators for violating air-pollution or water-pollution standards at some time during the previous five years. Not only are noncompliant plants allowed to keep operating, but they keep receiving their corporate pork from you and me.[444]

Why not use equipment that senses and automatically shuts down biomass plants when they violate their permits? Remote sensing and satellite technology can be used to better monitor and protect resources, detecting illegal pollution, logging, mining, poaching, or fishing. Ocean explorer and conservationist Jacques Cousteau pushed for satellite monitoring of the oceans four decades ago, realizing the power of these tools to protect our oceans.[445] Today, technology enables anyone with an Internet connection to track commercial fishing activity in the world's oceans in near real-time—for free.[446]

Epidemiology could be used to map disease occurrence—such as cancer clusters—to identify areas with elevated health risks that should be investigated for sources of toxic chemicals. We have wonderful tools we're not using to their full capacity.

RADICAL TRANSFORMATION

Human potential visionary Jean Houston believes humanity is ripe for radical transformation: "The vision of change I am describing is generally optimistic. It focuses on the emergence of patterns of possibility never before available to the Earth's people as a whole. This optimism is, paradoxically, based on the recognition that virtually every known institution and way of being is currently in a state of deconstruction and breakdown. Given the scientific, technological, cross-cultural, and social tools at hand, and given, too, that humanity is searching as never before to cooperate in so many areas, it seems feasible to me that we may be ready to integrate inner and outer dimensions of life in ways that infuse new depth into psychological and spiritual growth and new purpose and responsibility into social transformation." When a species "experiences enough ferment and stress," Houston asserts, it can suddenly "jump to a whole new order of being."[447]

Evolutionary thinker Barbara Marx Hubbard believes we could be experiencing the birth of a new species of humans as different from us as we are from Neanderthals. She says we are at a tipping point, "the greatest wakeup call in human history." Though it's natural that a successful, intelligent species would overpopulate, pollute, and wage war, the human species is realizing it does not want to preserve a world of inequality, injustice, environmental destruction, and war. We are waking up to what we want to create, with the opportunity to evolve by choice rather than by chance. Hubbard cautions, however, that there are no guarantees the birth of a new phase will be successful.[448]

Our hardwired urge to survive, honed over eons of evolution, pushes us to change. In many ways, not changing has become more difficult than changing. Enduring cancer, heart disease, severe weather events, disappearing resources, economic insecurity, separation, and/or depression is not exactly an easy road to travel. We grieve as things we hold dear and assumed would always be with us—elephants, coral reefs, and monarch butterflies—disappear before our eyes. Wendell Berry told Bill Moyers, "It's mighty hard right now to think of anything that's precious that isn't endangered. But maybe that's an advantage. The poet William Butler Yeats said somewhere, 'Things reveal themselves passing away.' And it may be that the danger we've now inflicted upon every precious thing reveals the preciousness of it and shows us our duty."[449]

In many ways, not changing has become more difficult than changing.

FROGS

Frogs have a lot to teach us. The "boiling frog" parable, though fictitious, holds that when you put a frog in room-temperature water and then slowly bring the water to a boil, the frog remains in the water until it dies. With its powerful leg muscles, the frog could easily jump out early on, but—lacking awareness—it doesn't. Like the frog, we already have the ability—clean energy technology, organic agriculture, contraception, and so much more—to address our crisis. But unlike the frog, many humans *are* aware of our predicament and its urgency. Even the president of the Flat Earth Society, a group of skeptical freethinkers, believes climate change is at least partially influenced by humans.[450] But so far, we're not jumping out of the pot. Too many of us avoid action, seemingly unconcerned, even about our own children, and essentially saying, "Let the kids deal with it." Politicians and CEOs aren't doing enough to fix the climate, so success or failure boils down to a question of citizens' will. If politicians and CEOs must fix the climate to win our votes and dollars, they will. Let's jump out of the warming pot and into their faces and say, "Turn off the heat and up your game on climate change, or we'll give you the boot." The longer the clock ticks, the harder it becomes to jump, and at some point, jumping may become impossible.

These times call on more of us to jump, despite naysayers around us. Consider another frog parable. Once upon a time, a community of frogs held a competition to climb to the top of a tall tower. Throngs gathered around the tower to watch. No one believed a frog could reach the top, and throughout the competition spectators said things like "it's impossible" and "they'll never make it." Sure enough, the climbers fell, one by one, and dropped out of the competition. But one frog persevered, taking step after difficult step, and finally reached the top—the frog that was deaf.[451]

Chorus of Frogs. On spring nights, I listen to a chorus of frogs singing in bass, alto, and soprano voices in a nearby wetland. I worry—will future springs be silent? Human destruction of their habitat and climate change kill frogs. Because amphibians are sensitive to environmental disruption and they reside in the middle of the food chain—eating smaller creatures and being eaten by larger ones—their health is often used as an indicator of ecosystem health.[452] One-third of amphibian species are globally threatened or extinct.[453] Scientist J. Alan Pounds writes that global warming is wreaking havoc on them and "will cause staggering losses of biodiversity if we don't do something fast."[454] I wish this were a parable.

As one door closes, another door opens. Whether we want it to or not, the era of "advanced" technology coupled with careless disregard for the natural world—and for ourselves—is coming to a close. A new era is trying to emerge, one of advanced technology coupled with stewardship of the natural world—including ourselves.

> *A new era is trying to emerge, one of advanced technology coupled with stewardship of the natural world.*

CHAPTER 9
GREEN TECHNOLOGY

We are drowning in information, while starving for wisdom.
The world henceforth will be run by synthesizers, people able
to put together the right information at the right time, think
critically about it, and make important choices wisely.

—*E. O. Wilson*

TECHNOLOGICAL ADVANCES PROPELLED OUR SUCCESS as our forebears moved from wood to stone to metal to electronic tools. Each advance added to our toolbox. Some tools we keep using, while others—such as slide rules—become obsolete. Our current need is to accelerate the transition to green technology already underway—with the greatest speed possible but without being reckless. Green technology promotes the collective health of our species and our environment the way good diet, exercise, and other beneficial lifestyle tools promote a person's basic health.

Our next level of technological sophistication involves meeting new and more challenging design criteria than in the past. Green technologies perform their intended functions *and* do so without damaging human or environmental health—here or there, now or later, without using resources at rates greater than their replenishment, and without generating unrecyclable wastes.

An output from a green process serves as a useful input to another process, using the same kind of circular and continuous "cradle to cradle" mode that nature uses. To green designers Michael Braungart and William McDonough, "waste equals food."[455] In 2013, Americans composted or recycled only about one-third of the municipal solid waste they generated.[456] It doesn't have to be this way. The City of San Francisco is well on its way to its goal of zero waste by 2020.[457]

There is no "away" any more, as in throwing waste away, because everywhere matters, now and later. Green designers see the Earth as a small spaceship—with parched, red Mars as a nearby reminder of what Earth could be like if we're not careful. Green design strives to prevent damage. That contrasts with our current reckless and destructive approach: trial and error, followed by damage control, and then lurching to the next ill-considered idea. Moving to green technology is a lot like a child moving into adulthood—and exercising greater skill, awareness, concern for others, and self-control.

Green is about greater sophistication and *enhanced* quality of life, not deprivation. We can have both high tech and high nature.[458] Instead of a lifeless, hot, black, barren roof on a city building, we can have a "green roof" (with living plants) that cools the air, insulates the building (lowering energy costs), reduces storm water runoff (reducing storm water management costs and flooding), and provides opportunities for gardening, wildlife, and human enjoyment. It can be a multiple win-win with no downside.

> *Green is about enhanced quality of life, not deprivation.*

Green technology lives by the "precautionary principle." This principle places the burden of proving that a proposed action is safe on the people who want to take the action, rather than placing the burden of proof on victims to show that someone else's action is harmful. Green design focuses on working "upstream" rather than "downstream"—for example, preventing air pollution rather than equipping people with respirators and treating them with lung cancer surgeries.

The most efficient use of resources often involves distributed rather than centralized systems. Our system of interconnected personal computers and smart phones is one example. Examples of distributed green technologies and practices include rooftop solar; rainwater collection; teleworking; mixed-use developments that put residences, stores, and workplaces in close proximity to one another; community-supported agriculture; community gardens; and farmer's markets. Locally produced goods and services can reduce environmental footprints, strengthen local economies, and provide greater reliability and independence. (Locally produced goods are less subject to transportation disruptions.)

We currently rely on an ecosystem of intertwined, unsustainable industries (see page 57). But we could just as easily rely on an ecosystem of green industries. We *need* corporations, but ones that work in the interests of citizens and the environment. Corporations have the organizational systems and processes to do things that individuals acting alone can't, such as making a car. Unfortunately, corporations are so adept they've managed to take over our government and make it work for them instead of for citizens, turning our world on its head.

Corporations try to succeed within whatever system they find themselves. Ultimately, citizens call the shots. If we take our current corporations, clean them up and "give them a haircut" (by closing the revolving door and taking away their ability to make political campaign contributions), and point them in the right direction (via enlightened government policies), they'll head in that direction and find ways to make profits under a new set of rules. If everyone wants to buy hybrid electric cars and no one wants to buy sport utility vehicles, car companies will make hybrids. They don't much care what kinds of cars they make—as long as they make sales and profits.

New approaches that address the long-term interests of citizens' health and their environment—among them, holistic medicine and organic agriculture— come with their own set of interrelated businesses. The integrated constellation of businesses connected to holistic medicine includes alternative health practitioners, testing laboratories, health food stores and co-ops, organic food producers and distributors, personal care products producers, nutritional supplements companies, health clubs, yoga and meditation centers, personal development companies, media companies, and more. Green businesses are prospering and growing—despite enjoying fewer government subsidies and political allies. Policy changes could accelerate their growth.

PUTTING IT ALL TOGETHER

We've done a great job of breaking problems into pieces and studying each one in detail. We are increasingly recognizing the need for integrators such as anthropologists, holistic medicine practitioners, and green architects and engineers to best navigate the weblike, interconnected nature of reality. Because Westerners are encouraged to work in one specialty area and leave everything else to others, we have plenty of specialists and not enough generalists. Few of us today grow our own food, build our own houses, sew our own clothes, or create our own entertainment, which until quite recently was standard.

Green practitioners put the pieces back together. One thing green architects do is harmonize the building envelope, the HVAC system, and the site. By contrast, in a conventional building, these systems might fight each other—poorly designed windows and overhangs perhaps letting in too much heat in the summer, forcing HVAC systems to work extra hard to cool the space.

We already have most of the technologies that can deliver a sustainable way of life. Therefore, creating a sustainable world may be easier than we think. We can further refine and optimize our toolbox as we proceed.

ORGANIC AGRICULTURE

A sustainable world depends on our return to organic agriculture for growing food and nonfood crops. A recent UN study advises that if we switch to eco-agricultural methods—which enhance soil productivity and protect crops against pests by relying on beneficial trees, plants, animals, and insects—we can double world food production in critical regions in ten years.[459]

People are starting to make the switch. Demand for organic food is growing.[460] Organic methods can be encouraged by requiring straightforward and comprehensive food labeling to inform consumers about all the synthetic chemicals industrial producers put in food.[461] Food labeling may be burdensome for industrial producers, but it is surely not so burdensome as it is for consumers to endure chronic disease caused by unhealthy food ingredients. As a society, we could also better regulate food safety and quality. We can ban unsafe chemicals and the routine use of antibiotics and place the burden of proof on food companies to demonstrate their foods are safe. We can require producers to keep food, air, water, and soil clean, avoid wildlife mortality, and treat farm animals ethically.

We can promote local agriculture, including community gardens, even on inner city rooftops and vacant lots.[462] Inspiring urban gardener Ron Finlay estimates that the City of Los Angeles owns 26 square miles of vacant lots, an area equivalent to 20 Central Parks, with enough space for 724,838,400 tomato plants.[463] We can teach kids about gardening, composting, food, and nutrition via hands-on experiences at school.

CLEANER ENERGY

We have developed numerous energy technologies that do not involve combustion, often referred to as "clean energy," including solar, wind, geothermal, hydro, wave, tidal, and fuel cell energy. In one hour, the sun beams onto Earth more than enough energy to satisfy global energy needs for an entire year.[464] Similarly, there is more than enough wind energy to more than satisfy global power demand.[465] Some technologies improve rapidly at the same time that their costs plummet, leading to fast growth and deployment. According to Bloomberg News, "solar and wind are crushing fossil fuels."[466] In Germany, a world leader in green technology, renewable sources accounted for 28 percent of power consumption in 2014, up from 6 percent in 2000. These sources are predominantly solar and wind but include some hydropower and, unfortunately, bioenergy.[467]

Clean energy is superior to combustion-based energy in other ways besides emitting less air pollution. Amory Lovins, chairman and chief scientist of Rocky Mountain Institute, compares fossil fuel energy and clean energy:

"The old fire was dug from below. The new fire flows from above. The old fire was scarce. The new fire is bountiful. The old fire was local. The new fire is everywhere. The old fire was transient. The new fire is permanent."[468]

Of course, any technology needs to be deployed intelligently and sited properly to be considered clean. Large hydropower projects devastate environments and societies around the world.[469] Energy developers and regulators in the United States site many solar and wind installations in inappropriate locations, destroying essential ecosystems such as wetlands and forests, and cramming projects down local citizens' throats.[470] Let's proceed calmly and rationally and implement green technology in a green way. Yes, it may be more lucrative to install solar on inexpensive pristine land—after clear-cutting it and selling the trees and maybe also selling the soil or sand and gravel. But solar has a much lighter environmental footprint when appropriately placed on roofs, highway rights-of-way, or closed landfills. Similarly, wind farms may be more suitably sited on farmland, offshore, or in locations other than on pristine land or next to houses where they are bound to create angry neighbors.

Solar Panels Have Been Around for Decades. People routinely used solar technology in homes and other buildings more than thirty-five years ago. In the late 1970s, I worked as the design department secretary for a company that designed and prefabricated solar houses, incorporating solar panels as well as passive solar features. The house orientation, windows, and eaves were designed to maximize solar gain in the winter and minimize it in the summer. Interiors were open to promote air circulation and let in natural light. Builders would prepare the location and assemble the homes, which the company would ship to the site in sections. The houses were cheery, comfortable, and gorgeous.

A clean energy imposter, however, must be rooted out: bioenergy. The main bioenergy technologies include burning wood for heat and electricity and making biofuels, including corn ethanol, cellulosic ethanol, and palm oil diesel. (Some other much less widely deployed bioenergy technologies, such as capturing and burning methane from landfill gas and anaerobic digesters at wastewater treatment plants, can be beneficial.) The primary bioenergy technologies could not be worse for the environment, yet many organizations and policies—even President Obama's Clean Power Plan—don't get it.[471] It's time to stop kidding ourselves that bioenergy is clean and green and stop going backwards with our technology. Effects of climate change warn us to stop burning things—period.

INTELLIGENT WATER MANAGEMENT

In the United States, we often waste water, largely because we pay peanuts for it. It's quite another story in other parts of the world, where fresh water is a cherished commodity. Basic strategies for better managing water can include the following:

- Price water appropriately instead of practically giving it away. People value what they pay for.

- Protect water quality to minimize the need for water treatment to remove contaminants.

- Use readily available technology to stop wasting water. Fix leaking pipes and redesign inefficient irrigation practices.[472]

- Maintain and upgrade water distribution systems to minimize leakage and protect water quality.

- Use low-flow showerheads, toilets, and other fixtures; reuse "grey water" from sinks for toilet flushing and landscape watering; and capture rainwater falling on roofs for landscape watering.

- Allow precipitation to soak into the ground on-site to replenish underground water supplies, rather than piping storm water off-site. Replenish aquifers with highly treated wastewater.[473]

- Meter water use, track water supplies, and modify behaviors to match the available supply—avoid growing "thirsty" crops, such as rice, in deserts, where irrigation may deplete aquifers.

- Adopt policies and realistic water management plans that result in sustainable water use, while sharing water with other species by maintaining adequate stream flows and water elevations.

- Educate people about why and how to protect water quality and quantity.

FOREST PROTECTION

Preserving, restoring, and expanding forests requires addressing the root causes of deforestation—which include undervaluing forests, wasteful use of forest products (such as single-use pallets), destructive agricultural practices, and corporate and government corruption.

A top priority is to preserve remaining old-growth forests, which takes many human lifetimes to grow back. Contrary to logging industry propaganda, old trees are especially effective at removing carbon dioxide from the atmosphere and storing carbon in live woody tissues and slowly decomposing organic matter in litter and soil.[474]

Joint efforts to protect forests are underway, including the 2014 New York Declaration on Forests. The agreement, which was signed by businesses, governments, and indigenous peoples, aims to cut tropical forest loss in half by 2020 and end it by 2030. And sustainable development goals adopted by 193 countries in 2015 call for advancing sustainable forest management, halting deforestation, restoring degraded forests, and planting more trees by 2020.[475]

Ecotourism can encourage forest preservation by, essentially, paying local people to not log. High agricultural yields and high biodiversity can be sustained in new, smart production systems. At one farm in Costa Rica, coffee and more than a dozen food crops are grown integrated with areas of rain forest. Up to one hundred species of birds have been identified on the farm and forest fragments, and hundreds of species of bees have been identified in the forests next to the farmed areas. Bats cover the night shift, consuming as much as their body weight in pests each night, carrying pollen, and scattering seeds.[476]

Governments at all levels, land trusts, and other entities can permanently protect more land. New national parks are being created in the United States.[477] However, many US public lands enjoy scant protection, if any.[478] Governments can stop destructive uses of public land—forests or otherwise—for logging, mining, ranching, drilling for oil or natural gas, water withdrawals, pipelines, bioenergy, and yes, solar and wind farms.

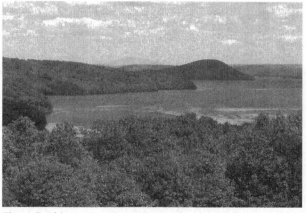

The Quabbin Reservation surrounding the Quabbin Reservoir, which provides drinking water for the metropolitan Boston area. This is the largest nearly intact forest in southern New England. However, commercial logging is allowed, including in some areas where people are not even allowed to walk. Photo credit: Chris Matera.

While reducing or eliminating corporations' access to the public's land, citizens deserve improved access to their own land for hiking, camping, and other benign activities. People will not only enjoy what is theirs and benefit from their time in nature, but their appreciation for the natural world will increase. Our kids' outdoor experiences will help grow the next generation of people who care about the natural world.

Most bioenergy projects should be rejected, as explained previously. Improved technology and programs to reduce, reuse, and recycle paper and wood could slash the need for logging. Logging that can't be eliminated can be done sustainably, taking trees selectively rather than rapaciously.[479]

We can also put people to work restoring the original biodiversity of forest ecosystems that have been logged. Tree-planting campaigns such as the Green Belt Movement can be remarkably effective.

CONTRACEPTION

The more of us there are, the larger our environmental impacts. Populations of humans and farm animals continue to grow, livestock numbers at twice the rate of humans.[480]

Newsweek magazine reports that in 2012, the estimated number of unintended pregnancies worldwide was 80 million and the world's population grew by 80 million. "In other words, if women all over the world had the ability to prevent the pregnancies they don't want, the world's population would stabilize." *Newsweek* estimates that the reduction in unwanted pregnancies would translate into an 8 percent to 15 percent reduction in global carbon emissions, improved health and quality of life, and economic growth due to women's greater participation in paid work. A stable human population would reduce habitat destruction, species extinction, and pollution. In the developing world, 222 million women want contraceptives but can't get them; meeting this need would have prevented 54 million unwanted pregnancies, 26 million abortions, 79,000 deaths of mothers, and 1.1 million infant deaths in 2012 alone. If only for human and environmental health reasons, women around the world should have access to the contraceptives they want. Providing contraceptives would also save money, $6 for every $1 spent, according to the US Agency for International Development.[481]

Contraceptives in My Life. I feel blessed to be one of the first women to have the option of saying "no thanks" to having children. It's an individual choice and there is no one right answer, but not having kids was definitely the right answer for me. I simply had no interest in having kids. Contraceptives enabled me to do things I preferred—going to school, working as an environmental consultant, doing pro bono environmental work, creating lots of art, taking workshops, and maintaining a healthy lifestyle.

Yes, I could have knocked myself out by raising children too. But I didn't want to and couldn't possibly have maintained the same level of these other activities—there are only so many hours in the day. A few of my female friends with kids envy my freedom. I wish for other women to have the freedom to do what they want.

Green Chemistry

A science revolution called "green chemistry" has ramped up in the United States since passage of the Federal Pollution Prevention Act of 1990. Its main goal is to design chemical products and processes that reduce or eliminate the generation of hazardous substances.[482]

The Presidential Green Chemistry Challenge Awards program recognizes innovations in cleaner, cheaper, and smarter chemistry. From 1996 through 2014, the ninety-eight award-winning technologies eliminated 826 million pounds of hazardous chemicals, saved more than 21 billion gallons of water, and eliminated 7.9 billion pounds of carbon dioxide emissions. The innovative technologies included the following:

- An environmentally safe marine antifoulant to control biological growth on the hulls of boats, to replace toxic and persistent tributyltin oxide

- Photographic film for medical imaging that uses heat instead of hazardous developer chemicals

- Detergents that allow for the use of nontoxic carbon dioxide, instead of hazardous chemical solvents and processes, as a solvent in many industrial applications, while conserving energy.[483]

In *Paradigms in Green Chemistry and Technology,* Angelo Albini and Stefano Protti write that "green chemistry will become an inseparable part of everyday chemistry and thinking the green way will become a natural habit for every chemical practitioner.... A sustainable future will become an actual possibility."[484]

Green chemistry, combined with controls to block the sale of chemicals before their health and environmental effects are known, will go a long way in cleaning up our act.

Health Care

Disease incidence goes down when people eat cleaner food, breathe cleaner air, drink cleaner water, and use fewer toxic products. Similarly, moving to a proactive health-care approach—focusing on maintaining good health to avoid disease—will also reduce disease incidence. We know prevention works.

In 1900, the three leading causes of death in the United States were influenza, tuberculosis, and gastrointestinal infections. The incidence of these diseases plummeted due to vaccines, drinking water and wastewater treatment, and other measures. But today, one-half of adult Americans have at least one chronic disease, such as heart disease, diabetes, or cancer. The incidence and severity of these conditions are reduced through healthy lifestyles that include good diet, physical activity, healthy weight, and avoidance of tobacco. A healthy lifestyle is associated with a 93 percent reduced risk of diabetes, 81 percent reduced risk of heart attack, 50 percent reduced risk of stroke, and 36 percent reduced risk of cancer.[485] Moreover, prevention can reduce illnesses and deaths from prescription drugs.

Taking back our health is becoming mainstream, with healthy lifestyle segments appearing even on network television and in conventional medical literature. Health care is moving away from a fee-for-service system toward one that pays doctors for preventing disease, a move that dramatically reduces health-care costs. In 2011, government agencies and private entities banded together in the first coordinated multipronged "Million Hearts" campaign aimed at preventing one million heart attacks and strokes over the next five years. Actions include reinforcing the preventive measures doctors should prescribe, helping patients take ownership for heart-attack prevention, making a heart-healthy lifestyle easier to follow, removing financial barriers to preventive care, working with chain restaurants to include nutrition information on menus, working with food manufacturers to replace trans fats with healthy oils, increasing public information about the dangers of smoking, and making more public places and workplaces smoke free.[486]

Taking back our health is becoming mainstream.

Though most doctors still practice "silo medicine"—in which doctors lack information beyond their narrow specialty—holistic medicine is on the increase. People increasingly want doctors to identify and fix the underlying causes of disease instead of just treating symptoms with "silver bullets" (drugs). Even one of America's top five hospitals, the Cleveland Clinic, now has a Center for Functional Medicine that is pioneering whole-patient-centered care.[487]

CONSERVATION AND EFFICIENCY

Conservation is the careful use of resources to prevent them from being lost or wasted—for example, driving a car fewer miles. Efficiency is the ability to do or produce something without wasting materials, time, or energy—

for example, driving an energy-efficient car. Progress in conservation and efficiency occurs relatively invisibly, in a multitude of small, incremental steps rather than via sweeping, headline-grabbing events. If we improved tracking of the costs and benefits of conservation and efficiency, we'd see what a good deal they are for both the environment and the economy. Vast opportunities for conservation and efficiency are overlooked in the United States.

Infrastructure is foundational to economic prosperity. Maintaining, conserving, and making more efficient all that we have includes paying attention to our often-neglected infrastructure—roads, bridges, dams, levees, ports, rail, transit, drinking water and wastewater systems, pipelines, electrical grids, parks, and schools.[488]

Vast opportunities for conservation and efficiency are overlooked in the United States.

Opportunities for reducing food waste are staggering. Americans throw out 40 percent of all the food we produce, and one-third of food produced worldwide is not eaten.[489] At the consumer level, this costs American families each about $150 per month.[490] Meanwhile, children go hungry. Injury and death of nontarget sea animals (bycatch) could be greatly reduced by the adoption of less wasteful fishing practices.[491]

Food is wasted during production, post-harvest handling and storage, processing and packaging, distribution and retail, and at the consumer and food service levels. Wasted food is the largest component of municipal waste sent to landfills, which is where most wasted food ends up. Food in landfills converts to methane, a potent greenhouse gas. Only 3 percent of food waste is composted. American families throw out about a quarter of all the food and beverages they buy. Most of it spoiled from not being used in time, improper storage, or surplus from what was cooked or served.

Food growers, distributors, and consumers can take actions to reduce food waste. The federal government could clear up confusion caused by "use by," "sell by," and "best by" dates, which often don't indicate when foods will no longer be fresh, prompting consumers to throw out food unnecessarily. Governments and businesses can expand markets for off-grade food, promote regional and local food distribution (reducing spoilage), and adopt policies that incentivize complete, rather than partial, harvest of crops. Food processors can improve their methods and put scraps to their highest use (such as for animal feed). Stores can better control their inventory, offer discounted items, and donate more food.[492]

In the realm of energy, "efficiency is the cheapest electricity resource," costing about one-third as much as new energy generation, according to the Massachusetts Division of Energy Resources.[493] Yet we often overlook conservation and efficiency. Controversial natural gas pipelines currently proposed in the Northeast and elsewhere would traverse pristine conservation lands and other sensitive habitats. Meanwhile, natural gas hemorrhages out of existing natural gas infrastructure.[494]

Efficiency is the cheapest electricity resource. —Massachusetts Division of Energy Resources

North Americans use twice as much energy as Europeans, with no appreciable difference in standard of living, 10 times more than the average Latin American, and more than 100 times that of a typical African.[495] Physicist Amory Lovins estimates energy efficiency can save 44 percent of projected 2050 US electricity needs, using proven building and industrial technologies that pay back far faster than any new source of supply.[496] According to the US Department of Energy, "Energy efficiency is one of the easiest and most cost-effective ways to combat climate change," while also cleaning the air we breathe, improving business competitiveness, and reducing energy costs for consumers.[497]

Many cell phone chargers continue to draw power even when not connected to a phone or after charging is complete—just one example of senseless waste. Manufacturers are starting to get on board. Energy Star devices reduce standby power consumption and generally use less power in all their functions.[498]

Other opportunities for energy conservation and efficiency include improvements in the efficiency of the electric grid; outdoor lighting that automatically turns off in daylight; more efficient transportation, buildings, appliances, and equipment; and conservation of water. Water heating alone accounts for 9 percent of US residential electricity use.[499]

Water conservation opportunities abound in every sector of our society. Agricultural water use is especially critical, since it accounts for most of the fresh water consumed in the United States. We can conserve water in homes, landscapes, businesses, industries, and farms using an array of technologies and practices too numerous to list here.[500] Just one small component of wasted water—household leaks—amounts to more than one trillion gallons of water wasted annually in the United States alone.[501]

We can conserve, restore, and expand forests. Conserving forests begins with reducing wasteful uses of wood and increasing reuse and recycling. We can permanently protect forests—for example, by creating new national parks and prohibiting damaging uses of our public land.[502]

We can manufacture higher-quality rather than shoddy products. Many items manufactured today fall apart quickly, generating senseless waste and squandering resources.

INFORMATION SHARING AND LEARNING

We're suddenly connected to each other and to information as never before via our new "global brain." Consider this: one Google search uses the computing power of the entire Apollo space mission.[503]

Of the global population of 7.4 billion people, 31 percent actively use social media, 46 percent use the Internet, and 51 percent use mobile phones.[504] By 2020, 90 percent of the world's population over the age of six may have a cell phone.[505] These technologies confer massive, decentralized power and tend to level the playing field. We can use them in creating a sustainable world—for communicating new ideas, planning actions, and tracking the condition of natural resources.

At the same time, privacy risks are real as increasing amounts of information are collected about us and shared—by governments in the name of national security and by companies in the name of commerce. The marketing giant Acxiom claims to have an average of 1500 pieces of information on each of more than 200 million Americans. Tim Sparapani of the American Civil Liberties Union thinks people would be stunned to learn what the trafficked information includes—information about religion, ethnicity, political affiliations, user names, incomes, debts, family history, medications, alcoholism, depression and other psychiatric problems, diseases and genetic problems, sexual orientation, and web browsing history. As you're searching the Internet, you've got a whole crowd following you. Your smartphone is a tracking device, and geo-location data on individuals has become a hot commodity. Peoples' contact lists can be downloaded from their phones without their knowledge.[506]

To preserve democracy and civil rights so we are free to create a sustainable world, our privacy needs to be protected while our access to information and communications is maintained, all while keeping up with rapid changes in technology. This currently is not happening.

CHAPTER 10
GREEN ECONOMY

*Reducing greenhouse gas emissions requires action in the very
same areas that throughout history have driven economic growth:
investment in efficiency, infrastructure, and innovation.*

—*Felipe Calderón, former President of Mexico*

THE ECONOMY HELPS GLUE OUR world together. Currently, our economic
system favors industrial agriculture, combustion-based energy, and forest
clear-cutting, among other technologies that liquidate or degrade natural
resources. Our system also discourages stewardship, which costs more under
our crude, incomplete, and, in some ways, corrupt economic system.

We have a global economy now. When China's economy suffers, the world
feels the reverberations. Our species needs collective financial health the same
way an individual needs financial health. We can replace our ecosystem of
destructive industries—big food, big energy, big timber, big pharma, big
disease management, and so on—with an ecosystem of human-friendly and
nature-friendly industries. Computers recently revolutionized our way of life
and our economy. Now, sustainability can do the same.

> *Computers recently revolutionized our way of life and our
> economy. Now, sustainability can do the same.*

OUR ECONOMY IS A HUMAN CREATION

Our economy is a human construct, so we can change it. One way is by
changing the tax code. Taxes are unavoidable. Without taxation, there could
be no government; without government, there could be no army; and without
an army, the country would be taken over by another country, and we'd have
to pay taxes to it.[507]

The US tax code favors corporations and the richest 1 percent of the population, at the expense of citizens and our environment. Corporations can even relocate from this country to foreign countries in order to skip out on paying taxes owed to the United States.

The tax code provides a powerful tool for implementing our intentions. Former US President Franklin D. Roosevelt improved the lives of ordinary citizens in The New Deal, which increased taxes to create Social Security, Wall Street regulation, and government-insured bank accounts. Every American president since, until Ronald Reagan, used tax revenue to fund some grand endeavor: for example, the Marshall Plan (Truman), the Interstate Highway System (Eisenhower), the space program (Kennedy), Medicaid (Johnson), the Environmental Protection Agency (Nixon), and the Department of Energy and Department of Education (Carter).[508]

We change the economy in other ways. The early economy of the United States relied on the labor of slaves, who were kept unfree, impoverished, overworked, unhealthy, uneducated, intimidated, isolated, and short-lived. In the 1800s, we changed the slave economy to one involving less brutalization of workers. The economy did not fail and our economy did not collapse, as many profiting from slavery insisted would happen.

A similar myth emerged more recently. It claimed we need to destroy the environment in order to fuel the economy and create jobs and that, conversely, helping the environment will hurt the economy, and with it, jobs. This is nonsense. The green paradigm recognizes the economy and environment prosper or suffer together. In the words of former US Senator Gaylord Nelson: "The economy is a wholly-owned subsidiary of the environment, not the other way around." An unhealthy environment can create poverty. If we continue to neglect climate change—unproductively spending ever-increasing amounts of our wealth responding to "natural" disasters, sea-level rise, crop failures, water scarcity, and other impacts—we'll have less to spend on productive pursuits such as education, and our economy will suffer.

Poverty likewise can damage the environment. A destitute person may by necessity cut down the last tree in an area because it is the only affordable source of energy for cooking. Poor people in many parts of the world face a choice: destroy their environment or starve.

Environmental, human, and economic health all rise and fall together, due to interconnections, and we're increasingly recognizing a green economy can promote all these areas. By changing our economic rules, we can take a system where greed runs wild—harming humans, their environment, and their economy—and transform it into one that works for people, the environment, and corporations. Corporations acting responsibly and intelligently need to be able to profit, grow, please shareholders, create jobs, and enjoy power and prestige.

Machines increasingly do the work humans once did. Robots replace factory workers, automatic teller machines replace bank employees, automatic tollbooths collect our tolls on the highway, machines harass us with phone calls at dinnertime, and on and on. Displaced workers can be put to work retrofitting and insulating buildings, restoring degraded ecosystems, planting trees, installing rooftop solar panels and water-efficient fixtures, recycling, promoting healthy lifestyles, growing organic food, monitoring and protecting resources, teaching children about nature, and building, maintaining, and upgrading green infrastructure.

Corporations and individuals alike will have to adapt to new kinds of work and changing conditions and rules, as always. We can phase in changes gradually to prevent shocks. Smart people and corporations see change as opportunity.

Creating a green economy can create an economic boom similar to the way The New Deal boosted the American people and World War II helped the country recover after the Great Depression. The New Deal, designed to relieve poverty, reduce unemployment, and speed economic recovery, put people to work planting trees and building reservoirs, bridges, roads, public buildings, parks, and airports.[509] The United States financed its World War II effort primarily by raising taxes. No one paid our country to engage in the space race. We simply decided to do it. These self-created activities created an economic boom that lasted until the early 1970s.

MIND THE GAPS

Our economic system is remarkably crude. A primary way we measure the health of the economy is with the gross domestic product, defined as the monetary value of all goods and services produced within a country's geographic borders in a given time period. We're happy when gross domestic product increases and sad when it decreases. However, gross domestic product ignores the nature of the goods and services and can make us think we're doing well when we're not. By this metric, spending money on emergency room visits for kids with asthma attacks caused by air pollution looks just as good as creating outdoor nature schools for kids, dollar for dollar. Gross domestic product can't tell right from wrong and thus is a terrible yardstick to use.

Also, our current economic system too often does not assign the costs of health and environmental damage to the people causing it. The costs are real, and people really pay them. Using the above example, power plant owners do not pay their share for children's emergency room visits necessitated by asthma attacks. Nor do they pay their share of costs for responding to worsening weather events caused by climate change. Because power plant owners don't pay these costs, they don't pass the costs along to us. Our artificially low electric bills may lead us to believe combustion-based energy is cheaper than solar. But we're paying more, maybe a lot more, elsewhere—in medical bills, medical insurance, taxes, and time lost from work and school, not to mention pain and suffering.

Our economic system is based on what activist David Bollier calls "private plundering of our common wealth," including forests, fisheries, farmland, and water. These gifts of the Earth must be managed for the survival and well-being of all.[510] Amory Lovins says that "so far, industrial capitalism has dealt seriously with only two forms of capital—money and goods—while liquidating and not valuing two even more important sources of capital: nature and people." He asserts that if we productively used and reinvested in all forms of capital, we would make more money and have more fun.[511] We see this phenomenon mirrored on the individual level, as well. Many of us focus on money and goods while neglecting our physical health or personal development, which are more or less analogous to "nature" and "people" on the collective level.

It's hard to place a value on things we don't pay cash for—such as air or a human life—and so much easier to simply ignore costs and benefits that are hard to quantify. However, these are often the most important ones, and an economic system that ignores them makes it cheaper to rape and run rather than to go to the trouble of protecting people and nature.

Policy-makers squirm at the idea of assigning a monetary value to a human life. However, this is unavoidable when policy-makers decide how much to spend to save a human life. Recent US government agency estimates of the value of a human life range from about $6 million to $9 million.[512]

Making intelligent decisions requires counting human lives and nature appropriately in economic analyses. Not doing so too often means our worth is estimated to be zero. As investor Jeremy Grantham points out, in our current system, "our grandchildren really do have no value."[513]

Difficult-to-Count Costs and Benefits. I know about these difficulties first-hand from my master's degree research. I conducted a cost-benefit analysis of two programs to find and fix leaks in water distribution systems. I analyzed two very different water systems—one in Kentucky drawing water from a river and the other in New York purchasing water from the New York City system. The Kentucky water was inexpensive, while the New York water was expensive. Both systems had good data on the costs of leak detection, leak repairs, and water purchase, pumping, and treatment costs. My research showed that detecting and fixing leaks saved both communities money because they didn't have to purchase, pump, and treat additional water.

I then realized I was leaving out other important benefits of fixing leaks—for example, increased availability of water for firefighting and other uses, fewer disruptive water main breaks, and more water left in ecosystems for use by plants and animals. These benefits were real and possibly even greater than the financial benefits I had quantified.

We also often ignore costs that *are* easy to quantify. Corporate representatives may argue that jobs will be lost if their project does not go forward. But the same representatives—as well as regulators—may ignore the jobs that will be lost if their dirty project *does* go forward, for example, due to decreased tourism in the area. Constructive and destructive projects alike create jobs.

Similarly, we ignore the true costs of war when we estimate the cost to wage the bloodbath but "forget" to factor in the costs of the aftermath. Concern grows over the lack of a long-term plan to pay for the care of thousands of US soldiers returning home from Iraq and Afghanistan with serious injuries requiring decades of care. Taking care of injured veterans is already the fifth largest expense of the federal government. Costs continue to mount and could ultimately exceed $1 trillion.[514]

Decision-making that serves the public interest would avoid cherry-picking the costs and benefits we are going to count. Lester Brown, founder of the Worldwatch Institute and the Earth Policy Institute, says our current system is like the corrupt and now defunct corporation, Enron, whose phony accounting kept liabilities off the books. We thought Enron was the seventh largest corporation, but in reality it was worth nothing.[515]

More comprehensive cost-benefit analyses are starting to be done. In one such analysis, which refuted spurious claims that USEPA regulations cost too much, the US Office of Management and Budget found the estimated benefits of USEPA regulations significantly exceeded the estimated costs. Benefits, totaling half a trillion dollars over ten years, were largely from reducing deaths from air pollution.[516]

Others, recognizing the folly of ignoring the value of ecosystem services, are starting to quantify them. In 1990, ecological economist Robert Constanza estimated the value of the services nature performs. He concluded nature performs services that would cost at least $33 trillion per year if we tried to do them, twice as much as global gross domestic product at that time. In other words, ecosystem services were worth twice as much as all the economies in the world.[517]

A more recent analysis put global ecosystem services at $100 trillion per year and found land degradation—for example, from logging and wetlands loss—cost $4 trillion to $20 trillion per year between 1997 and 2011. Another study cited in the same *Washington Post* article, titled "The Staggeringly Large Benefits of Conserving Nature," found an increase of eleven trees on a city block is comparable, in terms of improved human health, to raising people's annual income by $20,000 or making them 1.4 years younger.[518]

Another study estimated the value of ecosystem services forfeited due to land degradation—primarily by agriculture and forestry—at $6 trillion to $11 trillion annually, or the equivalent of 10 to 17 percent of global gross domestic product. The study notes that 52 percent of the world's agricultural land is "moderately to severely degraded" and estimates that within ten years, fifty million people may be forced to seek new homes and livelihoods due to land degradation. This many migrants collectively would constitute the world's twenty-eighth largest population. Furthermore, wise agricultural and forestry land use management, requiring no substantial capital, would be among the lowest-cost actions for reducing global warming.[519]

A 2014 report by the Global Commission on the Economy and Climate (GCEC) concludes that "countries at all levels of income now have the opportunity to build lasting economic growth at the same time as reducing the immense risks of climate change." The report states the necessary fixes may be effectively free. When the ancillary benefits of greener policies are taken into account, the fixes may wind up saving us money. The report adds that the longer we delay taking action, the more it will cost us to address the climate problem.[520] The GCEC's 2015 report similarly asserts that a prosperous and sustainable future is within our reach and provides ten practical recommendations that will boost economic growth and reduce climate risk.[521]

Politicians who complain about the cost of addressing environmental problems usually fail to consider the cost of *not* addressing them. Climate change imposes an array of costs. One study, by NextGen Climate and Demos, projects that, in a "no climate action" scenario, US gross domestic product will shrink by 5 percent by 2050 due to climate change, which is comparable to recessionary losses. It further projects that, again in a "no climate action" scenario, US gross domestic product will shrink by 36 percent by 2100 due to climate change, which is comparable to Great Depression-era losses.[522] Because greenhouse gas emissions—both from the end of pipes and from land abuse—come with real costs, it's time to put a price on greenhouse gas emissions as well as credit carbon dioxide uptake and storage by soil and plants.

Destruction of coastal wetlands, mangrove trees, and coral reefs made the Gulf Coast damage from Hurricane Katrina far worse. Restoration of wetlands in the upper portion of the Mississippi-Missouri watershed would have absorbed enough floodwater to substantially reduce the $16 billion in flood damages from the Great Midwest Flood of 1993.[523] Similarly, humans have ruined the oyster beds that once protected New Yorkers from storm surges such as those generated from Superstorm Sandy, which was the second deadliest hurricane in the northeastern United States in forty years and the second costliest in the nation's history.[524]

Another shortcoming is our habit of focusing on first costs, such as the cost to construct a facility, while paying too little attention to the operating and maintenance costs that follow. Life-cycle analysis, which considers both, leads to more beneficial decision-making over the longer term.

There is no reason we can't establish policies that require complete cost-and-benefit accounting. With such policies, we could pay as we go rather than stick future generations with the tab. Of course, it's easier and cheaper in the short term to act with no regard for consequences, just as it may be easier in the short term to charge everything to your credit card. This is what regulations are for—to avoid this kind of free-for-all.

As a result of failures on several levels, the US did not prosecute one single bank CEO who brought down the global economy in 2008. Consequently, the billions of dollars in penalties are borne by shareholders and taxpayers, as the banks write off the fines as a cost of doing business. Scholar, litigator, and prosecutor William Black told Bill Moyers he is certain a much larger disaster will happen because we've created the incentive structures to make it happen.[525]

Some policies lack teeth. US mine owners are allowed to ignore safety violations. As of 2014, some 2700 delinquent mine owners owed $70 million in safety fines. While they accumulated these debts, they generated 130,000 additional violations and 4000 additional injuries. However, the government has no legal authority to shut down a mine for not paying its penalties.[526] One coal company, Massey Energy, continued operating while it racked up 67,000 Clean Water Act violations. Meanwhile, democracy has been subverted, people have moved away, and West Virginia, in the heart of coal-mining country, is the next-to-poorest state in the country.[527] At least the CEO paid fines and went to jail for mine safety violations.[528]

We also fail to implement policies. The US Congress, contrary to President Obama's wishes, cut the budget of the Internal Revenue Service, even though each $1 cut causes tax revenue to fall by $10.[529]

Yet we're making some progress. Cooperatives may be the earliest modern structures to concern themselves about more than just monetary profit.

Starting in the mid-1800s, people formed these autonomous associations to meet their common economic, social, and cultural needs and wants through joint ownership and democratic control. Guiding principles typically include concern for community, which may or may not include the environment. In the United States, 30,000 cooperatives with 256 million members provide more than two million jobs. The cooperative movement brings together one billion of the world's people in the International Co-operative Alliance.[530]

The "triple bottom line" is a way for companies to consider people and the planet too, by preparing three different bottom lines—measuring financial profit, the company's social responsibility, and the company's environmental responsibility.[531] Profit still dominates in most applications, but at least people think more broadly with this kind of approach.

Benefit Corporations, or "B Corps," are a new class of corporations that voluntarily meet standards different from those of the traditional, profit-only, shareholder-driven model. B Corps are required to consider their impacts on workers, community, and the environment, in addition to shareholders. In most of the United States, they are required to report annually on their social and environmental performance against a third-party standard.[532] More than half the states allow the creation of B Corps. There are more than 1895 B Corps in at least fifty countries and 130 industries.[533]

The global Natural Capital Declaration expresses the financial sector's commitment to work toward integrating "natural capital criteria into financial products and services." Institutions that have signed the declaration promise to work with support organizations to help incorporate "natural capital factors" into their businesses.[534]

Similarly, the CEOs of some of the world's largest banks created the Banking Environmental Initiative, whose mission is to lead the banking industry in collectively directing capital towards environmentally and socially sustainable economic development. The Initiative's "Soft Commodities Compact" mobilizes the banking industry to combat deforestation.[535]

MAKE WAY FOR CLEAN TECHNOLOGY

Clean technology is becoming mainstream. New economic policies could accelerate this process, while discouraging reckless deployment as entrepreneurs clamor to cash in. Right now, we are thwarting clean, green technology in some ways and rolling it out destructively in other ways.

By subsidizing wasteful, polluting "dirty technology," we make it harder for clean technology to compete in the marketplace—and dirty technology already enjoys the advantages of larger market share and more years of experience. Special interests also use their money to expedite, or delay, or kill projects. While coal companies blow tops off mountains to get at underlying coal, dump the mountaintop soil and rock into rivers and streams, and never restore the land, the proposed Cape Wind project off the coast of Massachusetts underwent ten years of torturous permitting processes before gaining federal approval.[536] Billionaire industrialist William Koch fought the project for more than a decade, donating $5 million to, and leading, an adversarial group against the project. Other wealthy opponents also used their financial muscle to delay the project.[537]

Solar energy is often stymied by "net-metering caps." State net-metering programs allow certain energy customers with solar panels or other electrical generation to be paid for the electricity they contribute to the power grid. Limits on how much power can be sold back to the grid kills solar projects and rolls back or slows progress in expanding solar energy production.[538]

Perhaps the most important requirement for creating a sustainable world is getting money out of politics and thereby restoring our democracy. Philosopher Kathleen Dean Moore says the "one central social pathology" responsible for climate change, financial woes, pointless wars, and so many other problems today is "the buying and selling of elections and elected, mostly by corporations."[539] Spiritual teacher Marianne Williamson agrees: "Money in politics is the cancer underlying all the cancers."[540] Environmentalist Gus Speth explains: "The system is the problem. The system is at the root of the environmental ills.... The things that affect environmental outcomes are politics and the ascendancy of money power over people power."[541]

> *Money in politics is the cancer underlying all the cancers.*
> —*Marianne Williamson*

Economist Robert Reich describes the "giant vicious cycle" we find ourselves in economically. If lower and middle class people don't have money and benefits, they're afraid to spend. They cut back, which hurts the US economy, 70 percent of which consists of consumer spending. Poor economic performance leads to more insecurity, and so on. Everyone is acting rationally, given the rules of the game. "But the rules of the game are irrational," says Reich, and they do not generate a prosperous society. And the more uneven the playing field, the more income and wealth concentrate at the top. The more wealth concentrates at the top, the more susceptible a society is to corruption, to people using their money to buy rules that benefit them. "We want an economy that works for everyone, not just a small elite," he says.[542]

Unlimited campaign contributions allowed by the *Citizens United v. Federal Election Commission* Supreme Court decision, combined with the ever-widening chasm between rich and poor, make it nearly impossible for low–and middle-income people to run for office in the absence of public or small donor campaign finance programs. In 2014, winning candidates for the US House of Representatives had to raise about $1800 per day, and US Senate candidates had to raise about $3300 per day.[543]

Despite deep dissatisfaction, citizens have not pushed hard enough. Corporations have. Hedrick Smith wrote that corporate America blocks reform and keeps loopholes in place: "The flood of corporate campaign contributions into congressional races, so far little noticed by the media, is aimed largely at protecting the legal tax dodges of America's richest corporations."[544] However, a month later, he reported all but two of the major Presidential candidates—including Republicans—were now calling for reforms to get money out of politics.[545]

Corruption runs rampant in some industries. Peter Gøtzsche, in his book *Deadly Medicine and Organised Crime: How Big Pharma Has Corrupted Health Care,* exposes the pharmaceutical industry's "fraudulent behavior" and "morally repugnant disregard for human lives." He maintains that the "extraordinary system failure caused by widespread crime, corruption, bribery, and impotent drug regulation in need of radical reforms" is partly why drugs are the third leading cause of death, after heart disease and cancer, in the United States and Europe. "The main reason we take so many drugs is that drug companies don't sell drugs, they sell lies about drugs," writes Gøtzsche, and doctors "know very, very little about drugs that hasn't been carefully concocted and dressed up by the drug industry."[546]

Many reforms are needed throughout our system (see Chapter 12). Robert Reich says there is no economic system in global history that has worked as well as capitalism. But our capitalistic democracy must periodically save capitalism from its own excesses. This happened in the progressive era between 1901 and 1916, in the 1930s with the New Deal, in the 1960s with the war on poverty, and to some extent in the 1990s.[547] Based on this pattern, we are due for reform now and we can succeed again.

Restoring our capitalist democracy would decrease income inequality and improve upward mobility, giving people the money and confidence with which to buy more goods and services. With people buying more, corporations would make and sell more, creating more jobs and profits. And regular people doing better financially are likely to feel better emotionally too. Reacting to a greater sense of security and a feeling that they are getting a better deal, they may be inclined to devote more time to helping their community and the environment and actively participating in our democracy. People would be empowered, instead of feeling downtrodden by a corrupt system. Gus Speth says we need to implement deep reforms and drive them so deeply "that we emerge with a really different system ... that gives true and honest priority to people and place and planet, and not to profit and product."[548]

ECONOMIC CHANGES TO PROMOTE SUSTAINABILITY

Key sustainability-related areas are ripe for economic reforms. The following explores several of these areas.

FOOD AND AGRICULTURE

Feeding ourselves healthier food while keeping our planet clean begins with eliminating or redirecting the agricultural subsidies that make junk food cheap and real food expensive. Targeted subsidies for organic fruit and vegetable production might be a wise start. They could, among other benefits, promote clean food, environmental health, increased consumption of fruits and vegetables, local food production, community gardens, school gardens, and conversion of lawns to gardens. (According to Joel Salatin, our thirty-five million acres of lawn plus our thirty-six million acres used for housing and feeding "recreational" horses provide enough land to feed the entire United States without a single farm.[549])

The biggest hurdle for organics is the added cost of sustainable practices. If the negative impacts of industrial food production were factored in, industrial food would not enjoy a price advantage.[550] Journalist Dan Mitchell writes, "the true costs of producing a Quarter Pounder with Cheese are borne not only by McDonald's, but by all of us who have to deal with, among other things, environmental degradation caused by industrial farming and the bad public health outcomes of eating such meals. McDonald's doesn't pay much of those costs, and in fact draws a profit while the rest of us pay dearly."[551]

Americans spend 14 percent of gross domestic product on groceries and restaurants.[552] Apparently, most of us want others to provide our food. If consumers demand healthy, sustainably produced food, the food industry will provide it. The food industry, which just wants to make money, could thrive by providing healthy foods produced by sustainable, ethical methods. Whole Foods Market has done well by offering organic alternatives and adhering to higher standards for quality and disclosure than mainstream grocery store chains do.

Worldwide, consumers increasingly appreciate the benefits of eating organic food. "Organic food is one of the fasting growing segments of American agriculture," said Agriculture Secretary Tom Vilsack.[553] As the organic market share continues to expand, organic food prices should come down due to economies of scale.

ENERGY

The International Monetary Fund (IMF), with 188 member countries, estimated global subsidies for petroleum, coal, natural gas, and electricity for 2015 totaled $5.3 trillion.[554] This is equal to 6.5 percent of global gross domestic product and more than the total health spending of all the world's governments combined.

Eliminating subsidies would raise fossil fuel prices closer to their true costs. Reacting to the prices, consumers would increasingly conserve and opt for cleaner, greener sources. Increasing use of cleaner energy sources would bring down their costs, due to economies of scale, and make them even more attractive. The IMF calculates that eliminating energy subsidies would reduce global carbon dioxide emissions by 17 percent. This would be a huge boon for the climate. People would save money by being able to make informed decisions—with costs no longer hidden—and from improved human and environmental health. The IMF estimates premature deaths due to air pollution would be reduced by more than 50 percent. We'd also enjoy increased energy security by relying on unlimited energy sources such as sun and wind.[555]

> *Eliminating energy subsidies would reduce global carbon dioxide emissions by 17 percent. —International Monetary Fund*

People want clean energy. According to a 2015 Gallup poll, 79 percent of Americans say the United States should put more emphasis on producing domestic energy from solar, and 70 percent say the country should put more emphasis on producing energy from wind.[556]

WATER

Antiquated water policies in the United States—carried over from times when clean, fresh water seemed unlimited—can be modernized to help protect our water resources. Water is frequently sold at too a low price to promote careful use. What's more, backwards fee schedules sometimes provide a volume discount, charging lower rates for consuming more.[557] In the midst of a historic multiyear drought, underground pipes in water distribution systems in California lose enough water to supply the entire city of Los Angeles.[558] If water was priced higher, perhaps more leakage would be stopped. Half the homes in Sacramento lack water meters (which measure water use). Residents pay a flat fee, no matter how much they use—they could leave faucets running 24/7.

More than half the people on Earth suffer severe water scarcity for at least one month out of the year.[559] These people use water carefully because lack of clean water for drinking, irrigation, sanitation, and maintaining ecosystems causes infectious disease and death. Lack of access to safe water, combined with social norms, forces women and girls in developing countries to spend hours every day hauling water. This practice drains their energy, productive potential, and health and keeps them out of school. A UN report estimates that an annual investment of $0.84 trillion in water infrastructure could deliver more than $3 trillion annually in economic, environmental, and social benefits.[560]

FORESTS

A 2008 study commissioned by the European Union and conducted by a Deutsche Bank economist concluded the annual global cost of forest loss is between $2 trillion and $5 trillion. This figure comes from estimating the value of the various services forests perform, such as providing clean water and absorbing carbon dioxide.[561]

The 2014 Global Commission on Economy and Climate report recommended halting deforestation.[562] However, government subsidies drive deforestation around the world.[563] The elimination of logging subsidies would save taxpayers their money as well as their forests.

Corruption is killing many forests as government officials look the other way while forests are illegally clear-cut and indigenous societies are destroyed.[564] Forests can be protected by clamping down on illegal logging and restricting legal logging. Brazil uses satellite photography to detect illegal logging. Government officials go to the sites identified and confiscate the illegally cut logs, sell them, and use the proceeds to buy land for conservation. They put lawbreakers, including corrupt local officials, in jail.[565] Other countries could use this approach.

Andrew Mitchell of the Global Canopy Programme says, "Trashing forests and making money is great for investors—it's very profitable business." He calls for policy changes in import and export tariffs, taxation, subsidies, and government procurement policies. He says policy changes should make it possible for the supply chains of European and North America–based businesses to be forest-sustainable by 2020. He says supply chains for the rest of the world could be forest-sustainable by 2030.[566]

HEALTH

The World Health Organization predicts cardiovascular disease, chronic respiratory disease, cancer, diabetes, and mental health will cost the global economy a staggering $47 trillion over the next twenty years. This represents enough money to eradicate poverty among 2.5 billion people for more than fifty years.[567]

In the United States, health spending has been increasing faster than other sectors of the economy, and we spend significantly more per person on health care than any other country.[568] Yet the level of performance of the US health-care system ranked worst among eleven industrialized nations in 2014.[569]

This poor performance occurs because in the "byzantine world of American health care ... the real profit is made not by controlling chronic diseases like diabetes but by treating their many complications."[570] Funding for preventive medicine and public health is miniscule, and the specialty of preventive medicine comprises less than 1 percent of the physician workforce.[571] The Centers for Disease Control and Prevention reports that 86 percent of US health-care spending in 2010 was for people with chronic conditions, and chronic diseases are the leading cause of death and disability.[572] Health insurance will often pay for triple coronary bypass surgery but not for far cheaper nutritional counseling that could have prevented the need for it.

Globally, there are now 30 percent more obese people than people with not enough food to eat, and chronic, noncommunicable, lifestyle-driven disease kills more than twice as many people as infectious disease.[573] More than one-third of Americans are obese, and medical costs for obese people are more than $1,400 per year higher (on average) than for people who are not obese. Excess weight costs the United States around $147 billion in medical costs annually.[574]

In 2012, an Institute of Medicine report called for systemic policy changes to address the obesity epidemic in America. Changes include overhauling farm policies and the way food is marketed, building more walkable neighborhoods, and ensuring that children get at least one hour of physical activity a day.[575]

Dr. Hyman writes, "Perverse economic incentives drive policy and medical decisions, they are not in the best interest of the patients, and certainly do not have better health outcomes.... This quiet, dangerous set of forces in play in American society fuels the explosive and uncontrolled growth of disease in America." He observes that one-third of our "disease-creation economy" profits from making us fat and sick—namely, the food industry and the health-care industry. And industry drives medical education, research, and practice toward drugs and surgery and away from lifestyle solutions. The recent health-care reforms of the Affordable Care Act do not address the root problem of increasing chronic disease.[576]

Dr. Hyman has diagnosed and proposed a treatment plan for our sick medical system, identifying the root causes of its disease and prescribing solutions that address its causes rather than just suppress its symptoms. Hyman prescribes reclaiming what is rightfully ours—our food policy, our public airwaves, our schools, our health-care reform, and our medical education—and suggests actions in each of these areas—such as taxing sugar and creating school gardens.[577]

Decontaminating, safeguarding, and restoring our climate, air, water, and soil would also reduce health-care costs. The strengthened US Clean Air Act reduces health-care costs by trillions of dollars.[578]

Green Chemistry

Pike Research, a market research company, estimates green chemicals will save industry $65.5 billion by 2020.[579] This includes direct savings as well as avoided liability for environmental and social impacts. Green chemistry can result in economic advantages due to

- Higher yields for chemical reactions, requiring less raw material.

- Fewer steps for synthesis, resulting in less water and energy usage. Reduced use of petroleum, avoiding its hazards and effects of price fluctuations.

- Reduced waste, and thus lower costs for waste disposal and treatment and environmental cleanup.

- Replacement of purchased raw material by a waste product from some other process.

- Increased consumer sales due to reduced costs and greater product safety.[580]

Once we reform our system to count and assign to their rightful source all relevant costs and benefits—including health and environmental impacts—green chemistry, as the cheaper alternative, will become the norm.[581] A 2015 study estimates the cost of dealing with serious health problems due to endocrine-disrupting chemicals in Europe alone costs more than $175 billion per year.[582] Most of this is health-care cost for the effects of chemicals on children's developing brains. Similarly, the United States racks up $76 billion in children's health costs due to toxic chemicals and pollutants in air, food, water, and soil.[583] These expenditures are real, but they are not assigned to the chemicals that cause them. Green chemistry, by definition, will not come with such costs.

Green chemistry will also renew manufacturing jobs in the United States while protecting human and environmental health and reducing the chemical industry's pollution abatement costs. Environmental lawsuits and toxic releases reduce the value of the average US chemical company by almost one-third of total assets, or about $200 billion—losses that could be largely avoided with green chemistry. Overhauling the Toxic Substances Control Act could encourage green chemistry, benefitting citizens, the environment, and chemical manufacturers alike.[584]

GET MORE DONE AND HAVE MORE FUN

A green economy—one that counts all costs and benefits and promotes sustainability—will help prevent or solve many problems. Freed from spending so much money, time, and energy on damage control, we'll have more to spend on learning, the arts, and other enjoyable pursuits.

Corporations are composed of humans, and imagine how much happier those humans would be if the goals and actions of the corporations they worked for aligned with their own. And like the rest of us, most CEOs want the job satisfaction that comes from helping others and working toward a good future for our children. When Marion Stoddart led the cleanup of the Nashua River, the CEO of the largest polluter of the river got on board, telling her, "I want to wear a white hat. I'm tired of wearing a black hat."

British novelist Alexander McCall Smith calls "the business of kindness" a big movement in the twenty-first century, saying, "It's possible to do business in a way that isn't red in tooth and claw." Kindness runs through most of our relationships. If we took short-term advantage of our friends the way most corporations do, we wouldn't have any friends. Businesses are increasingly realizing that treating suppliers and customers well creates long-term arrangements, which are more profitable because they avoid the need to continually create new relationships, only to destroy them. Businesses can use the saved money, time, and energy on more desirable activities.[585]

CHAPTER 11
CONNECT AND COLLABORATE

There are only two superpowers left in the world. One is the rich and powerful that control huge military might and awesome weapons of both mass destruction and mass distraction. They number at most a few million. The other superpower is vast, numbering seven billion. I'm talking of all of you here and around the world. We have to recognize our collective superpower status that will only come when we work together.

—*Stephen Bezruchka, senior lecturer at the University of Washington*[586]

ON A MACRO LEVEL, THE overall pecking order has become reversed, in the United States at least, so the tail now wags the dog: corporations rule governments, governments rule citizens, and all try to rule nature. A sustainable world model acknowledges that nature rules everything, citizens rule governments, and governments rule corporations.

Developmental biologist Bruce Lipton, asks, "Are you in protection or do you grow?" When in protection against threats, growth stops and all of an organism's resources are directed to simply surviving. Lipton observes that if you believe you're a victim, you give up control.[587]

Many people today focus on protection and survival rather than citizenship and growth. Promoting equality, respect, and cooperation—with nature and among genders, races, generations, and societies—would free us up to live in growth rather than protection, better enabling us to create a sustainable world. This chapter describes promising efforts, in varying stages of development, moving us in this direction.

RIGHTS OF NATURE

Many indigenous cultures believe in the rights of nature, viewing plants, animals, and the Earth as relatives rather than resources and regarding people as responsible for taking care of their relatives. Their perception might be "my mother is in pain" rather than "the Earth is experiencing climate change."[588]

"Rights of nature" are beginning to be codified in the United States and other parts of the world. Some Pennsylvania townships have replaced the old notion of environmental protection, which views nature as property, with language in their ordinances that recognizes "that natural communities and ecosystems possess a fundamental right to exist and flourish, and that residents possess the legal authority to enforce those rights on behalf of the ecosystem."[589] More than two dozen US towns and cities have adopted local laws that recognize the rights of nature, and Pittsburgh, Pennsylvania, became the first major US city to do so.[590] The Community Environmental Legal Defense Fund (CELDF) partners with organizations in Australia, Colombia, Cameroon, India, Nepal, and other countries to develop rights of nature frameworks.[591]

The animal welfare movement is in different stages of development in different parts of the world. Successes have been achieved in Europe, Australia, New Zealand, Tanzania, and elsewhere.[592] Primatologist Jane Goodall has documented numerous heroic efforts to save endangered species from extinction.[593]

In 2014, an Argentinian court ruled that a twenty-nine-year-old Sumatran orangutan held in a Buenos Aires zoo was a "nonhuman person" who had been unlawfully deprived of her freedom and could be freed and transferred to a sanctuary. Paul Buompadre of the Association of Officials and Lawyers for Animal Rights said the landmark ruling "opens the way not only for other Great Apes, but also for other sentient beings which are unfairly and arbitrarily deprived of their liberty in zoos, circuses, water parks, and scientific laboratories."[594]

In 2008, Ecuador became the first country to recognize nature's rights in its constitution, which states nature in all its life forms has "the right to exist, persist, maintain, and regenerate its vital cycles." People have the right to enforce these rights on behalf of nature, and an ecosystem can be named as the defendant.[595] In 2012, Bolivia passed the first law on nature's rights, The Framework Law on Mother Earth and Integral Development for Living Well, which calls for "harmony and balance with nature, recovering and strengthening local and ancestral knowledge and wisdom." The law enshrines the legal rights of nature and requires efforts to avoid damage to the environment, biodiversity, human health, and cultural heritage.[596] In Colombia, more than 700,000 people have signed a petition calling for the adoption of Rights of Nature.[597]

The Global Alliance for the Rights of Nature is a worldwide movement of individuals and organizations. In December 2015, while the international conference on climate change was taking place in Paris, communities and organizations from all over the world formally established the International Tribunal for the Rights of Nature. The tribunal heard evidence on environmental issues such as climate change, hydraulic fracturing, and ecocide. The tribunal established that human rights and the rights of nature are being systematically violated as a result of the misconception that humans have the right and ability to dominate and exploit the Earth. Creation of the international tribunal opened the way for the creation of regional tribunals, to expand recognition of the rights of nature.[598]

HUMAN EQUALITY

As in Chapter 3, I have focused the following discussion of human inequality on gender discrimination, which affects the most people.

We can't afford to continue stifling half of the human population. Our challenges are too great to forego women's vast talents, capacities, and cooperative influence. Hillary Clinton, in her 1995 speech to the UN, said, "Women must enjoy the rights to participate fully in the social and political lives of their countries, if we want freedom and democracy to thrive and endure."[599]

Especially in the Western world, the gulf between men and women is narrowing, and it's increasingly acceptable for women to change their situations, such as by escaping bad marriages. Women who are free to push the boundaries to get to total equality almost have a duty to do so, because so many women in the world cannot, without risking their lives or the lives of their loved ones.

Jean Houston writes that women the world over are rising to full partnership with men in the entire domain of human affairs. She says we are "in the midst of the most massive shift of perspective that humankind has ever known.... The new values that are trying to arise are essentially women's values—holistic, syncretic, relationship and process-oriented, organic, and spiritual."[600]

The old "command and control" model is being replaced by a "connect and collaborate" model, wherein women excel.[601] The Dalai Lama says Western women will save the world. He believes women, with their nurturing instinct, are naturally more compassionate.[602] Western women generally have more freedom and resources at their disposal than women elsewhere. Previous generations of women, and many women throughout the world today, were and are for the most part consigned to a life of negating themselves and caring for family members.

The Dalai Lama says that Western women will save the world.

A recent Pew study indicates young women in the United States now place a higher importance on having a successful, high-paying career than young men do.[603] At the same time that options have opened up for women, so have options for men. According to the 2010 United States Census, the number of stay-at-home fathers in the country more than doubled in the prior ten years.[604] As Margaret Mead said, "Every time we liberate a woman, we liberate a man."[605]

Equal pay for equal work lies at the core of gender equality. The Institute for Women's Policy Research estimates that if women earned the same as comparable men—men who are of the same age, have the same level of education, work the same number of hours, and have the same urban/rural status—poverty among working women would be cut in half and the US economy would grow by $482 billion.[606] The pay gap has narrowed since the 1970s, but slowly, and has stalled in recent years.[607]

Similarly, equalizing access to financial and other resources would not only be just, but it would also help everyone. Former Secretary-General of the United Nations Kofi Annan explained that gender equality is central to providing food to the several billion people who don't have enough. He cited the UN Food and Agriculture Organization's estimate that if women farmers had the same access to productive resources as men, agricultural yields would increase by up to a third.[608] The World Bank is trying to expand women's access to financial services.[609]

One Billion Rising, the largest mass action to end violence against women in human history, holds events throughout the world to end violence against women. In 2015, millions of activists in most countries of the world gathered at rallies to change the paradigm and demand accountability, justice, and systematic change.[610]

Reproductive choice affects women's education, paid work, health, and length of life.[611] Hillary Clinton explains, "There is no one formula for how women should lead our lives. That is why we must respect the choices that each woman makes for herself and her family."[612]

Young women with reproductive freedom can receive more education. Furthermore, "education is the best contraception of all. A girl who gets into high school worldwide on the average is going to have two children. If she gets a degree, she's going to delay her childbearing until her college is over. She's going to have something very useful to both her family and her society," says journalist Alan Weisman.[613] Because creating a sustainable way of life requires curbing human population growth—if not reducing our numbers—empowering women should be seen as a matter of life and death.

Education can help women break through their "inner glass ceiling," the destructive social conditioning that says they don't belong, that they exist only to serve others and should be invisible.[614] Education can teach women about women leaders, the women's movement, and where women find themselves today in the larger context of history.[615]

At the same time, we can simultaneously alleviate men's suffering by teaching them they don't have to stifle their emotions or be aggressive and they can ask for help and reveal weakness and sensitivity. Author and coach John Lee writes that progress on this front enables former Speaker of the House John Boehner to weep before millions and for General Norman Schwarzkopf to say, "I wouldn't trust a man who couldn't cry."[616]

The prospects for gender equality are low as long as women are saddled with most of the work at home. To reduce gender gaps—and thereby significantly improve economic growth and standards of living—the International Labor Organization makes the following recommendations: improve infrastructure (for electricity, water, sanitation, and transportation) to reduce the burden of housework; provide care services, particularly childcare; and balance the gender division of paid and unpaid work.[617]

Collaborative organizations such as Rising Women Rising World train and develop women and men to balance feminine and masculine qualities in order to create a better world. Rising Women Rising World believes women "possess in abundance the capacities of compassion, creativity, courage, and sufficient consciousness to create a civilisation where all beings feel a sense of belonging and can fulfill their individual and collective purpose and potential, in harmony with the earth."[618] Founding member Rama Mani, international peace and security expert, writes, "My vision is to see the power of love replace the love of power."[619]

David Korten sees great hope for the world as half the human population comes out of the shadows to lead us. Women are "natural leaders ... and they are indeed rising to the challenge." The era of cooperation between men and women that is coming into being is critical to the peace, stability, and sustainability of our world.[620]

INTERGENERATIONAL SOLIDARITY

Many people want to reconnect the generations. Generations United lists more than 500 intergenerational programs in the United States alone.[621] Interest in genealogy has skyrocketed in recent years, and it is now the second most popular hobby in the United States, after gardening.[622] Part of Senator Bernie Sanders' appeal to young people may be his grandfatherly image. "I think Bernie is relatable, he's cozy; he's like your grandfather who tells the truth," explained a thirty-four-year-old architect.[623]

We need an "all hands on deck" approach to develop workable, long-term solutions to climate change. This presents a great opportunity for elders and "youngers" to collaborate, to bridge what climate scientist and "father of global warming" James Hansen calls the "geezer–young person gap."[624] Given that problems, solutions, costs, and benefits play out over timeframes spanning generations, climate change calls for intergenerational climate change activism.

Youngers around the world increasingly take action on climate change, partly out of concern about a long future of intensifying negative impacts.[625] Elders likewise increasingly take action, partly out of passion to protect their children and grandchildren. Halfdan Wiik of the Norwegian Grandparents Climate Campaign says, "For me, it's all about love and optimism. Elders of today have lived our lives in a world of great changes, for good and for bad. We know it can be changed once more."[626]

In the 1960s and early '70s, many of today's elders in the United States learned how to create change when they successfully demanded an end to the Vietnam War, expanded the civil rights and women's movements, and created the modern environmental movement. Environmentalist Bill McKibben calls on baby boomers to rally once again. He writes, "Now is the boomers' chance to reclaim their better, bolder natures and to end their run as it began."[627] Baby boomers began reaching the traditional retirement age of 65 in 2011. Retired boomers represent a huge, untapped resource that grows by 10,000 people every day in the United States alone.[628] Baby boomers wield enormous political and economic power, constituting more than a third of the US electorate and accounting for half of all US consumer spending.[629]

Throughout human history and in many cultures, elders have insisted on paying attention to the needs of succeeding generations. Pope Francis wrote in his 2015 encyclical, "Each community ... has the duty to protect the earth and to ensure its fruitfulness for coming generations.... We can no longer speak of sustainable development apart from intergenerational solidarity," he observes. "Intergenerational solidarity is not optional, but rather a basic question of justice, since the world we have received also belongs to those who will follow us."[630]

Elders and youngers bring different gifts, which, when united, yield a synergistic combination. Compared with youngers, many elders have more free time, financial resources, experience, economic and political clout, and sense of connection to nature. They have witnessed environmental changes over long time periods and take a long view, having observed repeated historical upheavals in their lifetimes. Aware they may have few years left, elders often work with a sense of urgency and willingness to take bold action.

And when they act, they have credibility because they are trying to benefit future generations, not just themselves.

Youngers likewise constitute a huge, untapped resource. They bring energy, idealism, eagerness to learn and grow, new knowledge, and proficiency with social media and the Internet. They provide "boots on the ground" at marches, rallies, and other events.

Elders and youngers both benefit from collaborating. Youngers appreciate elders who will hear them and back them up. With elders' encouragement, youngers may be more inclined to practice, test themselves, and lead. Youngers can learn from elders' experiences. Elders benefit from a sense of purpose and contribution as well as gratification that youngers value their knowledge and skills. Elders are inspired by the commitment and curiosity of youngers, and elders benefit from youngers' valuable expertise with communication technology.[631]

Numerous elders groups have recently formed to help address climate change, and their memberships are growing.[632] Elders and youngers attend events—such as the 2014 People's Climate March and 350.org workshops.[633] And several nonprofit organizations have an explicit mission to bring adults and children together in intergenerational action on climate change. Here are a few examples.

- Norwegian Grandparents Climate Campaign (NGCC) partners with Miljøagentene The Eco-Agents, an environmental organization for Norwegian children. Elders and youngers together write letters to government officials, speak to Parliament, rally, march, meet in schools, and educate the public. NGCC and The Eco-Agents jointly produced a four-page pamphlet and distributed it to members of Parliament and secondary school students and public libraries across Norway.[634]

- Suzuki Elders—a voluntary association of elders in Canada working with and through the David Suzuki Foundation—strives to "mentor, encourage, and support other elders and the younger generations in dialogue and action in the environment."[635] The group's intergenerational activities have included an Elders, Environment, and Youth Forum; participation in marches, rallies, conferences, and workshops; creation of an informational video; improvement of social media platforms; retreats on the theme "Elders and Youth: Listening to Each Other"; and workshops on intergenerational storytelling.[636] The association coaches elders to work effectively with youngers by going to where youngers are (such as public events and social media sites); connecting firmly with one or two who are eager to work with elders; scheduling events for times that work for youngers; providing refreshments; respecting youngers' social media prowess; supporting them without criticizing, directing, teaching, or holding expectations; listening; being patient; and understanding that youngers are busy with school and other activities.[637]

- No Planeta B, a sustainability consultancy organization of adults in Peru and the United States, launched the Cut the Red Tape Project to involve students, parents, and schools in climate change action. Participating schools sign a declaration committing to at least five climate change mitigation actions. These might include going paperless and having meatless Mondays. Schools in Peru, Brazil, Colombia, Ecuador, Mexico, Curaçao, Guyana, Argentina, the United States, and elsewhere have signed on.[638] Similarly, parents are invited to sign a declaration committing to at least five actions, such as reducing food waste and walking and bicycling more often.[639] No Planeta B brings together delegations of students, teachers, and school administrators at conferences.

- The Conscious Elders Network's Intergenerational Connections action team works to bring elders and youngers together to address critical issues of our time, including climate change.[640]

Our prospects for developing effective climate change solutions—as well as solutions to other problems we face—will improve if elders and youngers increasingly collaborate to combine their talents, skills, and perspectives. Elders and youngers working together not only can meet the challenge of climate change but also heal age divisions in Western societies. As Pope Francis writes, "The urgent challenge to protect our common home includes a concern to bring the whole human family together to seek a sustainable and integral development."[641]

> *The urgent challenge to protect our common home includes a concern to bring the whole human family together to seek a sustainable and integral development —Pope Francis*

REPLACE WAR WITH COOPERATION

Barbara Marx Hubbard and American politician Dennis Kucinich suggest creating a Department of Peace and a Peace Room, analogous to the Department of Defense and War Room, not only to resolve conflicts but to provide true security in the broadest sense of the term, including environmental. Hubbard says "the purpose of war is not to kill; the purpose is to provide security, and peace, actually" and that we can pursue these objectives more directly.[642] Peace becomes more imperative as our weapons become more deadly and numerous.

Prevention may provide the best answer to the challenging problems of war and violence. Sometimes, environmental, economic, or social problems—such as water scarcity, lack of jobs, or discrimination—drive war and violence, in which case solving these underlying problems can help. By strengthening international institutions such as the United Nations, we would render them more able to prevent and address conflicts.

Changing the way we think can end violence. Our outdated worldview of hierarchy and separate organisms pitted against each other in fierce competition over scarce resources can give way to a more scientifically accurate one, a view of connected organisms cooperating in order to survive. We can intentionally break the chain of violence through constructive education, media, and recreation.

Could war be an aberration similar to domestic violence or child abuse, which perpetuates itself by being handed down from generation to generation, each thinking this is "just the way things are," until someone decides to break the chain? Jean Houston writes, "For most of our history as a species, we lived in small communities, with little warfare, shared intent, and a basic agreement about how to live together."[643]

Houston describes a peaceful, complex society that prospered in recent history. The Iroquois Confederacy, originally established as early as 1142 or 1451, served as a model for American democracy and other governments around the world.[644] The Iroquois Confederacy united tribes after a period of violence and intertribal warfare. Houston describes it as "a radical change in consciousness that opens itself to a new order of health, justice, and creative power. This new order is expressed through dynamic conversation, intensive sharing of ideas, councils, ceremony, and cooperation." Women were considered equal to men in every way. White people adopted many of the principles of the Iroquois Confederacy, rejected others (such as gender equality), and then destroyed the Confederacy.[645]

Imagine freeing up the lives, labor, attention, and money spent on war to use instead on education, preventive medicine, clean energy, organic agriculture, environmental restoration and protection, and the arts. The US government allocates about half of all discretionary spending (the money the President and Congress have direct control over) to the military. By contrast, the next two highest categories of discretionary spending, education and health, each receive roughly one-tenth as much funding as the military.[646]

Our technology may be helping to propel us forward into a more cooperative mode. This applies not just to nuclear weapons technology, but also to dramatically increased communication and information sharing; new science such as the human genome project, which shows humans to be remarkably similar to other organisms and to each other; and technology that changes the basic way we see ourselves. Jean Houston observes, "People everywhere began feeling the current call to transformation when they first saw the Earth from outer space. Somehow that picture made all humans into family again, with one another and with the Earth…. It was then, in the late 1960s, that the ecology movement took off, as well as other movements for greater social responsibility."[647]

RESTORE AND EXPAND DEMOCRACY

Former US Vice President Al Gore says, bluntly, "Our democracy has been hacked."[648] Restoring and expanding democracy would clear up many problems. Then government would serve citizens rather than special interests.

In a knee-jerk reaction, many people think that since government is corrupt, we should just get rid of it or shrink it down. This seems easier to them than rooting out corruption. This response makes some corporate executives do cartwheels of joy—less government means more latitude for corporations to help themselves to the commons. Robert Reich says, "What the powerful moneyed interests would like in this country is for us all to get so cynical about politics that we basically give up…. Then they win everything."[649]

Robert Frank, management and economics professor at Cornell University, describes how some people spend enormous sums of money to spread the message that government is the problem. Multibillionaires Charles and David Koch have contributed more than $100 million to far-right-wing think tanks. Likewise, Rupert Murdoch's Fox News Channel; Richard Mellon Scaife, an heir to the Mellon fortune; and the John M. Olin Foundation spent huge sums to spread the message that government is the problem and "unfettered markets are the solution." According to Frank, they have successfully fostered "an inchoate but pervasive sense of anger that has made it all but impossible for government to act." Frank writes that countries whose citizens think most highly of their governments also have the highest income per capita and best public goods and services. Countries with weak governments have low income per capita, high crime and violence, and citizens who see government as ineffectual and corrupt.[650]

We need government because it can efficiently perform many functions individuals alone cannot—defense, building and maintaining infrastructure, protecting property rights, and protecting environmental and human health, to name a few. Only government can prevent liquidation of the commons. And only citizens can keep the government in check and protect it from corruption. Democracy, literally, is people governing themselves. The word means "people power"—from the Greek words *demos*, the people, and *kratia*, power.[651]

Unfortunately, citizens can never kick back and relax, which is what many of us have been doing. In 1787, when emerging from Independence Hall at the close of the Constitutional Convention, Benjamin Franklin was asked, "Well, Doctor, what have we got, a republic or a monarchy?" He replied, "A republic, Madam, if you can keep it." We are currently losing it.

While it's not perfect, because of the need for constant citizen oversight, democracy has proven to be better for the average person in a complex society than any other system thus far invented. Democracy gives us a middle class instead of just rulers and their slaves. The middle class is made possible by ordinary people having the rights to vote the bums out, speak, assemble, and enjoy protection from unreasonable search and imprisonment. As our democracy has been eroded recently, so has the middle class, as income inequality has soared. More and more people in the middle class have been pushed down into poverty. And a new threat to democracy, lack of privacy in the current age of digital surveillance, looms.[652]

Democracy gives us a middle class instead of just rulers and their slaves.

Democracy applies to humans universally. President Franklin Roosevelt's four freedoms—freedom of speech, freedom of worship, freedom from want, and freedom from fear—became part of the charter of the United Nations. Al Gore said that "an essential prerequisite for saving the environment is the spread of democratic government to more nations of the world.... The future of human civilization depends on our stewardship of the environment and—just as urgently—our stewardship of freedom. The powerful forces working against stewardship are the same in both cases: greed, self-involvement, and a focus on short-term exploitation at the expense of the long-term health of the system itself."[653]

The world is more democratic than ever, with the majority of countries under democratic control. Democracy is contagious, and once people have it, they are loath to give it up.[654]

For democracy to work, citizens have to push government to do the right things. Pushing can include voting, serving in government or on boards and committees, supporting candidates, signing petitions, participating in boycotts, attending rallies, crowdfunding, and writing, calling, and meeting with representatives.

As long as we have democracy, citizens rule. We must not turn away from our challenge in disgust or apathy. Robert Reich says, "Most Americans now are losing faith in our democracy ... our most precious gift, the most precious legacy that we have to hand down to future generations."[655]

Small-Town Democracy. I admire the way democracy is practiced in my small town, which has a population of about 800 people. I've spent many hours in the town hall during expertly moderated and often contentious debates that allow anyone and everyone to speak their minds.

On the walls of the town hall are several maps of the town, a photo of the river that runs beside it, and a giant quilt sewn by a group of loving women decades ago, with the name of the town in big letters and squares depicting features of the town, among them, a sand spring and an outhouse. The town hall is used for all kinds of community gatherings. An upright piano with a sewn cloth cover sits in the corner of the room. Weekly yoga classes are held in the town hall.

This past winter, a proposal for improving Internet service in the town attracted more voters to a special town meeting than could legally fit in the town hall, so the meeting had to be rescheduled and resited. While all this was being worked out, throngs of voters waited outside in the cold, reconnecting with friends and neighbors and having lively chats. The meeting was held a week or two later in a giant tent that had been set up in the parking lot next to the town hall. Though at times the discussion became heated, the meeting for the most part was almost festive, and people seemed to enjoy it. The proposal was voted down, and a group of citizens was formed at the meeting to explore other options.

I enjoy voting. The same dedicated and cheerful volunteers orchestrate the voting process. Recently, I noticed a container of strawberries on the voter check-in table. My neighbor had brought them along when he came to vote, as a treat for the volunteers.

In my town hall, I go to a little booth to mark my ballot with a short yellow pencil, and then I bring my ballot to the checkout table. After the volunteer crosses my name off a list, I slide my ballot into the slot of a worn wooden ballot box. The volunteer turns a crank and a little bell goes ding while a counter on the front of the box slowly advances the number of ballots cast. Often that number is in the double digits, making me feel that my vote really counts. I say good-bye to the volunteers by name and leave.

I love this small town—with its vibrant historical society and small town events such as town dinners and the annual "Penny Social," where you buy tickets to use to bid on donated items. A signboard on the main road advertises "Have a Great Thanksgiving, and Drive Safely" or "Please Vote on November 8." Our town even has its own monthly newsletter, which, among other things, lists birthdays and anniversaries and memorializes residents who have passed away. Each year, a Memorial Day celebration includes speeches followed by a parade from the historical society building to the town cemetery, a distance of about one-quarter mile. The parade includes a student marching band, the town's fire engines, and antique cars and trucks full of kids in the open cargo areas. Some people bring their dogs and horses as everyone walks to the cemetery and back, chatting amiably.

The library serves as a focal point for the town, even though it is open only three half-days per week. Nevertheless, cardholders can order just about any book, which is brought in via a "bookmobile." This feels very democratic and uplifting. Residents exhibit historical artifacts in the library and the historical society building. Residents volunteer to serve on the town boards and committees. I serve on at least one committee at any given time. A core group of devoted people contribute mightily to the town, and the rest of us are grateful to them.

EDUCATION

Education elevates people above the level of distraction and disempowerment. Educated people more often know when they're being exploited, see opportunities and feel capable of pursuing them, and support people working for rather than against their interests. A teacher inspired children living in slums in Calcutta, India, to cut their neighborhoods' malaria and diarrhea rates in half and turn garbage dumps into playing fields. The teacher helped children living outside of Calcutta break out of a stultifying life of making bricks and of girls having children at young ages.[656] Creating a sustainable world requires us to become more empowered, conscious, and focused on priorities. Education can facilitate this process.

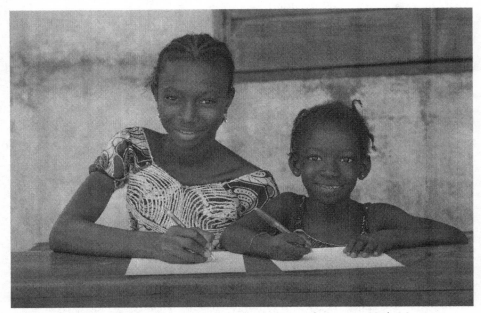

African school girls. Photo credit: ©Istockphoto.com/Riccardo Lennart Niels Mayer.

In their drive to improve gender equality and empower girls and women, the World Bank and other organizations focus on education. Both the Universal Declaration of Human Rights and the UN Convention on the Rights of the Child proclaim education to be a human right. According to the World Bank, "More educated women tend to be healthier, participate more in the formal labor market, earn more income, have fewer children, and provide better health care and education to their children, all of which eventually improve the well-being of all individuals and can lift households out of poverty. These benefits also transmit across generations, as well as to communities at large."[657]

Directly relevant education that is honest and empowering to kids (and adults) draws them in. Imagine a school that teaches students how to figure out what they want and how to get it. Or one that teaches them how to manage their money, protect their rights, or communicate effectively. Such education would create more powerful thinkers and doers.

Love

Ultimately, love for ourselves and others motivates us. It inspires us to stay or get healthy, restore the environment, green our technology and lifestyle, ensure equal rights, end war and cooperate, care for those who cannot defend themselves, educate and inform, and restore our democracy. Marianne Williamson says "there are only two emotions: love and fear" and "the relationship of love to fear is the same as the relationship of light to dark." Fear and darkness are not things; they are the absence of a thing, the absence of love and light. It doesn't work to focus on fighting fear. It works to focus on turning on the light, turning on the love. "When the mind is filled with love, literally fear cannot be."[658]

We choose moment by moment whether to live from fear or from love. Western society suffers from a deficit of love. Living from fear leads to hoarding, combativeness, and indifference.

Pope Francis writes, "Because all creatures are connected, each must be cherished with love and respect, for all of us as living creatures are dependent on one another." He adds, "Concern for the environment thus needs to be joined to a sincere love for our fellow human beings and an unwavering commitment to resolve the problems of society."[659]

Creating a sustainable world requires the efforts of individuals who love themselves and others enough to persevere in their actions despite opposition. With enough love we can create a cultural shift in our default response to the outside world, from one of fear, protection, and antagonism to cooperation, a desire to contribute, and observance of the Golden Rule, "do unto others as you would have them do unto you." Imagine a world in which corporations served customers, workers, shareholders, citizens, and the Earth.

CHAPTER 12

A HEALTH AND ENVIRONMENTAL REVOLUTION

It always seems impossible until it's done.

—*Nelson Mandela*

JUST AS AN INDIVIDUAL CREATES his or her life, the human species creates its life. Humans may be the first species to choose between conscious evolution and self-destruction. We're like a baby with a loaded gun—we're a species wielding awesome tools such as nuclear weapons and biotechnology. We need to grow up, and fast, before we get hurt.

The situation calls for nonviolent revolution—intentional, rapid, and radical change. I use the term "revolution," not "evolution," because "evolution" can suggest passivity and a slow pace. Some environmentalists wonder whether nonviolent protest and civil disobedience can bring about transformation quickly enough to save us. (Civil disobedience is the refusal to obey certain laws, demands, and commands by use of techniques such as boycotting, picketing, and nonpayment of taxes.) Kathleen Dean Moore says, "The reason nonviolent methods haven't worked is because we haven't really tried them yet. We haven't tried massive protests and civil disobedience. We haven't tried boycotts. We haven't harnessed the power of the global religions. Somewhere near half of us don't even vote. Here and there, sure, we've tried nonviolence, but not on the scale we need." She adds, "Let's give it a go."[660]

Addressing climate change requires global effort. We in America should lead the way because, cumulatively, the United States has dumped more greenhouse gases into the atmosphere than any other country.[661] Americans have the resources and freedom to take action. Others look to America for leadership and innovation. Winston Churchill, former Prime Minister of the United Kingdom, famously said, "You can always count on Americans to do the right thing—after they've tried everything else." Well, we have tried everything else—denial, procrastination, distraction, and finger-pointing—none of which has worked to reverse the ominous trends.

Recent performance of the US government shows it to be too corrupted, gridlocked, and dysfunctional to undertake the change that's needed on its own. Therefore, citizens must lead. If they do, government will follow—just as it did in the civil rights movement, women's movement, environmental movement, anti-war movement, Occupy Wall Street, and countless other examples. This is how democracy works.

Eco-philosopher Joanna Macy writes we are in "the third major watershed in humanity's journey, comparable in magnitude and scope to the agricultural and industrial revolutions."[662] Members of grassroots groups and nongovernmental organizations working for social justice, indigenous rights, and the environment number in the millions, in what environmentalist Paul Hawkens describes as the largest social movement in human history. He calls it "the movement with no name."[663]

Evolution results in the development of forms beyond what existed before, with added complexity and new capabilities. The new forms may be weak at first.[664] When mammals came along during the dinosaur age, they were small and pathetic—almost laughable—by comparison. American colonists may have seemed similarly weak—without authority, military strength, or money—when they declared independence from the King of England. Similarly, people who are pushing for human and environmental health may seem outnumbered and underpowered. But just wait! We *can* change course and create a sustainable world for ourselves and for others.

Now is Our Chance

The sooner we come to grips with our growing problems and take action, the easier our job will be. The time to act is now. Just because humans are overrunning the planet doesn't guarantee our dominance in the future. Species come and go, and most that ever lived have gone. The passenger pigeon was once the most abundant bird in America, if not the world. One in four birds in North America was a passenger pigeon—they were so numerous they would darken the sky. Their numbers went from billions to zero in 1914, after humans hunted them to extinction.

What will be our legacy? Will others in the future look back on us as the people who cleaned up their act and saved their environment, or as people who flamed out in a binge of hubris, apathy, greed, and fear?

We have everything to gain by acting and everything to lose by not acting. The status quo can no longer deliver a future that includes a stable climate, intact ecosystems containing diverse plant and animal species, a sound economy, upward mobility, decent food and health care, freedom and democracy, justice, and protection from nuclear catastrophe. But take heart. Because systems are so interconnected, restorative actions can compound and magnify in ways and at rates that astonish us. When conditions are ripe, anything can spark massive and rapid change—even a book *(Silent Spring)*, photograph (the Earth from space), or small action of one person—picking up a handful of salt, planting seven tree seedlings, or making the first chink in the Berlin Wall. Consider the rapidity and impacts of the revolution in communication and information technology.

In 2011, the United Nations declared that we need a technological revolution greater and faster than the Industrial Revolution to avoid "a major planetary catastrophe."[665] Massive change, of one kind or another, is surely coming.

EASIER THAN WE MAY THINK

Limiting beliefs fool us into thinking that creating a sustainable world will be difficult. If we focus instead on all we have going for us, we'll feel confident. Feeling confident, we'll try harder. Trying harder, we'll be more likely to succeed. Consider these assets:

- Humans have an awesome resumé. Our track record of evolutionary success extends back thousands, millions, or billions of years. Beyond physical survival, consider our astounding human achievements in language, mathematics, science, engineering, art, music, philosophy, and more.

- Humans have lived sustainably throughout the vast majority of human history. This bodes well for our prospects of doing so again. For Westerners, getting onto a sustainable path could be like turning on a light that hasn't been turned on in a while.

- We're hardwired to strive and care. All that evolutionary success leaves us with a compelling, built-in urge to survive and help our children survive. Teamwork provides humans with an evolutionary advantage, so the tendency to cooperate passes down from generation to generation. During a natural disaster or other calamity, humans display amazing acts of heroism and generosity (even though there may also be some looting and greed). A deep affiliation with nature is rooted in our biology.[666] We possess an innate propensity, refined over eons, to care for each other and for the natural world.

- We have a technology toolbox. We already have solutions to our problems, and we've already begun using them. We can increase the use of our green tools and refine them over time.

- Our lives are larger than ever before. We have more opportunities to live, learn, and act than ever. Average life expectancy in the United States has doubled since the 1700s. Our geographical reach has expanded, even extending beyond Earth for some explorers. Career opportunities have vastly expanded for many, especially women. With a computer and telephone, an entrepreneur can start a business.

- In the United States and elsewhere, we enjoy democracy and the authority to make changes. The Declaration of Independence guarantees equality; the rights to life, liberty, and the pursuit of happiness; and the right to alter, abolish, or institute any form of government. The Constitution confers additional freedoms, including freedom of speech and assembly. The Founding Fathers foresaw, and provided for, the need to "clean house" and make big changes from time to time.

- Humans are connected as never before, making it easier than ever to create a revolution. Rather than riding horses through the streets with lanterns to spread a message (like Paul Revere), we can simply e-mail, text, or post on social media.

- Intellectual freedom lets us decide. Not long ago, ideas like "you are a sorry sinner" were drummed into many of us on a regular basis. Now, many of us can opt out of such thinking and access ideas from all over the world, thinking whatever we choose.

- People want change. Polls indicate at least two-thirds of Americans are dissatisfied with the way things are going in the United States and at least one-third of Americans "worry a great deal" about drinking water pollution, surface water pollution, air pollution, species extinction, loss of tropical rain forests, and climate change.[667]

- Vision and experience can guide us. Many elders who are alive today created major change in the 1960s and 1970s. Elders can teach youngers about tactics and how to build on earlier achievements, and they can impart a broad intergenerational outlook. A large population of experienced elders, with available time and resources, stands at the ready.

- We live in an abundant universe. More energy than we could ever use avails itself to us from the sun. Nature provides plants, animals, and other natural resources, and it self-heals, restoring habitats and bringing species back from the brink of extinction when we stop our damaging behavior.

- Plenty of low-hanging fruit awaits easy picking, even in our everyday actions. For example, by wisely choosing the food we consume, we can propagate positive change throughout our world.

- Without denying the gravity of the challenges we face, we can still choose hope. A positive attitude may help our mental and physical health, and it is empowering, satisfying, and enjoyable.[668] Hope inspires positive actions and increases our chances of success.

> *For Westerners, getting onto a sustainable path could be like turning on a light that hasn't been turned on in a while.*

People profiting from the status quo want us to think it's hard to change things or change is not necessary. First they said there is no climate problem. Then they said there is a problem but it's not humans' fault. Now they say maybe there is a problem and humans may be partly responsible, but it will wreck the economy to solve it. They warn change will "cost jobs," "make our country less competitive," or "create a patchwork of regulations." Don't fall for this false logic. It will wreck the economy—and more—to *not* solve the problem. Such talk mimics our individual limiting beliefs, which tell us "it's too hard," or "it's too risky." Just as individuals evolve so as not to be ruled by their egos, our society can evolve so as not to be ruled by corporations. Furthermore, corporations can change. Corporations are comprised of individuals. When people in corporations evolve and think bigger, the corporations can evolve and think bigger. We by no means need to stay stuck in our current ways.

Not only big actions and choices, but also smaller ones can help us onto a sustainable path: What's for dinner? Do I shop for it at the supermarket or the food co-op? Do I buy a hybrid car, an average one, a truck, or a tank? We're all players.

Change, even for the better, can be scary or inconvenient at first, but we don't have to be uncomfortable for long. If you take a houseplant that has grown too large for its pot and transplant it to a larger pot so it can be healthier and grow well in the future, the roots are briefly exposed and disrupted during the transplanting process. But in no time, that plant is healthier in its new, larger, and more comfortable pot.

Sometimes efforts fail. But, as we've seen, *not* changing is becoming increasingly hard. All paths may be difficult now, so why not choose the one that's satisfying and helpful?

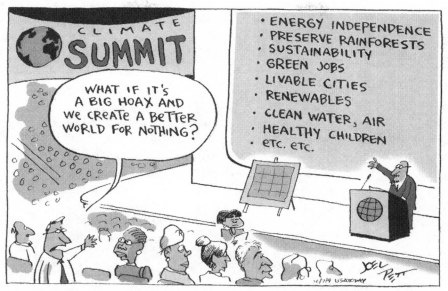

Used with permission. Joel Pett. http://www.kentucky.com/opinion/editorial-cartoons/joel-pett/.

THRIVING WHILE CREATING A SUSTAINABLE WORLD

Sustainability is about maximizing on a long-term basis—including the present!—our human, environmental, and economic health. Here are some ways we can thrive while creating a sustainable world:

- Adopt a lifestyle that enhances the health and well-being of ourselves, others, and the environment. Spend more time outdoors.

- Work in community with others. Celebrate wins, large and small. Inspire others to participate, thereby increasing momentum and energy. When more people share the work, it becomes easier.

- Make change-making as enjoyable as possible. Incorporate music, art, and food into rallies, marches, and other change-making gatherings.

- Take breaks from creating a sustainable world and do other things that give us pleasure to avoid burnout.

- Hold a vision of a beautiful, sustainable world and know absolutely that we can create it. Envision healthy, happy people and a planet teeming with plants and animals and blessed with clean air and water, a friendly climate, and thick, rich, intact soil. Choose positive thoughts: "I am excited to help out and protect the abundance we have. I'm grateful I live in a democracy where I have freedom and my opinions count. It will make me feel more alive to work to make things better."

- Use our gifts to advance what is truly important to us, out of a sense of purpose, responsibility, caring, and generosity. Knowing we're helping feels good.

My Experience Thriving, or Not, While Creating a Sustainable World. Much of the time I spent fighting the biomass industry did not feel enjoyable. But despite my outrage at injustice and the way the effort drained my time and energy, I experienced many enjoyable moments, especially when our side— consisting of concerned citizens, nonprofit organizations, elected officials, scientists, and physicians—achieved two victories. First, we brought to the Massachusetts State House enough citizen signatures to put a question on the ballot asking voters whether they wanted to subsidize bioenergy. Second, the state changed its regulations, cutting bioenergy subsidies in exchange for our not putting that question on the ballot.

I viewed this work, in community with others, satisfying and aligned with my values on a deep level. Fighting the biomass wars was a weird combination of extreme satisfaction and pain and irritation, but it made me feel alive. Our side enjoyed a lot of dinners and good times together (though, looking back, I wish we had celebrated small wins more).

Some people on our side suffered from burnout—they were not getting enough sleep, healthy food, and downtime. Witnessing this, I realized personal health and development are critical to success in creating a sustainable world, which requires purpose, commitment, strength, and stamina.

It's important to recognize that not all people are allowed to thrive while creating a sustainable world. Environmental advocates take huge risks and face violence in many parts of the world, and they are run ragged by the system elsewhere. The human rights watchdog group Global Witness reports that at least 908 environmental activists worldwide were murdered in retaliation for their work to protect wildlife and its habitats between 2002 and 2013.[669]

INDIGENOUS MOVEMENTS

Many indigenous people bravely fight against resource extraction by Westerners. Indigenous movements typically use nonviolent tactics: blockades, occupation of public spaces, and mass marches.

Indigenous peoples, knowing that "when you destroy the earth, you destroy yourself," go to lengths to protect nature in ways that strike many Westerners as extreme. Chief Phil Lane Jr. of the Ihanktowan Dakota and Chickasaw Nations describes how—despite desperate poverty, horrific living conditions, and 90 percent unemployment—Native Americans refused a $1 billion offer in exchange for allowing tar sands pipelines to go through their territories, insisting Mother Earth must be protected.[670]

Indigenous protests worldwide remind us that abuse of the environment also abuses people. As of this writing, more than one hundred Native American tribes are protesting the Dakota Access Pipeline project, making it the largest Native American mobilization in almost one hundred and fifty years. Indigenous people from as far away as the Amazon region travelled to North Dakota to support the protest. The pipeline threatens sacred lands and waters and would facilitate continued damage to the climate. The months-long protests show people of extremely limited means joining together to take strong action, using "boots on the ground" as well as social media to promote their cause.[671]

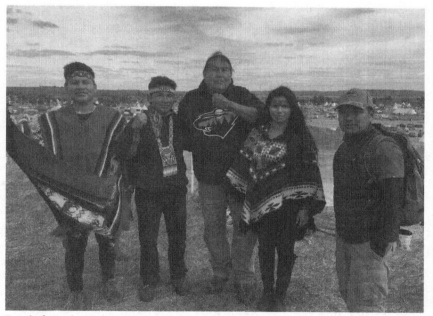

People from the Kichwa Nation in the Ecuadorian Amazon traveled by canoe, bus, and airplane to North Dakota to join in solidarity with the Standing Rock Sioux in protesting the Dakota Access Pipeline. For the past decade, the Kichwa visitors have been fighting efforts to drill for oil in their own community. Photo credit: ©Amazon Watch.

A network of indigenous movements is growing increasingly global, relevant and powerful. In 2005, Evo Morales was elected as Bolivia's first indigenous head of state. In 2010, he convened 30,000 international delegates for the World People's Conference on Climate Change and the Rights of Mother Earth. Anthropologist Maria Elena Garcia says that indigenous movements offer hope and "the importance of the imaginary. Of imagining a different world—imagining a different way of being in the world."[672] Indigenous people preserve and teach us humanity's ancient ways.

EMERGENCY RESPONSE

What do you do when the smoke alarm goes off due to a fire? You can fight the fire, or you can call in others to fight it, in an effort to save your family and home. Alternatively, you and your loved ones can seek protection, running away from the fire and letting it consume your home. Or you can pretend there is no fire, take the battery out of the smoke alarm, and carry on as usual, with potentially tragic results.

On a planetary level, we face similar choices now. We can seek protection—cocooning ourselves with water and air filters, information filters, gated communities, and so on. Or we can deny that a downward spiral is in process and go down in a fury of ecological unraveling, disease, and warfare. This latter option seems easiest—no action is necessary—but the outcome is the worst for all concerned. Or, we can take back our lives and our power and reverse the downward spiral. Kathleen Dean Moore says, "I think we have to find the time to be politically active. I don't want to cut anybody any slack on that. Are we going to let it all slip away—all those billions of years it took to evolve the song in a frog's throat or the stripe in a lily—because we're too busy?"[673]

Our future hinges on caring. Dr. Hyman writes, "The hardest part of being a doctor is helping people connect to why they want to heal…. What is it they treasure? What anchors them to life? Who and what is worth living for?"[674] This also applies to healing our world. If enough of us love enough and care enough—about ourselves, other people, and other species—we'll override inertia, distraction, and fear. We will take back control and heal our world.

And if we care enough, we'll persist despite inevitable resistance. Belgian Nobel laureate Maurice Maeterlinck wrote, "At every crossway on the road that leads to the future, each progressive spirit is opposed by a thousand men appointed to defend the past." Overcoming this opposition requires healthy, conscious, committed people who are willing to, in former First Lady Eleanor Roosevelt's words, "do the thing you think you cannot do."

There is a place for healthy outrage, outrage that drives us to take nonviolent actions. Outrage at injustice shows we're alive, paying attention, and caring. According to economist and lawyer William K. Black, "one of the major reasons we get intensifying crises, is we seem to have lost our capacity for outrage. And it's only people getting outraged that produces really positive social change."[675] Without outrage, we probably wouldn't have democracy, and white women and African Americans would still be the property of white men.

Stéphane Hessel writes, "It is high time that integrity, justice, and sustainable development be allowed to prevail." He adds, "What we need today … is for a segment of the population to rise up in protest. A minority is all we need, like yeast in a dough."[676]

According to social futurist Sara Robinson, a mass movement requires only about 15 percent of the population to be engaged and ready to take action. She points out that 15 percent of Americans participated in the American Revolution. Active Nazi Party members constituted only 15 percent of the population in prewar Germany! At 15 percent, almost everyone in the country knows someone in the group personally. And this is enough to win a few elections and put that 15 percent on the political map.[677] We'll never enlist everyone, but getting to 15 percent should be easier than ever now, thanks to telephones and the Internet.

We didn't get to 15 percent with the Occupy Wall Street movement.[678] Nevertheless, a 2011 poll found Americans overwhelmingly were aware of and supported the Occupy Wall Street protesters.[679] And Occupy Wall Street helped start a national conversation on income inequality, an issue all the 2016 presidential candidates then had to grapple with.

We can choose to obey our individual egos and our society's special interest groups. We can choose to indulge in limiting beliefs that warn us to stay within the confines of small, prescribed comfort zones. Or we can choose to override our egos and special interest groups, spending our time creating positive actions and bigger, more satisfying comfort zones.

According to a proverb, "If you want to go fast, go alone. If you want to go far, go together." Our climate emergency calls on us to go both fast and far, by taking action individually and collectively.

PROGRESS, NOW

We can build on actions people are already taking. They are considerable. The international climate agreement has been ratified.

Some people are pushing to get rid of "corporate personhood" and unlimited and secret campaign financing.[680] Others are fighting to require labeling of products containing GMOs. We're not there yet, but Martin Luther King Jr.'s dream of civil rights and racial equality for all *is* coming true—a black President, Barack Obama, led the United States for eight years. Special interests may be ravaging the environment, but citizens are fighting back. Democracy is spreading. Women's rights have advanced on some fronts, and birthrates may be starting to decrease.[681]

We can build on actions people are already taking. They are considerable.

At least eighty-one corporations signed President Obama's American Business Act on Climate pledge, indicating their support of efforts to address climate change. These corporations have wide potential impact. They operate in all fifty states, employ more than nine million people, and have more than $3 trillion in annual revenue.[682]

Many cities have pledged to convert to 100 percent clean energy, within varying time frames of up to thirty-five years. In the United States, they include Aspen, Colorado; San Diego, California; San Jose, California; and San Francisco, California. Outside the United States, they include Copenhagen, Denmark; Frankfurt and Munich, Germany; and the Isle of Wight, United Kingdom.[683] In "community rights" efforts in Pennsylvania, New Hampshire, Ohio, Colorado, Maine, and other locations in the United States, communities are passing laws asserting their authority for self-determination and to protect themselves from fracking, gravel extraction, water withdrawal, and other harmful projects.[684]

Many states and countries are acting on their own to promote sustainability. India plans to convert to 100 percent electric vehicles, charged without using fossil fuels, by 2030. Norway and the Netherlands have adopted similar goals.[685]

People around the world are restoring degraded lands and stopping desertification using simple reforestation and soil-conservation techniques. More farmers are integrating farming with preservation of forests and biodiversity.[686] In the Great Green Wall project in Africa, a mosaic of agricultural and tree-planting projects in "sustainable, climate-smart development" aims to eliminate poverty and halt and reverse the spread of the desert. People plant trees. Trees bring water—by creating clouds, slowing rainfall and runoff, helping soak water into the ground, and shading rivers and streams (thereby reducing evaporation). Water is the future in this arid environment.[687]

Bhutan—a small, isolated, Buddhist country between India and China—provides a successful example of sustainability.[688] Bhutan became a democracy in 2008, after the king gave up absolute rule at the end of a monarchy that had lasted more than one hundred years. The country preserves its forests in a network of national parks comprising 42 percent of the country's land area, and its constitution mandates that 60 percent of the country remain forested, indefinitely.[689] Low-impact hydropower from its abundant water resources provides most of Bhutan's energy as well as energy to neighboring countries, who can use it to offset millions of tons of carbon dioxide emissions.[690]

Bhutan embraces organic farming as a nationwide policy. Ecotourism policies limit the number of tourists.[691] Plastic bags and tobacco are banned, and one day a month all private vehicles are banned from Bhutan's roads.[692] The country places a high value on spirituality and gender equality.[693]

Bhutan offers free health care to its citizens and has invested in public health, including significantly improved access to safe drinking water and basic sanitation. The World Health Organization reports "a spectacular decrease in morbidity and mortality, with the average life expectancy increasing from 37 years in 1960 to over 68 years in 2012."[694]

Largely owing to its vast forests, abundant hydropower, sound land use, and modest energy consumption, Bhutan is one of only a handful of "carbon-negative" countries in the world. It absorbs three times more carbon than it emits—thereby helping rather than hurting the climate.[695]

The King of Bhutan determined in the 1970s that gross national product (later replaced by gross domestic product) inadequately measures progress because it leaves out a most important measure: happiness. Accordingly, Gross National Happiness was adopted as a metric of success, and it serves as the main guide for Bhutan's development and policies. Gross National Happiness has four pillars: good governance, equitable socioeconomic development, cultural preservation, and environmental conservation.[696]

Bhutan has a clean environment, strong culture, and modern technologies, including Internet access, cable TV, and cell phones.[697] Its economy, one of the smallest in the world, has grown consistently in recent years.[698] Its gross domestic product, a standard international measure of economic activity, does well even though Bhutan's main focus is on Gross National Happiness. Imagine a United States that preserved its forests and environment, used clean energy, grew food organically, practiced gender equality, and focused on Gross National Happiness, making decisions with the interests of citizens and the environment in mind.

FINDING FOCUS

We could exhaust ourselves trying to tackle, in single-issue efforts, everything that's wrong in our world. Fortunately, we don't have to. In 1970, groups that had been fighting various environmental issues—oil spills, polluting industrial facilities, raw sewage, toxic dumps, pesticides, wildlife extinction, and loss of wilderness—realized they shared common values. They got together and created Earth Day, which has evolved into an annual event that demonstrates and celebrates worldwide support for environmental protection.[699]

Everyone has a stake in climate change. Survival is a hard goal to argue against. Climate change provides the world with a common enemy— greenhouse gases—that the world can organize against, in unity. President Richard Nixon, no tree hugger but a savvy politician, believed focusing on the environment could heal deep divisions over the Vietnam War and civil rights. In his 1970 State of the Union address, he called on Americans to "make peace with nature and begin to make reparations for the damage we have done to our air, to our land, and to our water ... it has become a common cause of all the people in this country."

The health of the climate is foundational, just as basic as an individual's physical health. When the health of the individual or the climate is in trouble, getting well has to take priority. Al Gore wrote, "Modern industrial civilization, as presently organized, is colliding violently with our planet's ecological system.... As long as civilization as a whole, with its vast technological power, continues to follow a pattern of thinking that encourages the domination and exploitation of the natural world for short-term gains, this juggernaut will continue to devastate the earth no matter what any of us does. I have come to believe that we must take bold and unequivocal action: we must make the rescue of the environment the central organizing principle for civilization."[700] Similarly, E. O. Wilson wrote, "We need to think of our species as being in a race to save the living environment."[701]

Climate change reinforces our connection to nature. It forces us to acknowledge that nature runs the whole show and humans can't go their separate way. Pope Francis calls for "a spirit of generous care, full of tenderness" and "a loving awareness that we are not disconnected from the rest of creatures but joined in a splendid universal communion."[702]

Climate change is not the only problem we face on this planet, but it represents an "umbrella issue" that unifies and provides a framework for many other issues. For example, soil erosion impairs our ability to grow food, degrades water quality, *and* harms the climate. If we solve the problem of climate change, we will have solved many other problems, too.

US citizens in both major political parties view climate change as a critical problem and have called for action. For most of US history, environmental protection has not been a left-wing or right-wing issue. Corporate lawyer and fiscal conservative Frederic Rich said, "It breaks my heart to see that the conservative movement in America has really abandoned a century of tradition of support for conservation of the environment." Nevertheless, he is hopeful. Rich's prescriptions include reconnecting conservatives with conservation and reforming the green movement to change the perception that the green movement is against growth, business, capitalism, and people. He calls for the environmental movement to communicate messages of hope to inspire more people to participate. "People respond to a vision of hope," he observes.[703]

The climate situation requires immediate action. How much longer should we delay in the face of increasingly frequent and intense catastrophic events such as droughts, floods, hurricanes, tornadoes, tsunamis, wildfires, freezes, and heat waves? The creeping nature of climate change invites procrastination—unlike, say, a dropped bomb that creates sudden urgency.

Yet we don't have to change our entire way of life overnight. We can shift course gradually, through a series of steps. Consider this: if we phased out counterproductive subsidies and phased in beneficial subsidies by 10 percent per year for ten years, we would completely transform this system of economic incentives in just ten years, while avoiding sudden shocks.

Today, after the Great Recession, many Americans remain underutilized.[704] Globally, a shortfall of 1.8 billion good jobs creates societal stress and instability for a quarter of the world's population.[705] Here's an idea: why couldn't we put people to work with a massive green jobs program? Having more money to spend—on increasingly clean and green goods and services—they would contribute more tax revenue. Eliminating counterproductive subsidies and cleaning up the tax code could fund the effort. Other funding could be generated from cost savings on health and environmental damage control. We could simultaneously heal our environmental and health problems and boost the economy.

FIVE ACTIONS WILL SPUR THE MOVEMENT

Kathleen Dean Moore says, "Life is not something that we go through or that happens to us; it's something we create by our decisions."[706] We, you and I, decide what we want and then act on our decisions. One possible decision is to sit on the sidelines, let others make choices for us, and accept whatever consequences unfold. Another possibility is to resolve to do what it takes to create better lives for ourselves and others.

Just as exercise boosts an individual's mood and alleviates depression, taking action can boost our collective mood, alleviate our funk, and create momentum.[707] Collective actions at all levels—international, national, regional, state, and local—can augment individual actions such as those suggested in Chapter 7.

We can call on our governments to firmly commit to concrete actions and timetables to address climate change and related issues concerning biodiversity, rights of nature, indigenous rights, synthetic chemicals, agriculture, health, equality and human rights, corruption, trade and economics, security, and conflict resolution. We can adopt metrics such as Gross Domestic Happiness and Gross International Happiness.

Addressing climate change and creating a sustainable world will require five major actions: get money out of politics, green our way of life, green our economies, strengthen our democracies, and create social equality. Below are some specific ways we can go about it. We can each help advance one or more of these strategies, depending on our goals and preferences.

> *Creating a sustainable world will require five major actions: get money out of politics, green our way of life, green our economies, strengthen our democracies, and create social equality.*

Action 1: Get money out of politics.

- Reform campaign finance systems.
- Get rid of "corporate personhood."
- Slam shut the revolving door between government and industry.

Action 2. Green our way of life.

- Require proponents of technologies, products, and services to prove they are safe.
- Focus on resource conservation and efficiency, and upgrade our crumbling infrastructure.
- Stop the production of waste; ensure that outputs of one manufacturing process will be used as inputs to other processes.
- Designate plants, animals, and ecosystems as "persons" and codify rights of nature as law.
- Enforce laws and make new ones, as appropriate. Honor agreements, such as the global climate deal, and make new ones, if needed. Give laws and agreements effective enforcement mechanisms. Use satellite surveillance and other technology to protect the commons.
- Assign a person with authority and accountability, such as a Secretary of the Future in the President's cabinet, to lead efforts to develop and optimize long-term plans.
- Replace combustion-based energy with clean energy, deploying projects with care.

- Put carbon back into the ground by preserving, restoring, and expanding forests and using agricultural methods that regenerate soil and ecosystems.

- Preserve and expand other habitats—terrestrial, marine, and aquatic—and their plant and animal populations.

- Promote local, organic, and humane food production. Label all synthetic food ingredients.[708]

- Reduce meat consumption; educate the public about alternatives and the health and environmental impacts of meat consumption.

- Make contraception universally available.

- Provide infrastructure for safe, enjoyable, efficient, and green transportation, including walking, biking, and public transit.

- Phase out toxic chemicals while phasing in green chemistry.

Action 3. Green our economies.

- Eliminate perverse subsidies, such as those for combustion-based energy, industrial agriculture, and logging. Instead, use the money to promote green jobs and land protection.

- Eliminate other wasteful uses of taxpayers' money.

- Reform tax laws to remove loopholes and giveaways to the wealthy, and make sure corporations pay their fair share of taxes. End taxpayer-funded bailouts. Eliminate the ceiling on income subjected to Social Security taxes.[709]

- Impose meaningful fines and jail sentences for corporate executives who commit crimes.

- Prevent banks from becoming too large or treating the economy like a casino, betting with insured deposits.[710]

- Reject new international trade agreements that roll back environmental and worker protections, that put the interests of multinational corporations ahead of everything else, and that evade public scrutiny and participation. Rewrite old trade agreements.[711]

- Tax things we don't want, such as greenhouse gas emissions. Tax emissions not only from chimneys and pipes but also from agriculture, forestry, and other land use; credit carbon uptake by forests and farm fields.

- Charge the full costs associated with nonrecyclable wastes to those generating them.

- Count everything of value in our economic system, including items difficult to quantify, such as human lives and benefits derived from healthy ecosystems.

- Help indigenous peoples and others in developing countries survive sustainably—through ecotourism, ecosystem restoration work, payments for ecosystem benefits provided by their environments, and more.

- Subsidize research, development, and deployment of green technologies and practices.

Action 4. Strengthen our democracies.

- Foster democracy throughout the world. Democracy is foundational to everything else we want to accomplish.

- Strengthen international, national, and other institutions that can resolve conflicts and increase disarmament.

- Outlaw corrupt practices such as gerrymandering.

- Make it easier for people to vote.

- Protect citizens' privacy.

Action 5: Create social equality.

- Upgrade the status of women by providing them with education, family planning rights, voting rights, income equality, and legal protection.

- Institute and enforce equality for all on the basis of gender, race, ethnicity, and everything else, finally and forever—no more excuses.

- Improve and expand education for all children. In addition to a traditional curriculum, teach about democracy, human rights, equality, citizenship, self-empowerment, health, nature, environmental issues, food, gardening, finances, creativity, and the arts. Make education affordable and engaging, and give kids our best knowledge.

- Break up media conglomerates and restore diversity of viewpoints and opinions to the public's airwaves; expand public radio and television.

How to Engage

Change our way of life? That's a tall order. As Naomi Klein wrote, climate change "changes everything."[712] No one action is going to fix all that ails us—any more than one action could restore the health of a person with a long history of damaging habits. However, in both cases, consciousness, caring, and determination can begin the process.

Here are some easy steps you can take to participate in collective efforts to help create a sustainable world. (See also the individual efforts suggested in Chapter 7.)

- Make a "Priorities" list of a few things you really want. Make a "Preferences" list of a few things you really like to do. Make a "Why" list of reasons *why* creating a sustainable world is important to you.

- Select ways to contribute that align with your priorities, your preferences, and your whys. Focus on what *can* be done rather than on reasons why things "can't" be done. Join up with (or start) a group that is working on your priorities, and participate in ways you enjoy. Trust in your inherent value and intuition. Don't wait for permission, validation, or total confidence before stepping forward to take action. Know that we're all "stumbling forward," never "ready."

- Stay informed.

- Speak, write, and vote in a variety of venues to share your information, insights, opinions, and concerns—with friends, coworkers, neighbors, politicians, regulators, corporations, newspaper editors, and others. Demand that politicians and regulators take action. Tell municipal officials to green up municipal practices and facilities. Join marches, demonstrations, divestment efforts, and boycotts.

- Teach children about the natural world, environmental problems, and ways they can get involved.

- Serve on a committee in your town or city and advocate for sustainable solutions.

We can create an upward spiral by our actions. Tellus Institute President Paul Raskin says a culture of despair becomes "a self-fulfilling cause of the decline it foresees," but "a culture of hope, by inspiring collective engagement, can help realize the regenerative social transformation it embodies."[713] We can individually and collectively focus on our goals and our strengths, and resolve to be bigger than our problems.

Individuals, companies, governments, schools, nonprofit organizations, indigenous societies, and other groups are now leading the way toward a sustainable world. Success comes down to whether more individuals like you and me join in. We can act on our own, in groups, or both. Being a follower helps. Being a leader is even better.

Time is our scarcest resource. We absolutely can succeed if we accelerate the positive changes already underway, starting right now. What's more, you and I can thrive in the process.

NOTES

1. Meeker, Clare Hodgson. 2001. *I Could Not Keep Silent: The Life of Rachel Carson.* New York: McGraw-Hill Companies.

2. Chopak, Deepak. 2015. "Imagination, Imaginal Cells, and Evolutionary Leaps." *In the Rabbit Hole* .https://www.youtube.com/watch?v=6Ci59fWmc7g Jabr, Ferris. 2012. "How Does a Caterpillar Turn Into a Butterfly?" *Scientific American.* http://www.scientificamerican.com/article/caterpillar-butterfly-metamorphosis-explainer/; Lipton, Bruce. 2013. "Imaginal Cells in the Dying Caterpillar." https://www.youtube.com/watch?v=7DLokOQZlag.

3. *The New York Times.* 1964. "Rachel Carson Dies of Cancer; 'Silent Spring' Author Was 56." *The New York Times.* http://www.nytimes.com/learning/general/onthisday/bday/0527.html.

4. Smith, Kerri. 2009. "New Species Evolve in Bursts: Red Queen Hypothesis of Gradual Evolution Undermined." *Nature.* http://www.nature.com/news/2009/091209/full/news.2009.1134.html.

5. Ward, Peter D. and Donald Brownlee. 2002. *The Life and Death of Planet Earth: How the New Science of Astrobiology Charts the Ultimate Fate of our World.* New York: Macmillan.

6. BBC. 2016. "We Don't Know Which Species Should Be Classed as 'Human.'" http://www.bbc.com/earth/story/20160111-what-is-it-that-makes-you-a-human-and-not-something-else.

7. BBC. 2012. "History of Life on Earth." http://www.bbc.co.uk/nature/history_of_the_earth.

8. Leakey, Richard E. and Roger Lewin. 1995. *The Sixth Extinction: Patterns of Life and the Future of Mankind.* New York: Anchor Books.

9. D'Angelo, Chris. 2016. "In 20 Short Years, We've Wiped Out 10 Percent of Earth's Wilderness." *The Huffington Post.* http://www.huffingtonpost.com/entry/catastrophic-wilderness-loss-maps_us_57cde175e4b0e60d31dfccbf.

10. Jordan, David. 2008. *Apocalypse: Living Dangerously–Population and the Looming Disasters of the 21st Century.* Essex, UK: Chipmunk Publishing.

11. Harari, Yuval N. 2015. *Sapiens: A Brief History of Humankind.* New York: HarperCollins Publishers.

12. Diamond, Jared. 2005. *Collapse: How Societies Choose to Fail or Succeed.* New York: Viking Penguin.

13. Population Reference Bureau. Undated. "Human Population. Future Growth." Accessed October 6, 2016. http://www.prb.org/Publications/Lesson-Plans/HumanPopulation/FutureGrowth.aspx.

14. US Global Change Research Program. 2014. *National Climate Assessment.* http://nca2014.globalchange.gov/.

15. Blackadar, Clarke B. 2016. "Historical Review of the Causes of Cancer." *World Journal of Clinical Oncology 7*:1:54—86. http://www.ncbi.nlm.nih.gov/pmc/articles/PMC4734938/.

16. Williams, Jack. 2013. "U.S. Once Had Air Pollution to Match China's Today." *The Washington Post.* https://www.washingtonpost.com/news/capital-weather-gang/wp/2013/10/25/u-s-once-had-air-pollution-to-match-chinas-today/.

17. Carson, Rachel. 1962. *Silent Spring.* New York: Houghton Mifflin Co.; ATSDR. 2002. "Public Health Statement for DDT, DDE, and DDD." Atlanta: ATSDR. http://www.atsdr.cdc.gov/phs/phs.asp?id=79&tid=20.

18. Earth Day Network. 2016. "The History of Earth Day." www.earthday.org/about/the-history-of-earth-day.

19. Michigan Environmental Council. 2011. "When Our Rivers Caught Fire." *Michigan Environmental Report* http://www.environmentalcouncil.org/priorities/article.php?x=264.

20. USEPA. 2015. "TSCA Chemical Substance Inventory." https://www.epa.gov/tsca-inventory/about-tsca-chemical-substance-inventory.

21. Kollipara, Puneet. 2015. "The Bizarre Way the U.S. Regulates Chemicals—Letting Them on the Market First, Then Maybe Studying Them." *The Washington Post.* https://www.washingtonpost.com/news/energy-environment/wp/2015/03/19/our-broken-congresss-latest-effort-to-fix-our-broken-toxic-chemicals-law/.

22. ATSDR. 2009. "Health Consultation. Cornell Dubilier Electronics Incorporated, South Plainfield, Middlesex County, New Jersey." http://www.atsdr.cdc.gov/hac/pha/PHA.asp?docid=397&pg=1; USEPA. 2012. "Health Effects of PCBs." http://www.epa.gov/osw/hazard/tsd/pcbs/pubs/effects.htm.

23. Heintz, James and Robert Pollin. 2011. *The Economic Benefits of a Green Chemical Industry in the United States: Renewing Manufacturing Jobs While Protecting Health and the Environment.* Amherst, MA: University of Massachusetts. http://www.peri.umass.edu/publication/item/423-the-economic-benefits-of-a-green-chemical-industry-in-the-united-states-renewing-manufacturing-jobs-while-protecting-health-and-the-environment; Aguayo, Jose. 2015. "International Specialists Warn of Global Toll from Chemical Exposures." *Enviroblog.* http://www.ewg.org/enviroblog/2015/10/international-specialists-warn-global-toll-chemical-exposures; Grossman, Elizabeth. 2015. "Chemical Exposure Linked to Billions in Health Care Costs." *National Geographic.* http://news.nationalgeographic.com/news/2015/03/150305-chemicals-endocrine-disruptors-diabetes-toxic-environment-ngfood/; Vojdani, Aristo. 2014. "A Potential Link between Environmental Triggers and Autoimmunity." *Autoimmune Diseases.* http://www.hindawi.com/journals/ad/2014/437231/.

24. Brogan. Kelly. 2014. "Women's Health Issues and Toxicity." *The Detox Summit.* Interview by Deanna Minich. https://www.functionalmedicine.org/detoxsummit/.

25. Reinberg, Steven. 2014. "Worrisome Chemical May Lurk in Cash Register Receipts." *HealthDay.* http://www.cbsnews.com/news/bpa-chemical-in-plastics-cash-register-receipts/; Duke Medicine. 2012. "Plastics Linked to Severe Coronary Artery Disorder." *Duke Medicine Health News* 18:11:5.

26. Bilbrey, Jenna. 2014. "BPA-Free Plastic Containers May Be Just as Hazardous." *Scientific American.* https://www.scientificamerican.com/article/bpa-free-plastic-containers-may-be-just-as-hazardous/.

27. Deans, Bob and Robert Redford (preface by Sherwood Boehlert). 2012. *Reckless: The Political Assault on the American Environment.* Lanhan, MD: Rowman & Littlefield Publishers, Inc.

28. Public Affairs Television. 2012. "Encore: United States of ALEC." *Moyers & Company.* http://billmoyers.com/episode/encore-united-states-of-alec/.

29. Flynn, Dan. 2016. "Letter From the Editor: Mike Taylor Soon to Get Some Me-time." *Food Safety News.* http://www.foodsafetynews.com/2016/03/letter-from-the-editor-mike-taylor-soon-to-get-some-me-time/#.V0hCanb2aM8; Bittman, Mark. 2011. "Why Aren't G.M.O. Foods Labeled?" *The New York Times.* http://opinionator.blogs.nytimes.com/2011/02/15/why-arent-g-m-o-foods-labeled/?_r=0.

30. MacDonald, Christine C. 2008. *Green Inc.* Guilford, CT: The Globe Pequot Press.

31. Hiltzik, Michael. 2015. "Exposed: The Chemical Industry's Fake Grassroots Lobbying for Fire Retardants." *Los Angeles Times.* http://www.latimes.com/business/hiltzik/la-fi-mh-a-look-inside-the-chemical-industry-20150515-column.html.

32. Oreskes, Naomi and Erik M. Conway. 2011. *Merchants of Doubt: How a Handful of Scientists Obscured the Truth on Issues from Tobacco Smoke to Global Warming.* New York: Bloomsbury Press.

33. Women's International League for Peace and Freedom. Undated. "What Could Change if Corporate Personhood Were Abolished?" Accessed September 16, 2016. https://movetoamend.org/sites/default/files/MTA-WhatCouldChange_0.pdf.

34. Public Affairs Television. 2012. "On Winner-Take-All Politics." *Moyers & Company.* http://billmoyers.com/episode/on-winner-take-all-politics/; Smith, Hedrick. 2016. "Progress Report: Amend the Constitution." *Reclaim the American Dream.* http://reclaimtheamericandream.org/progress-amend/?utm_source=Individuals+-+Citizens+-+Audience+-+Donors&utm_campaign=f1921798c0-DC_Stuck_Individuals_EmailE-mail_6_2_2015&utm_medium=emaile-mail&utm_term=0_8cd20f7f75-f1921798c0-343584461.

35. Public Affairs Television. 2012. "David Stockman on Crony Capitalism." *Moyers & Company.* http://billmoyers.com/segment/david-stockman-on-crony-capitalism/.

36. Smith, Hedrick. 2016. "What Fires Anger in Grass Roots America?" *Reclaim the American Dream.* http://reclaimtheamericandream.org/2016/01/the-roots-of-anger/?utm_source=Individuals+-+Citizens+-+Audience+-+Donors&utm_campaign=5e00b71e6c-JohnsonControls_Individuals.1.29.16&utm_medium=email&utm_term=0_8cd20f7f75-5e00b71e6c-343584461.

37. Alperovitz, Gar. 2015. "Why Democratic Ownership Matters If We Care About Class." http://www.garalperovitz.com/2015/05/democratic-ownership-matters-care-class/.

38. Hacker, Jacob S. and Paul Pierson. 2010. *Winner-Take-All Politics*, New York: Simon & Schuster.

39. Public Affairs Television. 2012. "On Winner-Take-All Politics." *Moyers & Company.* http://billmoyers.com/episode/on-winner-take-all-politics/.

40. Public Affairs Television. 2012. "Inequality for All." *Moyers & Company.* http://billmoyers.com/episode/full-show-inequality-for-all/.

41. Federal Reserve Bank of St. Louis. 2016. "How Has Income Inequality Changed Over the Years?" https://www.stlouisfed.org/on-the-economy/2016/june/how-has-income-inequality-changed-years.

42. Public Affairs Television. 2012. "Inequality for All." *Moyers & Company.* http://billmoyers.com/episode/full-show-inequality-for-all/.

43. Smith, Hedrick. 2015. "Fixing Gerrymandering Could Fix Congress." *The Fayetteville Observer.* http://www.fayobserver.com/opinion/national_columns/hedrick-smith-fixing-gerrymandering-could-fix-congress/article_0ca87d79-0cc9-5965-bebd-97388603ba77.html.

44. WHO. 2016. "An Estimated 12.6 Million Deaths Each Year Are Attributable to Unhealthy Environments." http://www.who.int/mediacentre/news/releases/2016/deaths-attributable-to-unhealthy-environments/en/.

45. Hyman, Mark. 2010. "Is Being Healthy a Revolutionary Act?" http://drhyman.com/blog/2010/12/20/is-being-healthy-a-revolutionary-act/.

46. Prentice, Thomson. 2006. "Health, History and Hard Choices: Funding Dilemmas in a Fast-Changing World." Health and Philanthropy: Leveraging Change. University of Indiana. http://www.who.int/global_health_histories/seminars/presentation07.pdf.

47. Olshansky, S. J., Douglas J. Passaro, Ronald C. Hershow, Jennifer Layden, Bruce A. Carnes, Jacob Brody, Leonard Hayflick, Robert N. Butler, David B. Allison, and David S. Ludwig. 2005. "A Potential Decline in Life Expectancy in the United States in the 21st Century." *The New England Journal of Medicine* 352:1138—1145. http://www.nejm.org/doi/full/10.1056/NEJMsr043743#t=article.

48. Pappas, Stephanie. 2010. "A Third of 9-Month-Olds Already Obese or Overweight." *Live Science.* http://www.livescience.com/10367-9-month-olds-obese-overweight.html.

49. Centers for Medicare & Medicaid Services. 2014. "National Health Expenditure Data." https://www.cms.gov/Research-Statistics-Data-and-Systems/Statistics-Trends-and-Reports/NationalHealthExpendData/index.html?redirect=/nationalhealthexpenddata/02_nationalhealthaccountshistorical.asp.

50. Hyman, Mark. 2012. "New Cure for Chronic Disease Discovered." http://drhyman.com/new-cure-for-chronic-disease-discovered-8270/.

51. Porter, Eduardo. 2014. "Acceleration Is Forecast for Spending on Health." *The New York Times.* http://www.nytimes.com/2014/04/23/business/economy/forecasting-the-scale-of-health-spendings-climb.html?_r=0.

52. Bakalar, Nicholas. 2016. "Medical Errors May Cause Over 250,000 Deaths a Year." *The New York Times.* http://well.blogs.nytimes.com/2016/05/03/medical-errors-may-cause-over-250000-deaths-a-year/?_r=0.

53. PRI. 2010. "The Legacy of David Suzuki." *Living on Earth.* http://www.loe.org/shows/segments.html?programID=10-P13-00051&segmentID=6.

54. NASA. 2016. "A Blanket Around the Earth." http://climate.nasa.gov/causes/; USEPA. 2016. "Causes of Climate Change." https://www3.epa.gov/climatechange/science/causes.html.

55. Doyle, Alister. 2016. "Carbon Emissions Highest They Have Been in 66 Million Years." *Scientific American.* http://www.scientificamerican.com/article/carbon-emissions-highest-they-have-been-in-66-million-years/.

56. Hyman, Mark. 2009. *The UltraMind Solution.* New York: Scribner.

57. Chesler, Caren. 2016. "The Green Roller Coaster." *Slate.* http://www.slate.com/articles/technology/future_tense/2016/06/going_solar_isn_t_green_if_you_cut_down_tons_of_trees.html; Schultz, Matthias. 2013. "Mutiny in the Land of Wind Turbines." *Spiegel Online.* http://www.spiegel.de/international/germany/wind-energy-encounters-problems-and-resistance-in-germany-a-910816.html.

58. ASM International and Arthur C. Reardon. 2011. *Metallurgy for the Non-Metallurgist.* Second edition. Materials Park, OH: ASM International. http://www.google.com/url?sa=t&rct=j&q=&esrc=s&source=web&cd=11&cad=rja&uact=8&ved=0ahUKEwjWl5DrmJHPAhVFOj4KHf-JAZk4ChAWCBswAA&url=http%3A%2F%2Fwww.asminternational.org%2Fdocuments%2F10192%2F3212401%2F05306G_Sample_BuyNow.pdf%2Fab60c086-2c71-4de0-91f6-aad1112cf4dc&usg=AFQjCNF7GA8GyBOLEDyxN9_V_A0hBssw1g.

59. OPB. 2013. "New OPB Documentary Explores History of the Hanford Nuclear Site." http://www.opb.org/pressroom/pressrelease/new-opb-documentary-explores-history-of-hanford-nuclear-site/.

60. World Nuclear Association. 2016. "US Nuclear Power Policy." http://www.world-nuclear.org/information-library/country-profiles/countries-t-z/usa-nuclear-power-policy.aspx.

61. ATSDR. 2004. "Public Health Statement for Strontium." https://www.atsdr.cdc.gov/phs/phs. asp?id=654&tid=120; Schell, Jonathan. 2004. *The Jonathan Schell Reader: On the United States at War, the Long Crisis of the American Republic, and the Fate of the Earth.* New York: Nation Books.

62. Dean, Cornelia. 2009. "Mercury Found in Every Fish Tested, Scientists Say." *The New York Times.* http://www.nytimes.com/2009/08/20/science/earth/20brfs-MERCURYFOUND_BRF. html?_r=3&em.

63. Hyman, Mark. 2009. *The UltraMind Solution.* New York: Scribner.

64. Cone, Maria. 2012. "Is Cadmium as Dangerous for Children as Lead?" *Scientific American.* http://www.scientificamerican.com/article/is-cadmium-as-dangerous-for-children-lead/.

65. Powell, Alvin. 2014. "How Earth Was Watered." *Harvard Gazette.* http://news.harvard.edu/gazette/story/2014/02/how-earth-was-watered/.

66. Fishman, Charles. 2011. *The Big Thirst: The Secret Life and Turbulent Future of Water.* New York: Simon & Schuster, Inc.

67. The Editorial Board. 2015. "Watering California's Farms." *The New York Times.* http://www.nytimes.com/2015/04/05/opinion/sunday/watering-californias-farms.html?_r=1.

68. NASA. 2015. "Study: Third of Big Groundwater Basins in Distress." http://www.jpl.nasa.gov/news/news.php?feature=4626.

69. Brown, Lester R. 2011. *World on the Edge: How to Prevent Environmental and Economic Collapse.* New York: W.W. Norton & Company.

70. Dahl, Thomas E. and Gregory J. Allord. 1997. "Technical Aspects of Wetlands: History of Wetlands in the Conterminous United States." http://water.usgs.gov/nwsum/WSP2425/history.html.

71. Wearden, Graeme. 2016. "More Plastic Than Fish in the Sea By 2050, Says Ellen MacArthur." *The Guardian.* https://www.theguardian.com/business/2016/jan/19/more-plastic-than-fish-in-the-sea-by-2050-warns-ellen-macarthur.

72. Creeklife. Undated. "The Famous Flaming River of Cleveland—The Beautiful Cuyahoga!" Accessed September 15, 2016. https://creeklife.com/blog/cuyahoga-river-on-fire.

73. USEPA. 2016. "Hudson River Cleanup." https://www3.epa.gov/hudson/cleanup.html.

74. Fishman, Charles. 2011. *The Big Thirst: The Secret Life and Turbulent Future of Water.* New York: Simon & Schuster, Inc.; US Energy Information Administration. 2011. "Over Half the Cooling Systems at U.S. Electric Power Plants Reuse Water." *Today in Energy.* http://www.eia.gov/todayinenergy/detail.php?id=3950; Kenny, Joan F., Nancy L. Barber, Susan S. Hutson, Kristin S. Linsey, John K. Lovelace, and Molly A. Maupin. 2013. "Estimated Use of Water in the United States in 2005." *USGS Circular 1344.* http://pubs.usgs.gov/circ/1344/.

75. Fishman, Charles. 2011. *The Big Thirst: The Secret Life and Turbulent Future of Water.* New York: Simon & Schuster, Inc.

76. Environmental Working Group. 2005. "Body Burden: The Pollution of Newborns." http://www.ewg.org/research/body-burden-pollution-newborns.

77. Diamond, Jared. 2005. *Collapse: How Societies Choose to Fail or Succeed.* New York: Viking Penguin.

78. Miller, Daphne. 2013. "The Surprising Healing Qualities ... of Dirt." *Yes! Magazine.* http://www.yesmagazine.org/issues/how-to-eat-like-our-lives-depend-on-it/how-dirt-heals-us.

79. Hyman, Mark. 2009. *The UltraMind Solution.* New York: Scribner.

80. WWF-UK. 1999. *Chemical Trespass: A Toxic Legacy.*

81. Thirteen. 2013. "What Plants Talk About." *Nature.* http://www.pbs.org/wnet/nature/what-plants-talk-about-introduction/8228/; Wohlleben, Peter. 2016. *The Hidden Life of Trees: What They Feel, How They Communicate—Discoveries From a Secret World.* Vancouver, BC: Greystone Books.

82. Onti, T.A. and L.A. Schulte. 2012. "Soil Carbon Storage." *Nature Education Knowledge* 3:10:35. http://www.nature.com/scitable/knowledge/library/soil-carbon-storage-84223790.

83. Suzuki, David. 2012. *Everything Under the Sun: Toward a Brighter Future on a Small Blue Planet.* Vancouver, BC: Greystone Books.

84. NRDC. 2016. "Save the Forests or the Trees?" https://www.nrdc.org/onearth/save-forests-or-trees; FAO. 2006. "Deforestation Causes Global Warming." http://www.fao.org/newsroom/en/news/2006/1000385/index.html.

85. Executive Office of the President. 2013. "The President's Climate Action Plan." https://www.whitehouse.gov/sites/default/files/image/president27sclimateactionplan.pdf.

86. Nunery, Jared S. and William S. Keeton. 2010. "Forest Carbon Storage in the Northeastern United States: Net Effects of Harvesting Frequency, Post-Harvest Retention, and Wood Products." *Forest Ecology and Management* 29:1363-1375. http://www.uvm.edu/giee/pubpdfs/Nunery_2010_Forest_Ecology_and_Management.pdf; Sebastiaan Luyssaert, E. Detlef Schulze, Annett Börner, Alexander Knohl, Dominik Hessenmöller, Beverly E. Law, Phillippe Ciais, and John Grace. 2008. "Old-Growth Forests as Global Carbon Sinks." *Nature* 455:7210:213-5. http://www.nature.com/nature/journal/v455/n7210/abs/nature07276.html; Keeton, William S., Andrew A. Whitman, Gregory C. McGee, and Christine L. Goodale. 2011. "Late-Successional Biomass Development in Northern Hardwood-Conifer Forests of the Northeastern United States." *Forest Science* 57:6. https://www.uvm.edu/giee/pubpdfs/Keeton_2011_Forest_Science.pdf.

87. Moyer, Ellen. 2012. "The Power of Ordinary Citizens: Using Science to Stop Logging." *The Huffington Post.* http://www.huffingtonpost.com/ellen-moyer-phd/science-to-stop-logging_b_1799800.html. Maloof, Joan. 2016. *Nature's Temples: The Complex World of Old-Growth Forests.* Portland, OR: Timber Press; Foster, David R. and David A. Orwig. 2006. "Preemptive and Salvage Harvesting of New England Forests: When Doing Nothing Is a Viable Alternative." *Conservation Biology* 20:4:959—970.

88. Maloof, Joan. 2016. *Nature's Temples: The Complex World of Old-Growth Forests.* Portland, OR: Timber Press; Foster, David R. and David A. Orwig. 2006. "Preemptive and Salvage Harvesting of New England Forests: When Doing Nothing Is a Viable Alternative." *Conservation Biology* 20:4:959—970. http://harvardforest.fas.harvard.edu/publications/pdfs/Foster_ConservationBio_2006.pdf.

89. Crowther, T.W., H.B. Glick, K.R. Covey, C. Bettigole, D.S. Maynard, S.M. Thomas, J.R. Smith, G. Hintler, M.C. Duguid, G. Amatulli, M.-N. Tuanmu, W. Jetz, C. Salas, C. Stam, D. Piotto, R. Tavani, S. Green, G. Bruce, S.J. Williams, S.K. Wiser, M.O. Huber, G.M. Hengeveld, G.-J. Nabuurs, E. Tikhonova, P. Borchardt, C.-F. Li, L.W. Powrie, M. Fischer, A. Hemp, J. Homeier, P. Cho, A.C. Vibrans, P.M. Umunay, S.L. Piao, C.W. Rowe, M.S. Ashton, P.R. Crane, and M.A. Bradford. 2015. "Mapping Tree Density at a Global Scale." *Nature* 525:201-205. https://www.researchgate.net/publication/281532511_Mapping_tree_density_at_a_global_scale; Rowling, Megan. 2015. "How to Stop Deforestation? Make 'Good Stuff' Cheaper." *Reuters.* http://www.reuters.com/article/us-development-goals-forests-idUSKCN0RU0NF20150930.

90. The Huffington Post Canada. 2014. "Canada Largest Contributor to Deforestation Worldwide: Study." *The Huffington Post.* http://www.huffingtonpost.ca/2014/09/05/canada-deforestation-worst-in-world_n_5773142.html.

91. Carbon Trade Watch. 2013. "Protecting Carbon to Destroy Forests: Land Enclosures and REDD+." http://www.carbontradewatch.org/articles/protecting-carbon-to-destroy-forests-land-enclosures-and-redd.html.

92. Buchmann, Stepohen L. 2015. "Our Vanishing Flowers." *The New York Times*. http://www.nytimes.com/2015/10/17/opinion/our-vanishing-flowers.html.

93. Fuhrman, Joel. 2011. *3 Steps to Incredible Health, Volume 1*. Flemington, NJ: Gift of Health Press.

94. WGBH. 2001. "Roundtable: A Modern Mass Extinction?" http://www.pbs.org/wgbh/evolution/extinction/massext/.

95. Lamb, Eric. 2011. "Earth at a Glance." http://ecology.com/features/earthataglance/youarehere.html.

96. WWF. 2014. "Half of Global Wildlife Lost, Says New WWR Report." https://www.worldwildlife.org/press-releases/half-of-global-wildlife-lost-says-new-wwf-report.

97. Holldobler, Bert and Edward O. Wilson. 1990. *The Ants*. Cambridge, MA: Harvard University Press.

98. Conant, Eve. 2014. "As Dwindling Monarch Butterflies Make Their Migration, Feds Try to Save Them." *National Geographic*. http://news.nationalgeographic.com/news/2014/10/141010-monarch-butterfly-migration-threatened-plan/#close.

99. Sloan, Jacob. 2010. "Scientists Say Dolphins Should Be Considered 'Persons.'" http://disinfo.com/2010/01/scientists-say-dolphins-should-be-considered-persons/.

100. Brady, Diane and Christopher Palmeri. 2007. "The Pet Economy: Americans Spend an Astonishing $41 Billion a Year on Their Furry Friends." *Bloomberg*. http://www.bloomberg.com/news/articles/2007-08-05/the-pet-economy.

101. NASA and NOAA. 2016. "How Did Earth's Atmosphere Form?" http://scijinks.jpl.nasa.gov/atmosphere-formation/.

102. Biello, David. 2009. "The Origin of Oxygen in Earth's Atmosphere." *Scientific American*. http://www.scientificamerican.com/article.cfm?id=origin-of-oxygen-in-atmosphere.

103. Von Hippel, Frank N. 2011. "It Could Happen Here." *The New York Times*. http://www.nytimes.com/2011/03/24/opinion/24Von-Hippel.html?pagewanted=all.

104. ScienceDaily. 2016. "For the First Time, Air Pollution Emerges as a Leading Risk Factor for Stroke Worldwide." *ScienceDaily*. https://www.sciencedaily.com/releases/2016/06/160609222226.htm.

105. US Global Change Research Program. 2014. *National Climate Assessment*. http://nca2014.globalchange.gov/.

106. WHO. 2016. "Climate Change and Health." http://www.who.int/mediacentre/factsheets/fs266/en/.

107. Jamail, Dahr. 2016. "Global Climate Change: Agriculture on the Brink." *Truthout*. http://www.truth-out.org/news/item/35468-agriculture-on-the-brink.

108. Despommier, Dickson D. 2009. "A Farm on Every Floor." *The New York Times*. http://www.nytimes.com/2009/08/24/opinion/24Despommier.html.

109. Dennis, Brady and Chris Mooney. 2016. "Scientists Nearly Double Sea Level Rise Projections for 2100, Because of Antarctica." *The Washington Post*. https://www.washingtonpost.com/news/energy-environment/wp/2016/03/30/antarctic-loss-could-double-expected-sea-level-rise-by-2100-scientis ew Geography*. New York: Nation Books.

110. Parenti, Christian. 2011. *Tropic of Chaos: Climate Change and the New Geography*. New York: Nation Books.

111. NASA. 2016. "Global Fire Maps." https://lance.modaps.eosdis.nasa.gov/firemaps/; NASA. Undated. "Global Fire Monitoring." Accessed September 16, 2016. http://earthobservatory.nasa.gov/Features/GlobalFire/fire.php.

112. Grabmeier, Jeff. 2011. "Air Pollution Linked to Learning and Memory Problems, Depression." *Research News*. http://researchnews.osu.edu/archive/pollutionbrain.htm.

113. Hyman, Mark. 2009. *The UltraMind Solution*. New York: Scribner.

114. WHO. 2016. "Tobacco." http://www.who.int/mediacentre/factsheets/fs339/en/index.html.

115. Bomey, Nathan. 2015. "Thousands of Farmers Stopped Growing Tobacco After Deregulation Payouts." *USAToday.* http://www.usatoday.com/story/money/2015/09/02/thousands-farmers-stopped-growing-tobacco-after-deregulation-payouts/32115163/.

116. Lovelock, James E. and Lynn Margulis. 1974. "Atmospheric Homeostasis By and For the Biosphere: The Gaia Hypothesis." *Tellus.* http://tellusa.net/index.php/tellusa/article/view/9731.

117. National Humanities Center. 2006. "Enslaved Peoples." http://nationalhumanitiescenter.org/pds/amerbegin/settlement/text6/text6read.htm.

118. PBS. 2009. "Slaves Built the White House, U.S. Capitol." *PBS NewsHour Extra.* http://www.pbs.org/newshour/extra/daily_videos/slaves-built-the-white-house-u-s-capitol/.

119. Moore, Michael. 2007. *Sicko.* Dog Eat Dog Films, NY. https://freedocumentaries.org/documentary/sicko.

120. Guardian Readers and James Walsh. 2014. "10 of the Best Tony Benn Quotes—As Picked By Our Readers." *The Guardian.* http://www.theguardian.com/politics/2014/mar/15/10-of-the-best-tony-benn-quotes-as-picked-by-our-readers.

121. Gladstone, Rick. 2016. "Modern Slavery Estimated to Trap 45 Million People Worldwide." *The New York Times.* http://www.nytimes.com/2016/06/01/world/asia/global-slavery-index.html; Federer, Bill. 2016. "More Slaves Today Than At Any Time in History." *WND.* http://www.wnd.com/2016/02/more-slaves-today-than-at-any-time-in-history/.

122. Bangs, Richard. 2008. *New Zealand: Quest for Kaitiakitanga.* http://www.smarttravels.tv/AdventuresWithPurpose/site/shows_newzealand.html.

123. Suzuki, David. Undated. "The Declaration of Interdependence: A Pledge to Planet Earth." Accessed September 16, 2016. http://www.davidsuzuki.org/about/declaration/.

124. Survival International. 2000. *Disinherited Indians in Brazil.* London: Survival International. http://assets.survivalinternational.org/static/files/books/Disinherited.pdf.

125. Berkman, Michael and Eric Plutzer. 2010. *Evolution, Creationism, and the Battle to Control American Classrooms.* New York: Cambridge University Press. http://www.amazon.com/Evolution-Creationism-Control-Americas-Classrooms/dp/0521148863.

126. The World Bank. 2013. "Montreal Protocol." http://www.worldbank.org/en/topic/climatechange/brief/montreal-protocol.

127. McTaggart, Lynne. 2008. *The Field: The Quest for the Secret Force of the Universe.* New York: HarperCollins Publishers.

128. Hill, Napoleon. 2011. *Outwitting the Devil: The Secret to Freedom and Success.* New York: Sterling Publishing Co., Inc.

129. Cooper, Mark N. (Editor). 2007. "The Case Against Media Consolidation: Evidence on Concentration, Localism and Diversity." *McGannon Center Research Resources. Paper 1.* New York: Fordham University. http://fordham.bepress.com/mcgannon_research/1/?utm_source=fordham.bepress.com%2Fmcgannon_research%2F1&utm_medium=PDF&utm_campaign=PDFCoverPages.

130. Burgess, George H. 2015. "It's Time to Save Sharks, Not Destroy Them." *Fox News.* http://www.foxnews.com/opinion/2015/07/10/it-s-time-to-save-sharks-not-destroy-them.html.

131. Lipton, Bruce and Steve Bhaerman. 2010. *Spontaneous Evolution: Our Positive Future and a Way to Get There from Here.* Carlsbad, CA: Hay House, Inc.

132. National Institutes of Health. 2012. "NIH Human Microbiome Project Defines Normal Bacterial Makeup of the Body." https://www.nih.gov/news-events/news-releases/nih-human-microbiome-project-defines-normal-bacterial-makeup-body.

133. Perlmutter, David. 2015. *Brain Maker: The Power of Gut Microbes to Heal and Protect Your Brain—For Life.* New York: Little, Brown and Company.

134. Wilson, Kenneth. 2012. "Inflammatory Bowel Diseases: Advances in Treatment, Causes." *Duke Medicine Health News* 18:2:4-5.

135. Conley, Mikaela. 2011. "Overuse of Antibiotics May Cause Long-Term Harm." *ABC News.* http://abcnews.go.com/Health/antibiotics-bad-good-bacteria/story?id=14374547.

136. Gates, Donna. 2014. "Candida Cures." *The Natural Cures Movement.* Interview by Josh Axe, October 7, 2014.

137. O'Bryan, Tom. 2014. "Non-Celiac Gluten Intolerance and Toxicity." *The Detox Summit.* Interview by Deanna Minich, August 4-8, 2014.

138. Wade, Nicholas. 2005. "Your Body is Younger Than You Think." *The New York Times.* http://www.nytimes.com/2005/08/02/science/02cell.html?pagewanted=all&_r=0.

139. Weil, Andrew. 2011. *Spontaneous Happiness: A New Path to Emotional Well-Being.* New York: Little, Brown and Company.

140. National Public Radio. 2008. "Goodall Reflects on a Lifetime of Chimp Research." *Talk of the Nation.* http://www.npr.org/templates/story/story.php?storyId=97007902; Hollins University. 2015. "Jane Goodall Tells a Hollins Audience Why She Still Has Hope for Our Planet." https://www.hollins.edu/news/jane-goodall-tells-a-hollins-audience-why-she-still-has-hope-for-our-planet/.

141. Weil, Andrew. 2011. *Spontaneous Happiness: A New Path to Emotional Well-Being.* New York: Little, Brown and Company.

142. NIH National Human Genome Research Institute. 2016. "Frequently Asked Questions About Genetic and Genomic Science." http://www.genome.gov/19016904.

143. Popenoe, David. 1998. *Disturbing the Nest: Family Change and Decline in Modern Societies.* Piscataway, NJ: Aldine Transaction.

144. Social Security Administration. Undated. "Life Expectancy for Social Security." Accessed September 17, 2016. https://www.ssa.gov/history/lifeexpect.html; Pew Research Center. 2010. "Baby Boomers Retire." http://www.pewresearch.org/daily-number/baby-boomers-retire/.

145. NHS-UK. 2015. "Loneliness in Older People." http://www.nhs.uk/livewell/women60-plus/pages/loneliness-in-older-people.aspx; Hernandez, Carmen R. and Marta Z. Gonzelez. 2008. "Effects of Intergenerational Interaction on Aging." *Educational Gerontology* 34:292—305. https://keycenter.unca.edu/sites/default/files/Depression_among_Older_Citizens_Lessens.pdf.

146. BBC News. 2013. "Is Modern Life Making Us Lonely?"http://www.bbc.com/news/magazine-22012957.

147. Gallagher, Shaun. 2014. "The Cruel and Unusual Phenomenology of Solitary Confinement." *National Center for Biotechnology Information.* http://www.ncbi.nlm.nih.gov/pmc/articles/PMC4054665/.

148. Weil, Andrew. 2011. *Spontaneous Happiness: A New Path to Emotional Well-Being.* New York: Little, Brown and Company.

149. Public Affairs Television. 2013. "Sherry Turkle on Being Alone Together." *Moyers & Company.* http://billmoyers.com/segment/sherry-turkle-on-being-alone-together/.

150. BBC. 2009. "Depression Looms as Global Crisis." *BBC News.* http://news.bbc.co.uk/2/hi/health/8230549.stm.

151. Weil, Andrew. 2011. *Spontaneous Happiness: A New Path to Emotional Well-Being.* New York: Little, Brown and Company.

152. Amen, Daniel. 2013. *Unleash the Power of the Female Brain: Supercharging Yours for Better Health, Energy, Mood, Focus, and Sex.* New York: Harmony Books.

153. Hubbard, Barbara Marx. 1995. *The Revelation: A Message of Hope for the New Millennium.* Mill Valley, CA: Nataraj Publishing.

154. Mead, Margaret. 1935. *Sex and Temperament in Three Primitive Societies.* New York: William Morrow and Company.

155. Garrison, Laura T. 2012. "6 Modern Societies Where Women Literally Rule." *Mental Floss.* http://mentalfloss.com/article/31274/6-modern-societies-where-women-literally-rule.

156. Clinton, Hillary. 1995. "Hillary Rodham Clinton Remarks to the U.N. 4th World Conference on Women Plenary Session." http://www.americanrhetoric.com/speeches/hillaryclintonbeijingspeech.htm.

157. One Billion Rising. 2016. "What is One Billion Rising?" http://www.onebillionrising.org/about/campaign/one-billion-rising/.

158. Izadi, Elahe. 2014. "Nearly a Third of U.S. Women Have Experienced Domestic Violence." *The Washington Post.* https://www.washingtonpost.com/news/post-nation/wp/2014/09/08/nearly-a-third-of-u-s-women-have-experienced-domestic-violence?utm_term=.a78391148b0b.

159. Amin, Mohammad. 2009. "Do Banks Discriminate Against Women Entrepreneurs?" *The World Bank.* http://blogs.worldbank.org/psd/do-banks-discriminate-against-women-entrepreneurs.

160. Karp, Gregory. 2015. "Women Far Less Likely to be Approved for Mortgage in Chicago Area." *Chicago Tribune.* http://www.chicagotribune.com/business/ct-mortgage-lending-gender-0617-biz-20150616-story.html.

161. Ng, Christina. 2011. "JCPenney's 'Too Pretty to Do Homework' Shirt Pulled." *ABC News.* http://abcnews.go.com/blogs/headlines/2011/08/jcpenneys-too-pretty-to-do-homework-shirt-pulled/.

162. Steinem, Gloria. 2014. "Our Revolution Has Just Begun." *Ms. Magazine.* Winter/Spring 2014.

163. Kort, Michele. 2014. "Dr. Kenneth C. Edelin, 1939-2013." *Ms. Magazine.* Winter/Spring 2014.

164. Public Affairs Television. 2013. "Jessica González-Rojas and Lynn Paltrow on Abortion Rights Activism." *Moyers & Company.* http://billmoyers.com/segment/jessica-gonzalez-rojas-and-lynn-paltrow-on-abortion-rights-activism/.

165. Public Affairs Television. 2013. "Q&A: Going to Bed Hungry." http://billmoyers.com/2013/04/05/going-to-bed-hungry/.

166. CDC. 2015. "Suicide." http://www.cdc.gov/violenceprevention/pdf/suicide-datasheet-a.PDF.

167. Diamond, Jared. 2012. *The World Until Yesterday: What Can We Learn from Traditional Societies?* New York: The Penguin Group.

168. Perry, William J. 2015. *My Journey at the Nuclear Brink.* Stanford, CA: Stanford University Press.

169. Slavo, Mac. 2012. "Democide: Government Killed Over 260 Million in the 20th Century, Poised to Kill Billions More in the 21st." http://www.infowars.com/democide-government-killed-over-260-million-in-the-20th-century-poised-to-kill-billions-more-in-the-21st/.

170. Lucas, James A. 2015. "US Has Killed More Than 20 Million People in 37 Nations Since WWII." *Popular Resistance.* https://www.popularresistance.org/us-has-killed-more-than-20-million-in-37-nations-since-wwii/.

171. Bilmes, Linda J. 2013. "The Financial Legacy of Iraq and Afghanistan: How Wartime Spending Decisions Will Constrain Future National Security Budgets." *Harvard Kennedy School Faculty Research Working Paper Series RWP113-006.* https://research.hks.harvard.edu/publications/workingpapers/citation.aspx?PubId=8956.

172. Public Affairs Television. 2013. "Q&A: Blinding Us From Science." *Moyers & Company.* http://billmoyers.com/2013/05/18/blinding-us-from-science/; Public Affairs Television. 2013. "David Rosner and Gerald Markowitz on Toxic Disinformation." *Moyers & Company.* http://billmoyers.com/segment/david-rosner-and-gerald-markowitz-on-toxic-disinformation/.

173. National Geographic Society. 2013. "Genes Are Us. And Them." http://ngm.nationalgeographic.com/2013/07/125-explore/shared-genes.

174. PRI. 2013. "Tapir Scientist." *Living on Earth.* http://loe.org/shows/segments.html?programID=13-P13-00037&segmentID=5.

175. Kellert, Stephen R. 2012. *Birthright: People and Nature in the Modern World.* New Haven, CT: Yale University Press.

176. University of Cambridge. 2015. "World's Protected Natural Areas Receive Eight Billion Visits a Year." http://www.cam.ac.uk/research/news/worlds-protected-natural-areas-receive-eight-billion-visits-a-year.

177. Hetter, Katia. 2014. "Millions Flocked to National Parks Last Year, Despite Shutdown." *CNN.* http://www.cnn.com/2014/03/07/travel/national-parks-sites-most-visited-shutdown-impact-2013/.

178. Munandi, Aries. 2013. "Bird Watching is Growing in Popularity." *World of Birds.* http://newsofbird.com/2013/04/29/bird-watching-is-growing-in-popularity/.

179. US Fish & Wildlife Service. Undated. "For the Birds." Accessed September 17, 2016. http://publications.usa.gov/epublications/forbirds/forbird.htm; Sterba, James P. 2002. "American Backyard Feeders May Do Harm to Wild Birds." *The Wall Street Journal.* http://www.wsj.com/articles/SB104095070771926393.

180. PRI. 2016. "Beyond the Headlines." *Living on Earth.* http://loe.org/shows/shows.html?programID=16-P13-00024#feature2.

181. McTaggart, Lynne. 2008. *The Field: The Quest for the Secret Force of the Universe.* New York: HarperCollins Publishers; McTaggart, Lynne. 2011. *The Bond: Connecting Through the Space Between Us.* New York: Simon & Schuster, Inc.

182. McTaggart, Lynne. 2014. "Next Level Mind/Body Medicine: Interpersonal Connection." *The Evolution of Medicine Summit.* Interview by James Maskell, September 11, 2014.

183. Einstein, Albert. Undated. "Quotable Quote." *Goodreads.* Accessed September 18, 2016. http://www.goodreads.com/quotes/369-a-human-being-is-a-part-of-the-whole-called.

184. Hyman, Mark. 2010. "Cancer: New Science on How to Prevent and Treat It—A Report from TEDMED." http://drhyman.com/blog/2010/11/06/cancer-new-science-on-how-to-prevent-and-treat-it-a-report-from-tedmed/; Thomas, John P. "Cancer Makes Too Much Money to Cure." *Health Impact News.* http://healthimpactnews.com/2014/the-cancer-industry-is-too-prosperous-to-allow-a-cure/.

185. Jones, Toby C. 2012. "America, Oil, and War in the Middle East." *The Journal of American History* 99:1:208—218. http://jah.oxfordjournals.org/content/99/1/208.full.

186. Lipton, Bruce and Steve Bhaerman. 2010. *Spontaneous Evolution: Our Positive Future and a Way to Get There from Here.* Carlsbad, CA: Hay House, Inc.

187. Davey, Melissa, Adam Vaughan, and Amanda Holpuch. 2014. "People's Climate March: Thousands Demand Action Around the World—As It Happened." *The Guardian.* http://www.theguardian.com/environment/live/2014/sep/21/peoples-climate-march-live.

188. Edwards, Haley S. 2011. "We Are All Americans: The World's Response to 9/11." *Mental Floss.* http://mentalfloss.com/article/28724/we-are-all-americans-worlds-response-911.

189. The Institute for Functional Medicine. 2016. "Functional Medicine and Integrative Medicine." https://www.functionalmedicine.org/page.aspx?id=781.

190. Hyman, Mark. 2009. *The UltraMind Solution*. New York: Scribner.

191. Weil, Andrew. 2011. *Spontaneous Happiness: A New Path to Emotional Well-Being*. New York: Little, Brown and Company.

192. Wikipedia. 2016. "List of Environmental Organizations." http://en.wikipedia.org/wiki/List_of_environmental_organizations.

193. Tolle, Eckhart. 1999. *The Power of Now: A Guide to Spiritual Enlightenment*. Novato, CA: New World Library and Vancouver, BC: Namaste Publishing.

194. UN Regional Information Centre for Western Europe. 2016. "Indigenous People." http://www.unric.org/en/indigenous-people.

195. Duke Medicine. 2016. "Loneliness Can Have Severe Health Consequences." *Duke Medicine Health News* 22:6:2.

196. Diamond, Jared. 2012. *The World Until Yesterday: What Can We Learn from Traditional Societies?* New York: The Penguin Group.

197. Suzuki, David. 2012. "Pacific Underwater: Salmon Don't Grow on Trees, But Trees Grow on Salmon." http://www.davidsuzuki.org/blogs/healthy-oceans-blog/2012/10/-pacific-underwater-salmon-dont-grow-on-trees-but-trees-grow-on-salmon/.

198. Monbiot, George. 2014. "How Wolves Change Rivers." https://www.youtube.com/watch?v=ysa5OBhXz-Q.

199. USEPA. 2016. "Global Greenhouse Gas Emissions Data." http://www.epa.gov/climatechange/ghgemissions/global.html.

200. FAO. 2011. *Organic Agriculture and Climate Change Mitigation: A Report of the Round Table on Organic Agriculture and Climate Change*. Rome: FAO. http://www.fao.org/fileadmin/templates/organicag/pdf/11_12_2_RTOACC_23_webfiles.pdf.

201. Partnership for Policy Integrity. 2012. "New Survey Shows Americans Don't Support Biomass Energy." http://www.pfpi.net/new-survey-shows-americans-don%E2%80%99t-support-biomass-energy.

202. Wiltsee, G. 2000. *Lessons Learned from Existing Biomass Power Plants*. Boulder, CO: National Renewable Energy Laboratory. http://agris.fao.org/agris-search/search.do?recordID=US201300066564.

203. Partnership for Policy Integrity. 2011. "Biomass Electricity: Clean Energy Subsidies for a Dirty Industry." http://www.pfpi.net/biomass-electricity-clean-energy-subsidies-for-a-dirty-industry.

204. Green, Erin. 2015. "1,000 MW Generating Facility to Power One Million Homes." *Engineering.com*. http://www.engineering.com/DesignerEdge/DesignerEdgeArticles/ArticleID/10829/1000-MW-Generating-Facility-to-Power-One-Million-Homes.aspx.

205. *Harper's Magazine*. 2006. "Harper's Index." http://www.harpers.org/archive/2006/01/0080867.

206. Schulze, Ernst-Detlef, Christian Korner, Beverly Law, Helmut Haberl, and Sebastiaan Luyssaert. 2012. "Large-Scale Bioenergy from Additional Harvest of Forest Biomass Is Neither Sustainable Nor Greenhouse Gas Neutral." *Global Change Biology Bioenergy*. http://ncfp.files.wordpress.com/2012/04/biomass-energy-not-sustainable-or-carbon-neutral.pdf.

207. Partnership for Policy Integrity. 2011. "Carbon Emissions from Burning Biomass." http://www. pfpi.net/carbon-emissions; Schulze, Ernst-Detlef, Christian Korner, Beverly Law, Helmut Haberl, and Sebastiaan Luyssaert. 2012. "Large-Scale Bioenergy from Additional Harvest of Forest Biomass Is Neither Sustainable Nor Greenhouse Gas Neutral." *Global Change Biology Bioenergy*. http://ncfp. files.wordpress.com/2012/04/biomass-energy-not-sustainable-or-carbon-neutral.pdf.

208. The Australian News. 2011. "Forests Revealed as Climate Giants." http://www.theaustralian.com. au/news/world/forests-revealed-as-climate-giants/story-e6frg6so-1226095027486.

209. Partnership for Policy Integrity. 2014. "Federal Trade Commission Bioenergy Report." http://www. pfpi.net/federal-trade-commission-urged-to-investigate-biomass-power-industry.

210. Butler, Linda and Kurt Tidd. 2006. "Administrative Consent Agreement—Boralex Inc. et al." October 5, 2006. Maine Department of Environmental Protection.

211. Massachusetts Medical Society. 2009. "MMS Delegates Stand Firm in Opposing Biomass Plants." http://blog.massmed.org/index.php/2009/12/mms-delegates-stand-firm-in-opposing-biomass-plants/.

212. Massachusetts Department of Environmental Protection. 2011. "Palmer Renewable Energy, LLC-Conditional Approval for Comprehensive Plan Approval under Section 7.02 of the Commonwealth's Air Pollution Control Regulations"; USEPA. 2012. "What are Hazardous Air Pollutants." https://www.epa.gov/haps/what-are-hazardous-air-pollutants.

213. Partnership for Policy Integrity. 2011. "Biomass Electricity: Clean Energy Subsidies for a Dirty Industry." http://www.pfpi.net/biomass-electricity-clean-energy-subsidies-for-a-dirty-industry.

214. Humphrey, Dana N. 2005. *Fate of Dioxin and Arsenic from the Combustion of Construction and Demolition Debris and Treated Wood: A Study for Boralex Energy, Inc.* Orono, ME: University of Maine.

215. Kilian, Crawford. 2012. "High Levels of Cesium Found in Wood Stoves of Homes in Fukushima." *H5N1*. http://crofsblogs.typepad.com/h5n1/2012/01/high-levels-of-cesium-found-in-ash-in-wood-stoves-of-homes-in-fukushima.html; Ohno, Tsutomu and C.T. Hess. 1994. "Levels of ^{137}Cs and ^{40}K in Wood Ash-Amended Soils." *Science of the Total Environment* 152:2:199-23. http://www. sciencedirect.com/science/article/pii/004896979490491X.

216. WHO. 2014. "Dioxins and Their Effects on Human Health." http://www.who.int/mediacentre/factsheets/fs225/en/.

217. Ohno, Tsutomu and C.T. Hess. 1994. "Levels of ^{137}Cs and ^{40}K in Wood Ash-Amended Soils." *Science of the Total Environment* 152:2:199-23. http://www.sciencedirect.com/science/article/pii/004896979490491X.

218. Partnership for Policy Integrity. 2011. "Biomass Electricity: Clean Energy Subsidies for a Dirty Industry." http://www.pfpi.net/biomass-electricity-clean-energy-subsidies-for-a-dirty-industry.

219. Tighe & Bond. 2007. Letter on behalf of Russell Biomass to Massachusetts Department of Environmental Protection regarding Water Management Act Order to Complete Response. May 4, 2007.

220. Partnership for Policy Integrity. 2011. "Biomass Electricity: Clean Energy Subsidies for a Dirty Industry." http://www.pfpi.net/biomass-electricity-clean-energy-subsidies-for-a-dirty-industry.

221. Public Broadcasting System. 2009. "Taking Root: The Vision of Wangari Maathai." *Independent Lens*. http://www.pbs.org/independentlens/takingroot/.

222. Lappé, Frances Moore and Anna Lappé. 2011. "Wangari Maathai and the Real Work of Hope." *The Huffington Post*. http://www.huffingtonpost.com/frances-moore-lappe/wangari-maathai-died_b_982409.html.

223. PRI. 2011. "Replanting Kenya." *Living on Earth*. http://www.loe.org/shows/shows. html?programID=11-P13-00052.

224. Gettleman, Jeffrey. 2011. "Wangari Maathai, Nobel Peace Laureate, Dies at 71." *The New York Times*. http://www.nytimes.com/2011/09/27/world/africa/wangari-maathai-nobel-peace-prize-laureate-dies-at-71.html.

225. Lappé, Frances Moore and Anna Lappé. 2011. "Wangari Maathai and the Real Work of Hope." *The Huffington Post*. http://www.huffingtonpost.com/frances-moore-lappe/wangari-maathai-died_b_982409.html.

226. The Green Belt Movement. 2012. "Who We Are." http://www.greenbeltmovement.org/who-we-are.

227. Public Broadcasting System. 2009. "Taking Root: The Vision of Wangari Maathai." *Independent Lens*. http://www.pbs.org/independentlens/takingroot/.

228. PRI. 2011. "Replanting Kenya." *Living on Earth*. http://www.loe.org/shows/shows.html?programID =11-P13-00052.

229. Ibid.

230. PRI. 2011. "Replanting Kenya." *Living on Earth*. December 30, 2011. http://www.loe.org/shows/shows.html?programID=11-P13-00052.

231. Salatin, Joel. 2014. "Can You Earn a Living at Farming?" http://www.nytimes.com/2014/08/15/opinion/can-you-earn-a-living-at-farming.html?_r=2.

232. Cox, Jeff. 2006. *The Organic Cook's Bible*. Hoboken, NJ: John Wiley and Sons, Inc.

233. Charles, Dan. 2016. "Big Seed: How The Industry Turned From Small-Town Firms to Global Giants." *Morning Edition*. http://www.npr.org/sections/thesalt/2016/04/06/472960018/big-seed-consolidation-is-shrinking-the-industry-even-further.

234. Fox, Jennifer E., Jay Gulledge, Erika Engelhaupt, Matthew E. Burow, and John A. McLachlan. 2007. "Pesticides Reduce Symbiotic Efficiency of Nitrogen-Fixing Rhizobia and Host Plants." *Proceedings of the National Academy of Sciences* 104:24:10282-10287. http://www.pnas.org/content/104/24/10282.full.pdf.

235. Carson, Rachel. 1962. *Silent Spring*. New York: Houghton Mifflin Co.

236. Alavanja, Michael C.R. 2009. "Pesticides Use and Exposure Extensive Worldwide." *Reviews on Environmental Health* 24:4:303-309. http://www.ncbi.nlm.nih.gov/pmc/articles/PMC2946087/.

237. Hyman, Mark. 2009. *The UltraMind Solution*. New York: Scribner.

238. Mostafalou, Sara and Mohammad Abdollahi. 2013. "Pesticides and Human Chronic Diseases: Evidences, Mechanisms, and Perspectives." *Toxicology and Applied Pharmacology* 268:2:157-177. http://www.sciencedirect.com/science/article/pii/S0041008X13000549.

239. Quintos, Paul and Minerva Lopez. 2009. "The Globalization of Famine." *The Education for Development Magazine*. Quezon City, Philippines: IBON International; FAO. 2004. *What is Happening to Agrobiodiversity?* Rome: FAO. http://www.fao.org/docrep/007/y5609e/y5609e02.htm.

240. Harkness, Paul. 2010. "The High Cost of the 'Water Gap.'" https://www.atkearney.com.au/executive-agenda/full-article/-/asset_publisher/0HoTu01PO8ov/content/the-high-cost-of-the-water-gap/10192.

241. USGS. Undated. "Irrigation Water Use." Accessed September 18, 2016. http://water.usgs.gov/edu/wuir.html.

242. Brown, Lester R. 2011. "Growing Water Deficit Threatening Grain Harvests." http://www.earth-policy.org/book_bytes/2011/wotech2_ss2.

243. Suzuki, David. 1997. *The Sacred Balance: Rediscovering Our Place in Nature.* Vancouver, BC: Greystone Books.

244. WcP.Watchful.Eye. "Ocean Pollution. Sea 'Dead Zones', Oxygen-Deprived, Fishless: 1ˢᵗ Recorded in 1970, 417 in 2008, Largest Covers 70,000 Sq Km." 2010. *WcP.Watchful.Eye's Blog.* http://www. worldculturepictorial.com/blog/content/ocean-dead-zones-oxygen-deprived-fishless-1st-record.

245. Lang, Susan S. 2006. "'Slow, Insidious' Soil Erosion Threatens Human Health and Welfare as Well as the Environment, Cornell Study Asserts." *Cornell Chronicle.* http://www.news.cornell.edu/stories/2006/03/slow-insidious-soil-erosion-threatens-human-health-and-welfare.

246. Leu, Andre. 2013. "Scientific Studies Validate Sustainable Organic Agriculture." *Well Being Journal.* January/February 2013.

247. Foley, Jonathan. 2014. "A Five-Step Plan to Feed the World." *National Geographic* 225:5:26-57. http://www.nationalgeographic.com/foodfeatures/feeding-9-billion/#topskip.

248. PA/Huffington Post UK. 2013. "Food Waste: Half Of All Food Ends Up Thrown Away." *The Huffington Post.* http://www.huffingtonpost.co.uk/2013/01/10/food-waste-half-of-all-fo_n_2445022.html.

249. Oceana. 2014. *Wasted Catch: Unsolved Problems in U.S. Fisheries.* http://usa.oceana.org/reports/wasted-catch-unsolved-problems-us-fisheries.

250. Foley, Jonathan. 2014. "A Five-Step Plan to Feed the World." *National Geographic* 225:5:26-57. http://www.nationalgeographic.com/foodfeatures/feeding-9-billion/#topskip.

251. Hyman, Mark. 2013. "Occupy Wellness and Eat-In: The Power of the Fork—Part One." http://drhyman.com/blog/2013/03/09/occupy-wellness-and-eat-in-the-power-of-the-fork-part-one/#close; FAO. 2006. "Livestock a Major Threat to Environment." *FAO Newsroom.* http://www.fao.org/Newsroom/en/news/2006/1000448/index.html.

252. Walsh, Bryan. 2013. "The Triple Whopper Environmental Impact of Global Meat Production." *Time Magazine.* http://science.time.com/2013/12/16/the-triple-whopper-environmental-impact-of-global-meat-production/.

253. Monbiot, George. 2015. "There's a Population Crisis All Right. But Probably Not the One You Think." *The Guardian.* http://www.theguardian.com/commentisfree/2015/nov/19/population-crisis-farm-animals-laying-waste-to-planet.

254. Bureau of Land Management. 1994. *Rangeland Reform '94 Final Environmental Impact Statement.* Washington, DC: BLM.

255. FAO. 2006. "Livestock a Major Threat to Environment." *FAO Newsroom.* http://www.fao.org/Newsroom/en/news/2006/1000448/index.html.

256. FAO. 2006. *Livestock's Long Shadow.* Rome: FAO. https://fao.presswarehouse.com/books/BookDetail.aspx?productID=321690.

257. Brown, Jenny. 2012. *The Lucky Ones: My Passionate Fight for Farm Animals.* New York: Penguin Books.

258. Richardson, Jill. 2011. "Factory Farms Produce 100 Times More Waste Than All People In the US Combined and It's Killing Our Drinking Water." *AlterNet.* http://www.alternet.org/story/150993/factory_farms_produce_100_times_more_waste_than_all_people_in_the_us_combined_and_it's_killing_our_drinking_water?page=2.

259. Pollan, Michael. 2006. *The Omnivore's Dilemma.* New York: Penguin Group.

260. Mother Jones. 2013. "Gagged by Big Ag." *Mother Jones.* http://www.motherjones.com/environment/2013/06/ag-gag-laws-mowmar-farms.

261. Watts, Mark. 1996. "The Birth of BSE." *The Independent.* http://www.independent.co.uk/life-style/the-birth-of-bse-1344995.html.

262. Salatin, Joel. 2011. "Local Food." *Alternative Radio*. http://www.alternativeradio.org/products/salj001.

263. Walsh, Fergus. 2014. "Superbugs to Kill 'More Than Cancer' by 2050." *BBC News*. http://www.bbc.com/news/health-30416844.

264. Druker, Steven. 2015. *Altered Genes, Twisted Trust: How the Venture to Genetically Engineer Our Food Has Subverted Science, Corrupted Government, and Systematically Deceived the Public*. Salt Lake City: Clear River Press.

265. USDA. 2016. "Genetically Engineered Varieties of Corn, Cotton, and Soybeans Have Plateaued at More Than 90 Percent of U.S. Acreage Planted with Those Crops." https://www.ers.usda.gov/data-products/chart-gallery/gallery/chart-detail/?chartId=79096.

266. Center for Food Safety. 2012. "About Genetically Engineered Foods." http://www.centerforfoodsafety.org/issues/311/ge-foods/about-ge-foods.

267. Center for Food Safety. 2016. "Lawsuit Challenges FDA Approval of Genetically Engineered Salmon." http://www.centerforfoodsafety.org/press-releases/4317/lawsuit-challenges-fdas-approval-of-genetically-engineered-salmon.

268. Sustainable Pulse. 2015. "GMOs Now Banned in 38 Countries Worldwide—Sustainable Pulse Research." http://sustainablepulse.com/2015/10/22/gm-crops-now-banned-in-36-countries-worldwide-sustainable-pulse-research/#.V9__MpVSOhd.

269. Just Label It! 2016. "Labeling Around the World." http://justlabelit.org/right-to-know/labeling-around-the-world/; Label GMOs. Undated. "What Are We Eating?" Accessed October 11, 2016. http://www.labelgmos.org/the_science_genetically_modified_foods_gmo.

270. Center for Food Safety. 2016. "State Labeling Initiatives." http://www.centerforfoodsafety.org/issues/976/ge-food-labeling/state-labeling-initiatives#; Bass, Charles F. 2016. "President Obama Signs GMO Labeling Bill Into Law." *The National Law Review*. http://www.natlawreview.com/article/president-obama-signs-gmo-labeling-bill-law.

271. Kimbrell, Andrew. 2015. "Why the GMO Labeling Law President Obama Just Signed Into Law Is a Sham—And a National Embarrassment." *AlterNet*. http://www.alternet.org/food/why-gmo-labeling-bill-obama-just-signed-law-sham-and-national-embarrassment.

272. Kaskey, Jack. 2011. "Monsanto Corn May Be Failing to Kill Bugs in 4 States, EPA Says." *Bloomberg Businessweek*; Aris, A. and S. Leblanc. 2011. "Maternal and Fetal Exposure to Pesticides Associated to Genetically Modified Foods in Eastern Townships of Quebec, Canada." *Reproductive Toxicology* 4:528-33. http://www.ncbi.nlm.nih.gov/pubmed/21338670.

273. CBS News. 2011. "Mystery Science: More Details on the Strange Organism That Could Destroy Monsanto." http://www.cbsnews.com/news/mystery-science-more-details-on-the-strange-organism-that-could-destroy-monsanto/; Pieper, Kevin. 2012. "Farmers Must Spend More on Herbicides as Effectiveness Fades." *USA Today*. http://www.usatoday.com/money/industries/environment/story/2012-04-16/failing-herbicide/54319726/1.

274. IARC. 2015. "Evaluation of Five Organophosphate Insecticides and Herbicides." *IARC Monographs Volume 12*. https://www.iarc.fr/en/media-centre/iarcnews/pdf/MonographVolume112.pdf.

275. Newman, Bryan. 2007. *A Bitter Harvest: Farmer Suicide and the Unforeseen Social, Environmental, and Economic Impacts of the Green Revolution in Punjab, India*. Oakland, CA: Food First Institute for Food and Development Policy. http://www.foodfirst.org/en/node/1611; Sainath, P. 2007. "A Farmer is Committing Suicide Every 32 Minutes." *Counterpunch*. http://www.counterpunch.org/2007/11/17/a-farmer-is-committing-suicide-every-32-minutes/; The Guardian. 2014. "India's Farmer Suicides: Are Deaths Linked to GM Cotton?—In Pictures." https://www.theguardian.com/global-development/gallery/2014/may/05/india-cotton-suicides-farmer-deaths-gm-seeds.

276. Frazão, Elizabeth. 1999. *America's Eating Habits: Changes and Consequences*. Washington, DC: USDA. CDC. 2013. "Death in the United States." *NCHS Data Brief No. 115*. http://www.cdc. gov/nchs/data/databriefs/db115.htm; CDC. 2016. "Chronic Disease Overview." http://www. cdc.gov/chronicdisease/overview/; CDC. 2015. "Stroke Facts." http://www.cdc.gov/stroke/facts. htm; Skerrett, Patrick. 2011. "Is Fructose Bad for You?" *Harvard Health Blog*. http://www.health. harvard.edu/blog/is-fructose-bad-for-you-201104262425.

277. Hyman, Mark. 2009. *The UltraMind Solution*. New York: Scribner.

278. Fuhrman, Joel. 2011. *3 Steps to Incredible Health*. https://www.drfuhrman.com/connect/events/ pbs-television-programs.

279. Hyman, Mark. 2012. *The Blood Sugar Solution: The UltraHealthy Program for Losing Weight, Preventing Disease, and Feeling Great Now!* New York: Little, Brown and Company.

280. Longley, Robert. 2016. "Up to 75 Percent of US Youth Ineligible for Military Service." *About News*. http://usgovinfo.about.com/od/usmilitary/a/unabletoserve.htm.

281. United Nations. 2014. "Non-Communicable Diseases Deemed Development Challenge of 'Epidemic Proportions' in Political Declaration Adopted During Landmark General Assembly Summit." http://www.un.org/press/en/2011/ga11138.doc.htm.

282. Shah, Anup. 2011. "Health Care Around the World." http://www.globalissues.org/article/774/ health-care-around-the-world.

283. Zumbrun, Joshua. 2008. "Sugar's Sweet Deal." *Forbes*. http://www.forbes.com/2008/06/27/florida- sugar-crist-biz-beltway-cx_jz_0630sugar.html.

284. Salatin, Joel. 2011. "Local Food." *Alternative Radio*. http://www.alternativeradio.org/products/salj001.

285. Moss, Michael. 2014. *Salt Sugar Fat: How the Food Giants Hooked Us*. New York: Random House LLC.

286. Kenfield, Isabella. 2009. "Michael Taylor: Monsanto's Man in the Obama Administration." https:// www.organicconsumers.org/news/michael-taylor-monsantos-man-obama-administration; Hunt, Skip. 2012. "Do People Realize High Fructose Corn Syrup is Poison?" http://skiphuntphoto.com/ wonder/do-people-realize-high-fructose-corn-syrup-is-poison.

287. Heid, Markham. 2016. "Experts Say Lobbying Skewed the U.S. Dietary Guidelines." *Time Magazine*. http://time.com/4130043/lobbying-politics-dietary-guidelines/.

288. Environmental Working Group. Undated. "EWG's Farm Subsidy Database." Accessed July 11, 2016. http://farm.ewg.org/.

289. Stewart, James B. 2013. "Richer Farms, Bigger Subsidies." *The New York Times*. http://www. nytimes.com/2013/07/20/business/richer-farmers-bigger-subsidies.html?pagewanted=all&_r=0.

290. Buchheit, Paul and Max Fisher. 2015. "The Numbers are Staggering: US is 'World Leader' in Child Poverty (in 'Developed' Countries)." *Portside*. http://portside.org/2015-04-23/numbers-are- staggering-us-world-leader-child-poverty-developed-countries.

291. Juniper, Tony. 2014. "Apples and the Economic Impact of Birds." *Well Being Journal*. January/ February 2014.

292. Huff, Ethan A. 2011. "Study: Organic Farming Outperforms Conventional in Yields, Economic Viability, Conservation, and Health." *Natural News*. http://www.naturalnews.com/033925_ organic_farming_crop_yields.html; Lang, Susan S. 2005. "Organic Farms Produce Same Yields as Conventional Farms." *Cornell Chronicle*. http://www.news.cornell.edu/stories/2005/07/ organic-farms-produce-same-yields-conventional-farms.

293. Meyer, Nick. 2013. "UN Report Says Small-Scale Organic Farming Only Way to Feed the World." *TechnologyWater*. http://www.technologywater.com/post/69995394390/un-report-says-small -scale-organic-farming-only.

294. Scialabba, Nadia El-Hage and Caroline Hattam (Editors). 2002. *Organic Agriculture, Environment, and Food Security.* Rome: FAO. http://www.fao.org/docrep/005/y4137e/y4137e00.htm; Cook, Christopher D., Kari Hamerschlag, and Kendra Klein. 2016. *Farming for the Future: Organic and Agroecological Solutions to Feed the World.* Washington, DC: Friends of the Earth.

295. Lappé, Frances Moore. 2013. *EcoMind: Changing the Way We Think, to Create the World We Want.* New York: Nation Books.

296. Gardiner, Beth. 2016. "A Boon for Soil, and for the Environment." *The New York Times.* http://www.nytimes.com/2016/05/18/business/energy-environment/a-boon-for-soil-and-for-the-environment.html.

297. Scialabba. Nadia. 2009. "Agriculture and Climate Mitigation." *Beyond Kyoto.* Aarhus, Denmark. March 6, 2009. http://www.presentica.com/stephanie-cross/past-kyoto-aarhus-6-walk-2009-powerpoint-ppt-presentation.

298. Nightly Business Report. 2016. "Transcript: Nightly Business Report—May 19, 2016." http://nbr.com/2016/05/18/transcript-nightly-business-report-may-19-2016/; USDA. 2016. "Organic Market Overview." http://www.ers.usda.gov/topics/natural-resources-environment/organic-agriculture/organic-market-overview.aspx/.

299. Cox, Jeff. 2006. *The Organic Cook's Bible.* Hoboken, NJ: John Wiley and Sons, Inc.

300. Ibid.

301. Lappé, Frances Moore. 2011. *EcoMind: Changing the Way We Think, to Create the World We Want.* New York: Nation Books.

302. USDA. 2016. "State Fact Sheets." http://www.ers.usda.gov/data-products/state-fact-sheets/state-data.aspx?StateFIPS=00#Pbea937eb4dbe43a1bc692e1ac7b4cca5_4_499iT18C0x0.

303. *Whole Living Magazine.* 2012. "The Food Visionaries." November 2012. http://www.wholeliving.com/207807/food-visionaries#191900.

304. KPBS. 2011. "Growing Hope Against Hunger: A Sesame Street Special Presentation." http://www.kpbs.org/news/2011/oct/06/growing-hope-against-hunger-sesame-street-special-/.

305. Cox, Jeff. 2006. *The Organic Cook's Bible.* Hoboken, NJ: John Wiley and Sons, Inc.

306. Hubbard, Barbara Marx. 2007. *Gateway to Conscious Evolution.* (Set of seven compact disks.) Santa Barbara, CA: Foundation for Conscious Evolution.

307. Parenti, Christian. 2012. *Tropic of Chaos: Climate Change and the New Geography of Violence.* New York: Nation Books.

308. Speth, Gustave J. 2014. *Angels by the River: A Memoir.* White River Junction, VT: Chelsea Green Publishing.

309. Dyer, Wayne. 2009. *Excuses Begone!: How to Change Lifelong, Self-Defeating Thinking Habits.* Carlsbad, CA: Hay House, Inc.

310. Pandya, Haresh. 2013. "Shakuntala Devi, 'Human Computer' Who Bested the Machines, Dies at 83." *The New York Times.* http://www.nytimes.com/2013/04/24/world/asia/shakuntala-devi-human-computer-dies-in-india-at-83.html?_r=0.

311. WGBH. 2011. "How Smart Are Animals?" *Nova.* http://www.pbs.org/wgbh/nova/nature/how-smart-are-animals.html.

312. Emmert, J.M. 2009. "Rich Man, Poor Man: The Story of Napoleon Hill." *Success.* http://www.success.com/article/rich-man-poor-man.

313. Moyer, Ruthann D. 2008. *A Stolen Childhood: The Life and Times of David Earl Moyer: 1895-1987.* Bloomington, IN: Xlibris Corporation.

314. Canfield, Jack. 2015. *The Success Principles: How to Get from Where You Are to Where You Want to Be.* Second edition. New York: HarperCollins Publishers.

315. Johnson, Caitlin. 2006. "Cutting Through Advertising Clutter." *CBS News.* http://www.cbsnews.com/8301-3445_162-2015684.html; Hodgson, Kendra. Undated. *Killing Us Softly: Advertising Image of Women.* Accessed September 20, 2016. http://www.mediaed.org/assets/products/241/studyguide_241.pdf.

316. Dyer, Wayne. 2009. *Excuses Begone!: How to Change Lifelong, Self-Defeating Thinking Habits.* Carlsbad, CA: Hay House, Inc.

317. Tolle, Eckhart. 1999. *The Power of Now.* Vancouver: Namaste Publishing.

318. Lappé, Frances Moore. 2007. *Getting A Grip: Clarity, Creativity, and Courage in a World Gone Mad.* White River Junction, VT: Chelsea Green Publishing.

319. Siegel, Daniel J. 2011. *Mindsight: The New Science of Personal Transformation.* New York: Bantam Books.

320. WBGH. 2012. "How Smart Can We Get?" *Nova.* http://www.pbs.org/wgbh/nova/body/how-smart-can-we-get.html.

321. Jeffers, Susan. 1987. *Feel the Fear and Do It Anyway.* New York: Fawcett Books.

322. Eker, T. Harv. 2005. *Secrets of the Millionaire Mind: Mastering the Inner Game of Wealth.* New York: HarperCollins Publishing, Inc.

323. WGBH. 2014. "The Long Walk of Nelson Mandela." *Frontline.* http://www.pbs.org/wgbh/pages/frontline/shows/mandela/prison/.

324. Hubbard, Frank. 1965. *Three Centuries of Harpsichord Making.* Cambridge, MA: Harvard University Press.

325. Global Alliance for Transformational Entertainment. 2011. "Jean Houston." http://gatecommunity.org/s2houston/.

326. Wise, Jeff. 2010. "Yes, You Really Can Lift a Car Off a Trapped Child: The Science Behind Seemingly Impossible Feats of Strength." *Psychology Today.* http://www.psychologytoday.com/blog/extreme-fear/201011/yes-you-really-can-lift-car-trapped-child.

327. Hubbard, Barbara Marx. 2011. "Recap." *Healing with the Masters.* Interview by Jennifer MacLean. http://healingwiththemasters.com/barbara-marx-hubbard-recap/.

328. Twigg, Reg. 2013. *Survivor on the River Kwai: The Incredible Story of Life on the Burma Railway.* New York: Viking; Mercury, Leicester. 2013. "Death of PoW Who Endured Years of Hell on River Kwai." http://www.leicestermercury.co.uk/Death-PoW-endured-years-hell-River-Kwai/story-18924859-detail/story.html.

329. Neill, Michael. 2013. "Happiness and Success." *Hay House World Summit 2013.* Interview by Greg Sherwood, June 5, 2013. Carlsbad, CA: Hay House, Inc.

330. Siegler, M.G. 2010. "Eric Schmidt: Every 2 Days We Create As Much Information As We Did Up to 2003." *TechCrunch.* http://techcrunch.com/2010/08/04/schmidt-data/.

331. Bartmann, Bill. 2005. *Billionaire: Secrets to Success.* Dallas: Brown Books Publishing Group.

332. United Nations. 2013. "Malala Yousafzai Addresses United Nations Youth Assembly." http://www.youtube.com/watch?v=3rNhZu3ttIU.

333. Hill, Napoleon. 2007. *Think and Grow Rich.* Radford, VA: Wilder Publications.

334. Canfield, Jack. 2016. "Write a Book and Get It Published. (Yes, You!) Seven Key Strategies for Getting Started." http://jackcanfield.com/write-a-book/.

335. Weil, Andrew. 1995. *Spontaneous Healing.* New York: Ballantine Books.

336. Lustig, Robert H., Laura A. Schmidt, and Claire D. Brindis. 2012. "The Toxic Truth About Sugar." *Nature* 482:27-29. https://uhs.berkeley.edu/sites/default/files/wellness-toxictruthaboutsugar.pdf.

337. Fuhrman, Joel. 2011. *3 Steps to Incredible Health, Volume 1.* Flemington, NJ: Gift of Health Press.

338. Pollan, Michael. 2008. *In Defense of Food: An Eater's Manifesto.* New York: Penguin Books.

339. Ibid.

340. Klein, Sarah. 2010. "The Addictive Situation of Fatty Food." *The Situationist.* http://thesituationist.wordpress.com/2010/03/30/the-addictive-situation-of-fatty-food/.

341. Hyman, Mark. 2009. *The UltraMind Solution.* New York: Scribner.

342. Hyman, Mark. 2012. "Three Hidden Ways Wheat Makes You Fat." http://drhyman.com/blog/2012/02/13/three-hidden-ways-wheat-makes-you-fat/.

343. Cotman, C.W., N.C. Berchtold, and L.A. Christie. 2007. "Exercise Builds Brain Health: Key Roles of Growth Factor Cascades and Inflammation." *Trends in Neuroscience* 30:9:464-472. https://www.ncbi.nlm.nih.gov/pubmed/17765329.

344. Hyman, Mark. 2009. *The UltraMind Solution.* New York: Scribner.

345. Berkowitz, Bonnie and Patterson Clark. 2014. "The Health Hazards of Sitting." *The Washington Post.* https://www.washingtonpost.com/apps/g/page/national/the-health-hazards-of-sitting/750/.

346. Kilen, Brian. 2014. "Mayo Clinic Health Letter: Highlights from the October 2014 Issue." *Mayo Clinic News Network.* http://newsnetwork.mayoclinic.org/discussion/mayo-clinic-health-letter-highlights-from-the-october-2014-issue/.

347. Hyman, Mark. 2012. *The Blood Sugar Solution: The UltraHealthy Program for Losing Weight, Preventing Disease, and Feeling Great Now!* New York: Little, Brown and Company.

348. Crinnion, W.J. 2011. "Sauna as a Valuable Clinical Tool for Cardiovascular, Autoimmune, Toxicant-induced and other Chronic Health Problems." *Alternative Medicine Review* 16:3:215-225. https://www.ncbi.nlm.nih.gov/pubmed/21951023.

349. Dadd, Debra L. 1997. *Home Safe Home: Creating a Healthy Home Environment by Reducing Exposure to Toxic Household Products.* New York: Penguin Books.

350. Huffington, Ariana. 2016. *The Sleep Revolution: Transforming Your Life, One Night at a Time.* New York: Harmony Books.

351. Bogard, Paul. 2013. *The End of Night: Searching for Natural Darkness in an Age of Artificial Light.* New York: Little, Brown and Company.

352. Konnikova, Maria. 2014. "Goodnight. Sleep Clean." *The New York Times.* http://www.nytimes.com/2014/01/12/opinion/sunday/goodnight-sleep-clean.html?_r=0.

353. CDC. 2016. "1 in 3 Adults Don't Get Enough Sleep." *CDC Newsroom.* http://www.cdc.gov/media/releases/2016/p0215-enough-sleep.html.

354. Portage Path Behavioral Health. 2003. "The Portage Path Behavioral Health Reference Guide to: Stress in the Workplace." www.portagepath.org/wp-content/uploads/2015/04/WorkPlaceStress.pdf.

355. Lipton, Bruce. 2005. *The Biology of Belief: Unleashing the Power of Consciousness, Matter & Miracles.* Carlsbad, CA: Hay House, Inc.

356. Mind of Success.com. 2012. "T. Harv Eker Quotes: Success Is Easy." http://www.mindofsuccess.com/t-harv-eker-quotes/.

357. Orman, Suze, 2013. "Your Relationship with Your Money Begins with Your Relationship with Yourself." *Hay House World Summit 2013.* Interview by Reid Tracy, June 8, 2013. Carlsbad, CA: Hay House, Inc.

358. Twist, Lynne and Theresa Barker. 2003. *The Soul of Money: Reclaiming the Wealth of Our Inner Resources*. New York: W.W. Norton & Company, Inc.

359. Orman, Suze, 2013. "Your Relationship with Your Money Beings with Your Relationship with Yourself." *Hay House World Summit 2013*. Interview by Reid Tracy, June 8, 2013. Carlsbad, CA: Hay House, Inc.

360. WGBH. 2013. "What Does the American Dream Mean to You?" *Frontline*. http://www.pbs.org/wgbh/pages/frontline/business-economy-financial-crisis/two-american-families/what-does-the-american-dream-mean-to-you/.

361. HubPages. 2014. "Making a Quantum Leap." http://hubpages.com/literature/making-a-quantum-leap.

362. The Chopra Center. 2016. "The Law of Giving and Receiving." http://www.chopra.com/articles/the-law-of-giving-receiving.

363. McTaggart, Lynne. 2013. "How Understanding Our True Human Bond Can Lead to a Happier You and a Healthier Planet." *Hay House World Summit 2013*. Interview by Greg Sherwood, June 4, 2013. Carlsbad, CA: Hay House, Inc.

364. Smith, Emily Esfahani. 2013. "Meaning is Healthier Than Happiness." *The Atlantic*. August 2013.

365. Shimoff, Marci. 2008. *Happy for No Reason: 7 Steps to Being Happy from the Inside Out*. New York: Free Press; Chopra, Deepak. 2009. *The Ultimate Happiness Prescription: 7 Keys to Joy and Enlightenment*. New York: Harmony Books.

366. Canfield, Jack. 2015. *The Success Principles: How to Get from Where You Are to Where You Want to Be*. Second edition. New York: HarperCollins Publishers.

367. Steiner, Susan. 2012. "Top Five Regrets of the Dying." *The Guardian*. http://www.theguardian.com/lifeandstyle/2012/feb/01/top-five-regrets-of-the-dying.

368. Shimoff, Marci. 2008. *Happy for No Reason: 7 Steps to Being Happy from the Inside Out*. New York: Free Press.

369. Attwood, Janet Bray, and Chris Attwood. 2008. *The Passion Test: The Effortless Path to Discovering Your Life Purpose*. New York: Penguin Group.

370. Bartmann, Bill. 2005. *Billionaire: Secrets to Success*. Dallas: Brown Books Publishing Group.

371. Covey, Stephen. 1989. *The Seven Habits of Highly Effective People*. New York: Fireside.

372. Eker, T. Harv. 2015. "Two Ways to Avoid Overwhelm and Remain Productive Throughout Your Day." http://www.harveker.com/2015/02/24/two-ways-to-avoid-overwhelm-and-remain-productive-throughout-your-day/.

373. Schwartz, David. 1987. *The Magic of Thinking Big*. New York: Simon & Schuster, Inc.

374. Gawain, Shakti. 1978. *Creative Visualization: Use the Power of Your Imagination to Create What You Want in Your Life*. Novato, CA: Nataraj Publishing.

375. Poneman, Debra. 2013. *Seeds for Your Soul*. (Set of six compact disks.) http://yestosuccess.com/seedsforyoursoul/.

376. Hay, Louise. Undated. "Affirmations." Accessed September 25, 2016. http://www.louisehay.com/affirmations/.

377. Childre, Doc and Howard Martin. 1999. *The HeartMath Solution*. New York: HarperCollins Publishers.

378. Shimoff, Marci. 2010. *Love For No Reason: 7 Steps to Creating a Life of Unconditional Love*. New York: Free Press.

379. Public Affairs Television. 2013. "Wendell Berry, Poet & Prophet." *Moyers & Company*. http://billmoyers.com/episode/full-show-wendell-berry-poet-prophet/.

380. Public Affairs Television. 2014. "Time to Get Real on Climate Change." *Moyers & Company.* http://billmoyers.com/episode/full-show-time-to-get-real-on-climate-change/.

381. PRI. "Agony and Ivory." *Living on Earth.* http://www.loe.org/shows/shows.html?programID=11-P13-00029.

382. Jensen, Derrick. 2006. "Beyond Hope." *Orion Magazine.* May/June 2006. http://www.orionmagazine.org/index.php/articles/article/170/.

383. Demartini, John. 2002. *The Breakthrough Experience: A Revolutionary New Approach to Personal Transformation.* Carlsbad, CA: Hay House, Inc.

384. Conner, Cheryl. 2012. "Employees Really Do Waste Time at Work, Part II." *Forbes.* http://www.forbes.com/sites/cherylsnappconner/2012/11/15/employees-really-do-waste-time-at-work-part-ii/#49d89edd27ad.

385. Linn, Denise. 2013. "Spiritual Secrets to Activate Fabulous Abundance." *Hay House World Summit 2013.* Interview by John Holland, June 2, 2013. Carlsbad, CA: Hay House, Inc.

386. Lovgren, Stefan. 2005. "Animals Laughed Long Before Humans, Study Says." *National Geographic.* http://news.nationalgeographic.com/news/2005/03/0331_050331_animallaughter.html.

387. Fortune. 2015. "Why Americans Just Won't Take Time Off." *Fortune.* http://fortune.com/2015/05/01/paid-time-off-vacation/; Fottrell, Quentin. 2015. "Americans Take Half of Their Paid Vacation, but Chinese Take Less." *MarketWatch.* http://www.marketwatch.com/story/americans-only-take-half-of-their-paid-vacation-2014-04-03.

388. Chopra, Deepak. 2013. "Who Am I?: Breaking Free from the Conditioned Mind." *Hay House World Summit 2013.* Interview by Greg Sherwood, June 10, 2013. Carlsbad, CA: Hay House, Inc.

389. Ibid.

390. Tolle, Eckhart. 1999. *The Power of Now: A Guide to Spiritual Enlightenment.* Novato, CA: New World Library and Vancouver, BC: Namaste Publishing.

391. Moore, Kathleen Dean. 2011. *Moral Ground: Ethical Action for a Planet in Peril.* San Antonio, TX: Trinity University Press.

392. Democker, Mary. 2012. "If Your House Is On Fire: Kathleen Dean Moore On The Moral Urgency of Climate Change." *The Sun.* http://thesunmagazine.org/issues/444/if_your_house_is_on_fire.

393. Hessel, Stéphane. 2010. *Time for Outrage: Indignez-vous!* New York: Twelve? Hachette Book Group.

394. Goldman Environmental Foundation. 2016. "The Goldman Environmental Prize." http://www.goldmanprize.org/.

395. Caldicott, Helen. 2011. "Hiroshima to Fukushima." *Flag in Distress: Rants for a Better America.* http://flagindistress.com/2011/08/hiroshima-to-fukushima/.

396. Kouzes, James M. and Barry Z. Posner. 2012. *The Leadership Challenge: How to Make Extraordinary Things Happen in Organizations.* Fifth edition. San Francisco: Jossey-Bass.

397. The World Bank. 2016. "Household Final Consumption Expenditure, Etc. (% of GDP)." http://data.worldbank.org/indicator/NE.CON.PETC.ZS.

398. Moyer, Ellen. 2016. "Meat Eating—What Should We Do?" *The Huffington Post.* http://www.huffingtonpost.com/ellen-moyer-phd/meat-eating-what-should-we-do_b_9284862.html.

399. USDOE. 2015. "Are Energy Vampires Sucking You Dry?" http://energy.gov/articles/are-energy-vampires-sucking-you-dry.

400. Lawrence Berkeley National Laboratory. 2016. "Standby Power." http://standby.lbl.gov/summary-table.html.

401. CatalogChoice. 2016. "Simplify Your Life: Stop Junk Mail For Good." https://www.catalogchoice.org/.

402. USFW. 2016. "Pollinators." http://www.fws.gov/pollinators/; National Wildlife Federation. 2016. "Garden for Wildlife." http://www.nwf.org/How-to-Help/Garden-for-Wildlife/Gardening-Tips/Using-Native-Plants.aspx.

403. Environmental Working Group. 2016. "Know Your Environment. Protect Your Health." www.ewg.org.

404. Canfield, Jack. 2015. *The Success Principles: How to Get from Where You Are to Where You Want to Be.* Second edition. New York: HarperCollins Publishers.

405. Insight Seminars Worldwide. 2016. "Insight II: The Opening Heart." http://www.insightseminars.org/insight-ii.html.

406. DeSilver, Drew. 2016. "US Voter Turnout Trails Most Developed Countries." *Pew Research Center.* http://www.pewresearch.org/fact-tank/2016/08/02/u-s-voter-turnout-trails-most-developed-countries/.

407. Landau, Elizabeth. 2014. "Subway to Remove 'Dough Conditioner' Chemical from Bread." *CNN.* http://www.cnn.com/2014/02/06/health/subway-bread-chemical/.

408. Lutkehaus, Nancy C. 2008. *Margaret Mead: The Making of an American Icon.* Princeton, NJ: Princeton University Press.

409. Houston, Jean. 2004. *Jump Time: Shaping Your Future in World of Radical Change.* Second edition. Boulder CO: Sentient Publications.

410. Center for Biological Diversity. Undated. "Our Story." Accessed September 25, 2016. http://www.biologicaldiversity.org/about/story/.

411. McSpadden, Russ, Lydia Millet, Mike Stark, and Kieran Suckling. 2015. *A Wild Love: The Center for Biological Diversity's First 25 Years.* Tuscon, AZ: Center for Biological Diversity/Arizona Lithographers.

412. Center for Biological Diversity. Undated. "Support the Center." Accessed September 25, 2016. http://www.biologicaldiversity.org/support/.

413. Foster, David R. and David A. Orwig. 2006. "Preemptive and Salvage Harvesting of New England Forests: When Doing Nothing is a Viable Alternative." *Conservation Biology* 20:4:959-970. http://www.sierraforestlegacy.org/Resources/Conservation/FireForestEcology/SalvageLoggingScience/Salvage-Foster06.pdf.

414. Moyer, Ellen. 2012. "The Power of Ordinary Citizens: Using Science to Stop Logging." *The Huffington Post.* http://www.huffingtonpost.com/ellen-moyer-phd/science-to-stop-logging_b_1799800.html.

415. Klaft, Lynne. 2009. "Savior of the Nashua River." *Worcester Telegram & Gazette.* http://www.telegram.com/article/20090628/NEWS/906280422/0.

416. Edwards, Susan and Dorie Clark. 2010. *Marion Stoddart: The Work of 1000.* Documentary Educational Resources. http://www.der.org/films/work-of-1000.html.

417. Nashua River Watershed Association. 2012. "River Classroom: A Day of Science and Adventure." http://www.nashuariverwatershed.org/what-we-do/provide-education/for-schools-and-groups/river-classroom.html.

418. Nashua River Watershed Association. 2012. "Protecting the Nashua River Greenway." http://www.nashuariverwatershed.org/what-we-do/protect-water-and-land/riverside-greenway-protection-overview.html.

419. Nashua River Watershed Association. 2012. "NRWA's Mission and History: Leadership and Success." http://www.nashuariverwatershed.org/who-we-are/mission-and-history.html.

420. National Geographic Society. 1993. "Water: The Power, Promise, and Turmoil of North America's Fresh Water." *National Geographic Magazine* 184:5A. http://www.amazon.com/National-Geographic-Special-Edition-November/dp/B004PHS98O; Cherry, Lynne. 2002. *A River Ran Wild: An Environmental History.* New York: HMH Books for Young Readers.

421. National Women's History Project. Undated. "2010 Partners." Accessed September 25, 2016. http://www.nwhp.org//?s=stoddart&x=13&y=10.

422. Stoddart, Marion. 2010. *Commit! A Leadership Handbook.* https://www.createspace.com/3412514; Edwards, Susan and Dorie Clark. 2010. *Marion Stoddart: The Work of 1000.* Documentary Educational Resources. http://workof1000.org/host-a-screening.

423. Houston, Jean. 2012. *The Wizard of Us: Transformational Lessons from Oz.* New York: Atria Books and Hillsboro, OR: Beyond Words.

424. Stoddart, Marion. 2010. *Commit! A Leadership Handbook.* https://www.createspace.com/3412514.

425. Perez, Ines. 2013. "Climate Change and Rising Food Prices Heightened Arab Spring." *Scientific American.* http://www.scientificamerican.com/article/climate-change-and-rising-food-prices-heightened-arab-spring/.

426. Ryan, Tim. 2013. *A Mindful Nation: How a Simple Practice Can Help Us Reduce Stress, Improve Performance, and Recapture the American Spirit.* Carlsbad, CA: Hay House, Inc.

427. NASA. 2009. "NASA Spinoff: Technology Transfer Program." https://spinoff.nasa.gov/Spinoff2009/Intro_2009.html.

428. Greene, Brian. 2011. "How 'Occupy Wall Street' Started and Spread." *U.S. News & World Report.* http://www.usnews.com/news/washington-whispers/articles/2011/10/17/how-occupy-wall-street-started-and-spread.

429. Doniger, David. 2012. "Ozone Success Gives Hope for Climate." *USA Today.* http://usatoday30.usatoday.com/news/opinion/forum/story/2012-09-28/ozone-layer-montreal-protocol/57850784/1.

430. BBC. 2011. "An Asbo in 14th Century Britain." *BBC News Magazine.* http://www.bbc.com/news/magazine-12847529.

431. BBC. 2011. "Filthy Cities—Eps 1 Medieval London." *Filthy Cities.* http://www.pbs.org/show/filthy-cities/.

432. BBC. 2011. "Filthy Cities Paris." *Filthy Cities.* http://vimeo.com/23405739.

433. BBC. 2011. "Filthy Cities: Industrial New York." *Filthy Cities.* https://vimeo.com/45101348.

434. Satran, Joe. 2012. "FDA Food Inspections Fail to Catch Vast Majority of Pathogens, 'Bloomberg Markets' Finds." *The Huffington Post.* http://www.huffingtonpost.com/2012/10/11/fda-food-regulation_n_1955074.html.

435. Brancaccio, David and Katie Long. 2016. "What If We Had a Secretary of the Future?" *Marketplace.* http://www.marketplace.org/2016/02/29/elections/secretary-future/secretary-future.

436. Abel, David. 2016. "SJC Rules Mass. Failed to Issue Proper Regulations to Cut Emissions." *The Boston Globe.* http://www.bostonglobe.com/metro/2016/05/18/sjc-rules-that-state-failed-issue-proper-regulations-cut-emissions/N6rAAeeGAr4LrjqF8K71JJ/story.html.

437. Korten, David C. 2006. *The Great Turning: From Empire to Earth Community.* Bloomfield, CT: Kumarian Press, Inc. and San Francisco: Berrett-Koehler Publishers, Inc.

438. Tyson, Neil D. and Avis Lang. 2013. *Space Chronicles: Facing the Ultimate Frontier.* New York: W.W. Norton & Company, Inc.

439. Beckwith, Michael B. 2008. *Spiritual Liberation: Fulfilling Your Soul's Potential.* New York: Atria Paperback, and Hillsboro, OR: Beyond Words Publishing.

440. Public Affairs Television. 2014. "The New Robber Barons." *Moyers & Company*. http://billmoyers.com/episode/steve-fraser-new-robber-barons/.

441. Schwartz, Nelson D. 2004. "Inside the Head of BP He Doesn't Like Red Meat. He Thinks Green. What is John Browne Doing Running the World's Largest Oil Company?" *Fortune Magazine*. http://archive.fortune.com/magazines/fortune/fortune_archive/2004/07/26/377141/index.htm.

442. Banerjee, Neela. 2011. "Auto Industry Fights MPG Upgrade." *Chicago Tribune*. http://articles.chicagotribune.com/2011-07-20/business/sc-biz-0720-fuel-economy-20110720_1_fuel-efficiency-sales-of-fuel-efficient-vehicles-electric-vehicle-mandate; Tuttle, Brad. 2012. "How the New MPG Standards Will Affect Drivers, Automakers, Car Dealerships & More." *Time*. http://business.time.com/2012/08/30/how-the-new-mpg-standards-will-affect-drivers-automakers-car-dealerships-more/.

443. Winston, Andrew. 2011. "Weak Environmental Regulations Show Little Faith in U.S. Business." *Harvard Business Review*. https://hbr.org/2011/09/weak-environmental-regulations.html.

444. Koehler, Matthew. 2012. "WSJ Analysis: 80% of Wood-Burning Biomass Plants Generate Violations." *The Wall Street Journal*. http://forestpolicypub.com/2012/07/24/wsj-analysis-80-of-wood-burning-biomass-plants-generate-violations/.

445. Cousteau, Jacques. 1976. "Jacques Cousteau at NASA Headquarters." http://www.nss.org/settlement/nasa/CoEvolutionBook/JCOUST.HTML.

446. Oceana. Undated. "Global Fishing Watch—About the Project." Accessed October 1, 2016. http://globalfishingwatch.org/the-project.

447. Houston, Jean. 2004. *Jump Time: Shaping Your Future in a World of Radical Change*. Boulder, CO: Sentient Publications.

448. Hubbard, Barbara Marx. 2015. *Conscious Evolution: Awakening the Power of Our Social Potential*. Novato, CA: New World Library; Hubbard, Barbara Marx. 2011. "Recap." *Healing with the Masters*. Interview by Jennifer MacLean. http://healingwiththemasters.com/barbara-marx-hubbard-recap/.

449. Public Affairs Television. 2013. "Wendell Berry on His Hopes for Humanity." *Moyers & Company*. http://billmoyers.com/segment/wendell-berry-on-his-hopes-for-humanity/.

450. LoGiurato, Brett. 2013. "Obama's Climate Joke About A 'Flat Earth Society' Actually Referenced A Real Group." *Business Insider*. http://www.businessinsider.com/flat-earth-society-to-obama-climate-change-speech-georgetown-2013-6.

451. Hill, Napoleon. 2009. *Napoleon Hill's Golden Rules: The Lost Writings*. Hoboken, NJ: John Wiley & Sons, Inc.

452. USGS. 2013. "Frogs, Salamanders and Climate Change." *ScienceDaily*. http://www.sciencedaily.com/releases/2013/05/130518153747.htm.

453. Borrell, Brendan. 2009. "Is the Frog-Killing Chytrid Fungus Fueled by Climate Fluctuations?" *Scientific American*. http://www.scientificamerican.com/article/frog-killing-chytrid-fungus-climate-fluctuations/.

454. Handwerk, Brian. 2006. "Frog Extinctions Linked to Global Warming." *National Geographic News*. http://news.nationalgeographic.com/news/2006/01/0112_060112_frog_climate.html.

455. Braungart, Michael and William McDonough. 2002. *Cradle to Cradle: Remaking the Way We Make Things*. New York: North Point Press.

456. USEPA. 2016. "Municipal Solid Waste." https://archive.epa.gov/epawaste/nonhaz/municipal/web/html/index.html.

457. SF Environment. 2016. "Zero Waste by 2020." http://www.sfenvironment.org/zero-waste/overview/goals.

458. Louv, Richard. 2011. *The Nature Principle: Reconnecting with Life in a Virtual Age*. Chapel Hill, NC: Algonquin Books of Chapel Hill.

459. De Schuttler, Olivier. 2011. "News Release: Eco-Farming Can Double Food Production in 10 Years, Says New UN Report." http://www.srfood.org/images/stories/pdf/press_releases/20110308_agroecology-report-pr_en.pdf.

460. USDA. 2016. "Organic Market Overview." http://www.ers.usda.gov/topics/natural-resources-environment/organic-agriculture/organic-market-overview.aspx; IFOAM EU. 2016. *Organic in Europe: Prospects and Developments 2016*. http://www.ifoam-eu.org/en/news/2016/04/05/new-publication-organic-europe-increased-demand-organic-food-production-not-moving.

461. Moyer, Ellen. 2013. "Telling the Truth About Food Ingredients Helps the Consumer, the Economy and the Environment." *The Huffington Post*. http://www.huffingtonpost.com/ellen-moyer-phd/gmo-labeling_b_2619074.html.

462. Fulton, April. 2015. "A Farm, Tended by Tweens, Grows on a Brooklyn Rooftop." *National Geographic*. http://theplate.nationalgeographic.com/2015/11/03/a-farm-tended-by-tweens-grows-on-a-brooklyn-rooftop/.

463. Hochman, David. 2013. "Urban Gardening: An Appleseed with Attitude." *The New York Times*. http://www.nytimes.com/2013/05/05/fashion/urban-gardening-an-appleseed-with-attitude.html?_r=0.

464. National Geographic Society, Undated. "Solar Energy: Here's What You Need to Know About the Warming Planet, How It's Affecting Us, and What's at Stake." *National Geographic*. Accessed October 2, 2016. http://environment.nationalgeographic.com/environment/global-warming/solar-power-profile/.

465. Myers, Andrew. 2012. "Wind Could Meet Many Times World's Total Power Demand by 2030, Stanford Researchers Say." *Stanford News*. http://news.stanford.edu/news/2012/september/wind-world-demand-091012.html.

466. Randall, Tom. 2016. "Wind and Solar Are Crushing Fossil Fuels." *Bloomberg*. http://www.bloomberg.com/news/articles/2016-04-06/wind-and-solar-are-crushing-fossil-fuels.

467. Phillips, Art. 2015. "Germany Just Got 78 Percent Of Its Electricity From Renewable Sources." *ThinkProgress*. http://thinkprogress.org/climate/2015/07/29/3685555/germany-sets-new-renewable-energy-record/.

468. Lovins, Amory. 2013. *Reinventing Fire: Bold Business Solutions for the New Energy Era*. White River Junction, VT: Chelse Green Publishing.

469. Gies, Erica. 2015. "Heading Off Negative Impacts of Dam Projects." *The New York Times*. http://www.nytimes.com/2015/12/09/business/energy-environment/heading-off-negative-impacts-of-dam-projects.html.

470. Hladky, Gregory B. 2016. "Environmentalists Worried About Energy Projects Cutting Down Key Woodlands." *Hartford Courant*. http://www.courant.com/business/hc-energy-versus-forests-20160815-story.html.

471. Moyer, Ellen. 2012. "Burning Trees to Make Electricity—What Are They Thinking?" *The Huffington Post.* http://www.huffingtonpost.com/ellen-moyer-phd/burning-trees-to-make-ele_b_1601275.html; Moyer, Ellen. 2015. "Biomass, Biofuel, Biopower, and Bioenergy: Sound So Cool But Wreck the Climate and Rip Us Off." *The Huffington Post.* http://www.huffingtonpost.com/ellen-moyer-phd/biomass-biofuel-biopower-_b_8680774.html; The Editorial Board. 2016. "An Energy Bill in Need of Fixes." *The New York Times.* http://www.nytimes.com/2016/04/21/opinion/mixed-signals-on-energy.html?action=click&pgtype=Homepage&clickSource=story-heading&module=opinion-c-col-left-region&region=opinion-c-col-left-region&WT.nav=opinion-c-col-left-region&_r=1; The Editorial Board. 2016. "Dear Congress: Burning Wood is Not the Future of Energy." *The Washington Post.* https://www.washingtonpost.com/opinions/burning-wood-is-not-the-future-of-energy/2016/04/28/9cd9376c-08b9-11e6-bdcb-0133da18418d_story.html; Porter, Eduardo, 2016. "Next 'Renewal Energy': Forests, If Senators Get Their Way." *The New York Times.* http://nyti.ms/2d0nmU8.

472. Moyer, Ellen. 2015. "Liquidating Our Water Resources—California Drought Highlights Unsustainable Agricultural Practices." *The Huffington Post.* http://www.huffingtonpost.com/ellen-moyer-phd/liquidating-our-water-res_b_7692180.html.

473. Theobald, Daniel. 2015. "Options to Replenish Depleting Groundwater." *Water Online.* http://www.wateronline.com/doc/options-to-replenish-depleting-groundwater-0001.

474. Luyssaert, Sebastian, E. Detlef Schulze, Anett Börner, Alexander Knohl, Dominik Hessenmöller, Beverly E. Law, Philippe Ciais, and John Grace. 2008. "Old-Growth Forests as Global Carbon Sinks." *Nature* 455:213–215. http://web.natur.cuni.cz/fyziol5/kfrserver/gztu/pdf/Luyssaert_et_al_2008.pdf.

475. Rowling, Megan. 2015. "How to Stop Deforestation? Make 'Good Stuff' Cheaper." *Reuters.* http://www.reuters.com/article/us-development-goals-forests-idUSKCN0RU0NF20150930.

476. PBS. 2013. "Using 'Nature as an Asset' to Balance Costa Rica's Farming With Preservation." *PBS NewsHour.* http://www.pbs.org/newshour/bb/world-jan-june13-costarica_06-10/.

477. Undiscovered America. 2016. "Proposed National Parks." http://www.undiscoveredamerica.org/proposed-national-parks/.

478. Schleeter, Ryan. 2015. "Not Even National Parks Are Safe From Fracking." *Greenpeace.* http://www.greenpeace.org/usa/not-even-national-parks-are-safe-from-fracking/.

479. Peter. 2016. *The Hidden Life of Trees: What They Feel, How They Communicate—Discoveries From a Secret World.* Vancouver, BC: Greystone Books.

480. Monbiot, George. 2015. "There's a Population Crisis All Right. But Probably Not the One You Think." *The Guardian.* http://www.theguardian.com/commentisfree/2015/nov/19/population-crisis-farm-animals-laying-waste-to-planet.

481. Schlanger, Zoë and Elijah Wolfson. 2014. "How to Defuse the Population Bomb." *Newsweek.* http://www.newsweek.com/2014/12/26/fixing-crowded-earth-293024.html.

482. USEPA. 2016. "Green Chemistry." http://www.epa.gov/greenchemistry.

483. USEPA. 2015. *Presidential Green Chemistry Challenge Award Recipients 1996-2014.* http://www.epa.gov/sites/production/files/2015-02/documents/award_recipients_1996_2014.pdf.

484. Albini, Angelo and Stefano Protti. 2016. *Paradigms in Green Chemistry and Technology.* New York: Springer.

485. Chopra, Deepak. 2015. "A Hidden Solution to America's Health-Care Crisis." *The Huffington Post.* http://www.huffingtonpost.com/deepak-chopra/a-hidden-solution-to-amer_b_7664564.html.

486. Patel, Mahesh J. 2011. "Initiative Launched to Prevent One Million Heart Attacks and Strokes." *Duke Medicine Health News* 17:12:3.

487. Comarow, Avery and Ben Harder. 2016. "2016-17 Best Hospitals Honor Roll and Overview." *U.S. News & World Report.* http://health.usnews.com/health-news/best-hospitals/articles/2015/07/21/best-hospitals-2015-16-an-overview.

488. American Society of Civil Engineers. 2013. "Report Card for America's Infrastructure." http://www.infrastructurereportcard.org/a/#p/home.

489. Ferdman, Roberto A. 2014. "Americans Throw Out More Food Than Plastic, Paper, Metal, and Glass." *The Washington Post.* https://www.washingtonpost.com/news/wonk/wp/2014/09/23/americans-throw-out-more-food-than-plastic-paper-metal-or-glass/.

490. Gunders, Dana. 2012. "Wasted: How America Is Losing Up to 40 Percent of Its Food from Farm to Fork to Landfill." *NRDC Issue Paper IP:12-06-B.* https://www.nrdc.org/food/files/wasted-food-ip.pdf.

491. Oceana. 2014. "Wasted Catch: Unsolved Problems in U.S. Fisheries." Washington, DC: Oceana. http://usa.oceana.org/reports/wasted-catch-unsolved-problems-us-fisheries.

492. Gunders, Dana. 2012. "Wasted: How America Is Losing Up to 40 Percent of Its Food from Farm to Fork to Landfill." *NRDC Issue Paper IP:12-06-B.* https://www.nrdc.org/food/files/wasted-food-ip.pdf.

493. Massachusetts Division of Energy Resources. 2007. "Massachusetts Saving Electricity: A Summary of the Performance of Electric Efficiency Programs Funded by Ratepayers Between 2003 and 2005." http://ma-eeac.org/wordpress/wp-content/uploads/1_Saving-Electricity_A-Summary-of-the-Performance-of-Electric-Efficiency-Programs-Funded-by-RatePayers.pdf.

494. Schwartz, John. 2015. "Methane Leaks in Natural-Gas Supply Chain Far Exceed Estimates, Study Says." *The New York Times.* http://www.nytimes.com/2015/08/19/science/methane-leaks-in-natural-gas-supply-chain-far-exceed-estimates-study-says.html?_r=1.

495. Penna, Anthony N. 2014. *The Human Footprint: A Global Environmental History.* Second edition. Hoboken, NJ: Wiley-Blackwell.

496. Lovins, Amory. 2013. "Climate Change: No Breakthroughs Needed, Mr. President." *The Huffington Post.* http://www.huffingtonpost.com/amory-lovins/climate-change-no-breakth_b_2654248.html.

497. USDOE. Undated. "Energy Efficiency." Accessed October 3, 2016. http://energy.gov/science-innovation/energy-efficiency.

498. USEPA. Undated. "Energy Efficiency." *Energy Star.* Accessed October 6, 2016. https://www.energystar.gov/.

499. US Energy Information Administration. 2016. "How is Electricity Used in U.S. Homes?" https://www.eia.gov/tools/faqs/faq.cfm?id=96&t=3.

500. Vickers, Amy. 2001. *Handbook of Water Use and Conservation.* Amherst, MA: WaterPlow Press.

501. USEPA. 2016. "Fix A Leak Week." http://www3.epa.gov/watersense/pubs/fixleak.html.

502. Undiscovered America. 2016. "Proposed National Parks." http://www.undiscoveredamerica.org/proposed-national-parks/.

503. Olanoff, Drew. 2012. "Fun Fact: One Google Search Uses the Computing Power of the Entire Apollo Space Mission." *The Next Web.* http://thenextweb.com/google/2012/08/28/fun-fact-one-google-search-uses-computing-power-entire-apollo-space-mission/#gref.

504. Kemp, Simon. 2016. "Digital in 2016." *We Are Social.* http://wearesocial.com/special-reports/digital-in-2016.

505. Woods, Ben. 2014. "By 2020, 90% of World's Population Aged Over 6 Will Have a Mobile Phone: Report." *The Next Web.* http://thenextweb.com/insider/2014/11/18/2020-90-worlds-population-aged-6-will-mobile-phone-report/#gref.

506. Kroft, Steve. 2009. "The Data Brokers: Selling Your Personal Information." *60 Minutes*. http://www.cbsnews.com/news/the-data-brokers-selling-your-personal-information/.

507. Frank, Robert H. 2011. *The Darwin Economy: Liberty, Competition, and the Common Good*. Princeton, NJ: Princeton University Press.

508. Dubose, Lou. 2014. "Ignoring Obama's Record Rewards the Party of No." *The Washington Spectator*. October 1, 2014.

509. WGBH. Undated. "The New Deal." *American Experience*. Accessed October 6, 2016. http://www.pbs.org/wgbh/americanexperience/features/general-article/dustbowl-new-deal/.

510. Bollier, David. 2014. "These Days, It's Cool to Be a Commoner." *Yes! Magazine*. Summer 2014.

511. Gold, Jordan. 2011. "Loving the Challenge." Pushing the Limits Interview with Amory Lovins (Part I). *Corporate Knights*. July 6, 2011.

512. Partnoy, Frank. 2012. "The Cost of a Human Life, Statistically Speaking." *The Globalist*. http://www.theglobalist.com/the-cost-of-a-human-life-statistically-speaking/.

513. Farzad, Roben. 2012. "Shortcomings of Capitalism: 'Our Grandchildren Have No Value.'" *Bloomberg*.

514. Leonard, Abby. 2011. "Paying For War: The Cost of Caring for America's Wounded Vets." *Need to Know on PBS*. http://www.pbs.org/wnet/need-to-know/security/video-paying-for-war-the-cost-of-caring-for-americas-wounded-vets/9652/.

515. Brown, Lester. 2008. "The 'Invisible Hand' is Blind to Climate Externalities and the Value of NaturalResources." *Grist*. http://grist.org/article/a-massive-market-failure/.

516. PRI. 2013. "Saving Money with Environmental Regulation." *Living on Earth*. http://loe.org/shows/shows.html?programID=13-P13-00019.

517. Gold, Jordan. 2005. "David Suzuki: No Sacrifice Needed." Pushing the Limits Interview with David Suzuki. *Corporate Knights*. Issue 11.

518. Mooney, Chris. 2015. "The Staggeringly Large Benefits of Conserving Nature." *The Washington Post*. https://www.washingtonpost.com/news/energy-environment/wp/2015/07/13/were-finally-starting-to-realize-what-nature-is-really-worth/.

519. Zara, Christopher. 2015. "World Loses Trillions of Dollars Worth of Nature's Benefits Each Year Due to Land Degradation." *ScienceDaily*. September 15, 2015.

520. GCEC. 2014. *Better Growth Better Climate*. http://newclimateeconomy.report/2014/; Gillis, Justin. 2014. "Fixing Climate Change May Add No Costs, Report Says." *The New York Times*. http://www.nytimes.com/2014/09/16/science/earth/fixing-climate-change-may-add-no-costs-report-says.html.

521. GCEC. 2015. *Seizing the Global Opportunity*. http://newclimateeconomy.report/2015/.

522. NextGen Climate and Demos. 2016. *The Price Tag of Being Young: Climate Change and Millennials' Economic Future*. http://www.demos.org/publication/price-tag-being-young-climate-change-and-millennials-economic-future.

523. Postel, Sandra. 2010. "Five Years After Katrina, An Important Lesson Goes Unheard." *National Geographic*. http://voices.nationalgeographic.com/2010/08/30/five_years_after_katrina_an_im/.

524. Greenberg, Paul. 2012. "An Oyster in the Storm." *The New York Times*. http://www.nytimes.com/2012/10/30/opinion/an-oyster-in-the-storm.html?_r=0; Associated Press. 2013. "Sandy Was USA's 2nd-Costliest Hurricane." *USA Today*. http://www.usatoday.com/story/weather/2013/02/12/hurricane-sandy-weather-katrina/1912941/.

525. Eisinger, Jesse. 2014. "Why Only One Top Banker Went to Jail for the Financial Crisis." *The New York Times.* http://www.nytimes.com/2014/05/04/magazine/only-one-top-banker-jail-financial-crisis.html; Public Affairs Television. 2014. "Too Big to Jail?" *Moyers & Company.* http://billmoyers.com/episode/too-big-to-jail/.

526. NPR. 2014. "Coal Mines Keep Operating Despite Injuries, Violations and Millions In Fines." *All Things Considered.* http://www.npr.org/2014/11/12/363058646/coal-mines-keep-operating-despite-injuries-violations-and-millions-in-fines.

527. Goodman, Amy, Robert F. Kennedy, Jr., and Bill Haney. 2011. "The Growing Political War Surrounding Coal Mining Is a Fight About Democracy." *AlterNet.* http://www.alternet.org/story/151054/the_growing_political_war_surrounding_coal_mining_is_a_%27fight_about_democracy%27.

528. Blinder, Alan. 2016. "Donald Blankenship Sentenced to a Year In Prison in Mine Safety Case." *The New York Times.* http://www.nytimes.com/2016/04/07/us/donald-blankenship-sentenced-to-a-year-in-prison-in-mine-safety-case.html?_r=0.

529. Ohlemacher, Stephen. 2011. "GOP Looks to Cut IRS Budget Despite Returns." *The Washington Post.* http://www.washingtonpost.com/wp-dyn/content/article/2011/03/01/AR2011030104721.html.

530. International Co-operative Alliance. 2015. "Co-operative Facts & Figures." http://ica.coop/en/whats-co-op/co-operative-facts-figures.

531. Hindle, Tim. 2009. "Triple Bottom Line." *The Economist.* http://www.economist.com/node/14301663.

532. B Lab. 2016. "What is a Benefit Corporation?" http://benefitcorp.net/what-is-a-benefit-corporation.

533. B Lab. 2016. "B Corporations." https://www.bcorporation.net/.

534. UNEP. Undated. "Natural Capital Declaration." Accessed October 3, 2016. http://www.naturalcapitaldeclaration.org/.

535. Cambridge Institute for Sustainability Leadership. 2015. "Banking Environment Initiative." http://www.cisl.cam.ac.uk/business-action/sustainable-finance/banking-environment-initiative.

536. LeBlanc, Steve. 2011. "Feds Approve Cape Wind Power Project Off Massachusetts Coast." *USA Today.* http://usatoday30.usatoday.com/money/industries/energy/2011-04-19-cape-wind-power-electric.htm.

537. Seelye, Katharine. 2013. "Koch Brother Wages 12-Year Fight Over Wind Farm." *The New York Times.* http://www.nytimes.com/2013/10/23/us/koch-brother-wages-12-year-fight-over-wind-farm.html.

538. Eisenstadter, Dave. 2015. "State's Net-Metering Caps Threaten to Stymie Solar Projects, Advocates Say." *Daily Hampshire Gazette.* http://www.gazettenet.com/home/17844593-95/solar-projects-may-be-stymied-by-states-net-metering-caps-advocates-say.

539. Democker, Mary. 2012. "If Your House Is On Fire: Kathleen Dean Moore On The Moral Urgency of Climate Change." *The Sun.* http://thesunmagazine.org/issues/444/if_your_house_is_on_fire.

540. Ennis, John W. Undated. "Money in Politics A to Z Guide." *Pay 2 Play: Democracy's High Stakes.* Accessed October 3, 2016. http://www.pay2play.tv/a_to_z.

541. PRI. 2015. "Gus Speth Calls for a 'New' Environmentalism." *Living on Earth.* http://loe.org/shows/segments.html?programID=15-P13-00007&segmentID=6.

542. Public Affairs Television. 2012. "Inequality for All." *Moyers & Company.* http://billmoyers.com/episode/full-show-inequality-for-all/.

543. Levy, Gabrielle. 2015. "How Citizens United Has Changed Politics in 5 Years." *U.S. News & World Report.* http://www.usnews.com/news/articles/2015/01/21/5-years-later-citizens-united-has-remade-us-politics.

544. Smith, Hedrick. 2016. "What Fires Anger in Grass Roots America?" *Reclaim the American Dream.* http://reclaimtheamericandream.org/2016/01/the-roots-of-anger/?utm_source=Individuals+-+Citizens+-+Audience+-+Donors&utm_campaign=5e00b71e6c-JohnsonControls_Individuals.1.29.16&utm_medium=e-mail&utm_term=0_8cd20f7f75-5e00b71e6c-343584461.

545. Smith, Hedrick. 2016. "Will Campaign Reform Make It to the White House?" *Reclaim the American Dream.* http://reclaimtheamericandream.org/2016/02/a-stunning-watershed/#continue.

546. Gøtzsche, Peter. 2013. *Deadly Medicine and Organised Crime: How Big Pharma Has Corrupted Health Care.* London: Radcliffe Publishing Ltd.

547. Public Affairs Television. 2012. "Inequality for All." *Moyers & Company.* http://billmoyers.com/episode/full-show-inequality-for-all/.

548. PRI. 2015. "Gus Speth Calls for a 'New' Environmentalism." *Living on Earth.* http://loe.org/shows/segments.html?programID=15-P13-00007&segmentID=6.

549. Salatin, Joel. 2014. "We Can Feed the World!" *Common Ground.* http://commonground.ca/2014/03/we-can-feed-the-world/.

550. Scheer, Roddy and Doug Moss. 2016. "Why People Aren't Buying into Organic Food Products." *Scientific American.* http://www.scientificamerican.com/article/organic-still-a-small-slice-of-the-pie/.

551. Mitchell, Dan. 2016. "Calculating the Hidden Cost of Industrial Farming." *Civil Eats.* http://civileats.com/2016/07/20/this-study-could-help-us-numbers-on-the-true-cost-of-food/.

552. Jacobson, Louis. 2014. "Do Americans Pay More in Taxes Than in Food, Clothing and Housing?" *PolitiFact.* http://www.politifact.com/truth-o-meter/statements/2014/apr/23/tax-foundation/do-americans-pay-more-taxes-food-clothing-and-hous/.

553. USDA. 2016. "USDA Reports Record Growth in U.S. Organic Producers, $1 Billion in USDA Investments Boost Growing Markets for Organic Products and Local Foods." https://www.ams.usda.gov/press-release/usda-reports-record-growth-us-organic-producers-1-billion-usda-investments-boost.

554. Coady, David, Ian Parry, Louis Sears, and Baoping Shang. 2015. "How Large Are Global Energy Subsidies?" *IMF Working Paper WP/15/105.* https://www.imf.org/external/pubs/ft/wp/2015/wp15105.pdf.

555. Carrington, Damian. 2015. "Fossil Fuels Subsidised by $10M a Minute, Says IMF." *The Guardian.* http://www.theguardian.com/environment/2015/may/18/fossil-fuel-companies-getting-10m-a-minute-in-subsidies-says-imf.

556. Riffkin, Rebecca. 2015. "U.S. Support for Nuclear Energy at 51%." *Gallup.* http://www.gallup.com/poll/182180/support-nuclear-energy.aspx.

557. Porter, Eduardo. 2014. "The Risks of Cheap Water." *The New York Times.* http://www.nytimes.com/2014/10/15/business/economy/the-price-of-water-is-too-low.html?_r=0.

558. Dryden, Carley and Mike Reicher. 2014. "California's Water Agencies Lose Millions of Gallons Underground Due to Leaky Pipes." *The Daily Breeze.* http://www.dailybreeze.com/environment-and-nature/20141021/californias-water-agencies-lose-millions-of-gallons-underground-due-to-leaky-pipes.

559. News Wire Publications. 2016. "Four Billion People Affected by Severe Water Scarcity." *Homeland Security News Wire.* http://www.homelandsecuritynewswire.com/dr20160218-four-billion-people-affected-by-severe-water-scarcity.

560. Goonetilleke, Ashantha. 2015. "UN Report Investing In Water Could Yield 3 Trillion Annually." *The Water Network.* https://thewaternetwork.com/article-FfV/un-report-investing-in-water-could-yield-3-trillion-annually-0-AzDbSoRZhqkF73NbP7aQ.

561. Black, Richard. 2008. "Nature Loss 'Dwarfs Bank Crisis.'" *BBC News.* http://news.bbc.co.uk/2/hi/7662565.stm.

562. GCEC. 2014. *Better Growth Better Climate.* http://newclimateeconomy.report/2014/.

563. Burger, Andrew. 2015. "How Government Subsidies Drive Deforestation and Inequality." *Triple Pundit.* http://www.triplepundit.com/2015/04/subsidies-driving-deforestation-socioeconomic-exclusion/.

564. Chamberlain, Gethin. 2012. "'They're Killing Us': World's Most Endangered Tribe Cries for Help." *The Guardian.* http://www.theguardian.com/world/2012/apr/22/brazil-rainforest-awa-endangered-tribe.

565. Azevedo, Tasso. 2014. "Hopeful Lessons From the Battle to Save Rainforests." *TED Talks.* http://www.ted.com/talks/tasso_azevedo_hopeful_lessons_from_the_battle_to_save_rainforests.

566. Rowling, Megan. 2015. "How Can We Stop Deforestation?" *World Economic Forum.* http://www.weforum.org/agenda/2015/10/how-can-we-stop-deforestation.

567. Bloom, D.E., E.T. Cafiero, E. Jané-Llopis, S. Abrahams-Gessel, L.R. Bloom, S. Fathima, A.B. Feigl, T. Gaziano, M. Mowafi, A. Pandya, K. Prettner, L. Rosenberg, B. Seligman, A. Stein, and C. Weinstein. 2011. *The Global Economic Burden of Non-communicable Diseases.* Geneva: World Economic Forum. http://apps.who.int/medicinedocs/en/d/Js18806en/.

568. Kane, Jason. 2012. "Health Costs: How the U.S. Compares With Other Countries." *PBS NewsHour The Rundown.* http://www.pbs.org/newshour/rundown/health-costs-how-the-us-compares-with-other-countries/.

569. Hellmann, Melissa. 2014. "U.S. Health Care Ranked Worst in the Developed World." *Time.* http://time.com/2888403/u-s-health-care-ranked-worst-in-the-developed-world/.

570. Urbina, Ian. 2006. "In the Treatment of Diabetes, Success Often Does Not Pay." *The New York Times.* http://www.nytimes.com/2006/01/11/nyregion/nyregionspecial5/11diabetes.html?pagewanted=all&_r=0.

571. Chopra, Deepak. 2015. "A Hidden Solution to America's Health-Care Crisis." *The Huffington Post.* http://www.huffingtonpost.com/deepak-chopra/a-hidden-solution-to-amer_b_7664564.html.

572. CDC. 2016. "Chronic Disease Overview." http://www.cdc.gov/chronicdisease/overview/.

573. Hyman, Mark. 2012. "Three Hidden Ways Wheat Makes You Fat." *The Huffington Post.* http://www.huffingtonpost.com/dr-mark-hyman/wheat-gluten_b_1274872.html.

574. CDC. 2016. "Adult Obesity Facts." http://www.cdc.gov/obesity/data/adult.html.

575. PBS. 2012. "Will Obesity Reverse Rise in U.S. Life Expectancy?" *PBS NewsHour.* http://www.pbs.org/newshour/bb/health-jan-june12-obesity_05-08/.

576. Hyman, Mark. 2012. "Money, Politics, and Health Care: A Disease-Creation Economy—Part I." http://drhyman.com/blog/2012/09/06/money-politics-and-health-care-a-disease-creation-economy-part-i/.

577. Hyman, Mark. 2012. "Money, Politics, and Health Care: A Disease-Creation Economy—Part II." http://drhyman.com/blog/2012/09/12money-politics-and-health-care-a-disease-creation-economy-part-ii/.

578. Trust for America's Health, Environmental Defense Fund, and David Gardiner & Associates. 2011. *Saving Lives and Reducing Health Care Costs: How Clean Air Act Rules Benefit the Nation.* http://healthyamericans.org/assets/files/EDF%20TFAH%20Report%20on%20CAA%20health%20care%20savings%20-%20FINAL.pdf.

579. Navigant Research. 2011. "Green Chemicals Will Save Industry $65.5 Billion by 2020." *Newsroom.* http://www.navigantresearch.com/newsroom/green-chemicals-will-save-industry-65-5-billion-by-2020.

580. USEPA. 2016. "Benefits of Green Chemistry." http://www.epa.gov/greenchemistry/benefits-green-chemistry.

581. Heintz, James and Robert Pollin. 2011. "The Economic Benefits of a Green Chemical Industry in the United States: Renewing Manufacturing Jobs While Protecting Health and the Environment." http://www.peri.umass.edu/publication/item/423-the-economic-benefits-of-a-green-chemical-industry-in-the-united-states-renewing-manufacturing-jobs-while-protecting-health-and-the-environment.

582. Grossman, Elizabeth. 2015. "Chemical Exposure Linked to Billions in Health Care Costs." *National Geographic.* http://news.nationalgeographic.com/news/2015/03/150305-chemicals-endocrine-disruptors-diabetes-toxic-environment-ngfood/.

583. Aguayo, Jose. 2015. "International Specialists Warn of Global Toll From Chemical Exposures." *EWG.* http://www.ewg.org/enviroblog/2015/10/international-specialists-warn-global-toll-chemical-exposures.

584. Heintz, James and Robert Pollin. 2011. "The Economic Benefits of a Green Chemical Industry in the United States: Renewing Manufacturing Jobs While Protecting Health and the Environment." http://www.peri.umass.edu/publication/item/423-the-economic-benefits-of-a-green-chemical-industry-in-the-united-states-renewing-manufacturing-jobs-while-protecting-health-and-the-environment.

585. Markuson, Lisa. 2015. "Kindness in Business." *Likeable Local.* http://blog.likeablelocal.com/kindness-in-business.

586. Bezruchka, Stephen. 2011. "Toward A Healthy Society." *Alternative Radio.* http://archives.evergreen.edu/webpages/curricular/2011-2012/occupysymposium/files/2012/03/BEZS7-TowardHealthierSociety-11.pdf.

587. Lipton, Bruce. 2007. *The Biology of Belief: Unleashing the Power of Consciousness, Matter, & Miracles.* Carlsbad, CA: Hay House, Inc.

588. U.S. Global Change Research Program. 2014. *National Climate Assessment.* http://nca2014.globalchange.gov/report/sectors/indigenous-peoples.

589. Cienfuegos, Paul. 2010. "Corporations vs. People." *Alternative Radio.* http://www.alternativeradio.org/products/ciep001.

590. Global Alliance for the Rights of Nature. 2016. "Frequently Asked Questions." http://therightsofnature.org/frequently-asked-questions/.

591. Community Environmental Legal Defense Fund. 2016. "International Center for the Rights of Nature." http://celdf.org/how-we-work/education/rights-of-nature/.

592. World Animal Net. 2016. "The Animal Welfare Movement." http://worldanimal.net/our-programs/strategic-advocacy-course-new/module-1/social-change/the-animal-welfare-movement.

593. Goodall, Jane. 2009. *Hope for Animals and Their World: How Endangered Species Are Being Rescued from the Brink.* New York: Hachette Book Group.

594. Lough, Richard. 2014. "Court Rules Orangutan Held in Argentina Zoo is 'Non-Human Person' And Can Be Freed." http://www.huffingtonpost.com/2014/12/21/orangutan-argentina_n_6363582.html.

595. Global Alliance for the Rights of Nature. 2016. "Ecuador Adopts Rights of Nature in Constitution." http://therightsofnature.org/ecuador-rights/.

596. Chávez, Franz. 2014. "Bolivia's Mother Earth Law Hard to Implement." *Inter Press Service News Agency.* http://www.ipsnews.net/2014/05/bolivias-mother-earth-law-hard-implement/.

597. Pachamama Alliance. 2016. "Petition" *Pachamama Hub.* http://pachamamahub.org/petition/.

598. Ecosocialist Horizons. 2015. "International Rights of Nature Tribunal Constituted in Paris." http://ecosocialisthorizons.com/2015/12/international-rights-of-nature-tribunal-constituted-in-paris/.

599. Clinton, Hillary. 1995. "Hillary Rodham Clinton Remarks to the U.N. 4th World Conference on Women Plenary Session." http://www.americanrhetoric.com/speeches/hillaryclintonbeijingspeech.htm.

600. Houston, Jean. 1998. *A Passion for the Possible: Guide to Realizing Our True Potential.* New York: HarperOne; Peyser, Randy. 2015. "Dr. Jean Houston Women Changing the World." *Awaken Teachers.* http://www.awaken.com/2015/02/women-changing-the-world/.

601. Friedman, Thomas L. 2007. *The World is Flat 3.0: A Brief History of the Twenty-first Century.* New York: Picador.

602. Chan, Victor. 2010. "Western Women Can Come to the Rescue of the World." *The Dalai Lama Center.* http://dalailamacenter.org/blog-post/western-women-can-come-rescue-world.

603. Patten, Eileen and Kim Parker. 2012. "A Gender Reversal On Career Aspirations: Young Women Now Top Young Men in Valuing a High-Paying Career." *Pew Social & Demographic Trends.* http://www.pewsocialtrends.org/files/2012/04/Women-in-the-Workplace.pdf.

604. Alfonsi, Sharyn and Claire Pedersen. 2012. "Is Dad the New Mom? The Rise of Stay-At-Home Fathers." *ABC News.* http://abcnews.go.com/US/stay-home-dads-dad-mom/story?id=16596365#.UZYlC_rD-M8.

605. Lewis, Jone Johnson. Undated. "Margaret Mead Quotes." Accessed October 5, 2016. http://womenshistory.about.com/cs/quotes/a/qu_margaretmead.htm.

606. Institute for Women's Policy Research. 2016. "5 Things to Know in Advance of Tonight's Debate." *FemChat.* https://femchat-iwpr.org/.

607. American Association of University Women. 2016. "The Simple Truth About the Gender Pay Gap (Fall 2016)." http://www.aauw.org/research/the-simple-truth-about-the-gender-pay-gap/.

608. Annan, Kofi. 2012. "Unjust Global Systems, Their Impact on Worldwide Hunger and Undernutrition and Necessary Changes to be Undertaken by Relevant Actors." *Kofi Annan Foundation.* http://www.kofiannanfoundation.org/speeches/unjust-global-systems-their-impact-on-worldwide-hunger-and-undernutrition-and-necessary-changes-to-be-undertaken-by-relevant-actors/.

609. Isaac. John. 2014. "Expanding Women's Access to Financial Services." *The World Bank.* http://www.worldbank.org/en/results/2013/04/01banking-on-women-extending-womens-access-to-financial-services.

610. 1 Billion Rising. 2016. "What is One Billion Rising?" http://www.onebillionrising.org/about/campaign/one-billion-rising/.

611. Steinem, Gloria. 2014. "Our Revolution Has Just Begun." *Ms. Magazine.* Winter/Spring 2014.

612. Clinton, Hillary. 1995. "Hillary Rodham Clinton Remarks to the U.N. 4th World Conference on Women Plenary Session." http://www.americanrhetoric.com/speeches/hillaryclintonbeijingspeech.htm.

613. Weisman, Alan. 2014. *Countdown: Our Last, Best Hope for a Future on Earth?* New York: Little, Brown and Company; PRI. 2013. "Counting Down the Planet." *Living on Earth.* http://loe.org/shows/shows.html?programID=13-P13-00041.

614. Stone, Sidra. 2000. *The Shadow King; The Invisible Force That Holds Women Back.* Lincoln, NE: iUniverse.

615. Kunhardt McGee Productions, Storyville Films, and WETA-TV. 2013. "Makers: Women Who Make America." http://www.pbs.org/show/makers-women-who-make-america/.

616. Lee, John. 2013. "A New Man in Town." *The Center Post.* Fall/Winter 2013-2014.

617. ILO News. 2012. "Labour Market Gender Gap: Two Steps Forward, One Step Back." *International Labour Organization.* http://www.ilo.org/global/about-the-ilo/newsroom/news/WCMS_195445/lang--en/index.htm.

618. Rising Women Rising World. 2016. "Vision and Values." http://risingwomenrisingworld.com/vision-values/.

619. Rising Women Rising World. 2016. "Dr. Rama Mani." http://risingwomenrisingworld.com/portfolio-items/dr-rama-mani/.

620. Korten, David C. 2007. *The Great Turning: From Empire to Earth Community.* Bloomfield, CT: Kumarian Press, Inc. and San Francisco: Berrett-Koehler Publishers.

621. Generations United. 2016. "Directory." http://www.gu.org/OURWORK/Programs/Directory.aspx.

622. Rodriquez, Gregory. 2014. "How Genealogy Became Almost as Popular as Porn." *Time.* http://time.com/133811/how-genealogy-became-almost-as-popular-as-porn/.

623. Levenson, Michael. 2016. "Bernie Sanders Becomes Unlikely Leader of a Youth Movement." *The Boston Globe.* https://www.bostonglobe.com/metro/2016/01/18/bernie-sanders-unlikely-appeal-college-students/muC3jazXBjXv7myW1wKOtL/story.html.

624. McGrath, Matt. 2013. "NASA's James Hansen Retires to Pursue Climate Fight." *BBC News.* http://www.bbc.com/news/science-environment-22000810; Hansen, James. 2015. "Bridging the Geezer-Young Person Gap." http://csas.ei.columbia.edu/2015/07/15/bridging-the-geezer-young-person-gap/.

625. UN Joint Framework Initiative on Children, Youth and Climate Change. 2012. *Growing Together in a Changing Climate: The United Nations, Young People, and Climate Change.* http://unfccc.int/cc_inet/files/cc_inet/information_pool/application/pdf/growingtogether.pdf.

626. Moyer, Ellen. 2015. "Bridging the Geezer-Young Person Gap to Drive Climate Change Solutions." *The Huffington Post.* http://www.huffingtonpost.com/ellen-moyer-phd/bridging-the-geezeryoung-_b_8015554.html.

627. McKibben, Bill. 2008. *The Bill McKibben Reader: Pieces from an Active Life.* New York: Macmillan.

628. Pew Research Center. 2010. "Baby Boomers Retire." http://www.pewresearch.org/daily-number/baby-boomers-retire/.

629. Newport, Frank, Jeffrey M. Jones, and Lydia Saad. 2014. "Baby Boomers to Push U.S. Politics in the Years Ahead." *Gallup.* http://www.gallup.com/poll/167012/baby-boomers-push-politics-years-ahead.aspx; NPR. 2015. "For Advertisers, Baby Boomers Are A Market Hiding In Plain Sight." *Weekend Edition Saturday.* http://www.npr.org/2015/05/02/403766871/for-advertisers-baby-boomers-are-a-market-hiding-in-plain-sight.

630. Pope Francis. 2015. "Encyclical Letter Laudato Si' of the Holy Father Francis On Care for Our Common Home." http://w2.vatican.va/content/francesco/en/encyclicals/documents/papa-francesco_20150524_enciclica-laudato-si.html.

631. Ellis, Diana. 2015. "Elders, Youth and the Environment—We Are In This Together." *Suzuki Elders.* http://www.suzukielders.org/elders-youth-and-the-environment-we-are-in-this-together/.

632. Moyer, Ellen. 2015. "Elders Take Action on Climate Change." *The Huffington Post.* http://www.huffingtonpost.com/ellen-moyer-phd/elders-take-action-on-climate-change-_b_7309578.html.

633. Fields, Liz. 2014. "Thousands Rally in New York for the People's Climate March." *Vice News.* https://news.vice.com/article/thousands-rally-in-new-york-for-the-peoples-climate-march.

634. Grandparents Climate Campaign. Undated. "Co-operation for Change." Accessed October 5, 2016. http://www.besteforeldreaksjonen.no/?page_id=1493.

635. David Suzuki Foundation. Undated. "Suzuki Elders." Accessed October 5, 2016. http://www. davidsuzuki.org/about/people/suzuki-elders/.

636. David Suzuki Foundation. Undated. "Working Groups." *Suzuki Elders*. Accessed October 5, 2016. http://www.suzukielders.org/home/working-groups/.

637. Ellis, Diana. 2015. "Elders, Youth and the Environment—We Are In This Together." *Suzuki Elders*. http://www.suzukielders.org/elders-youth-and-the-environment-we-are-in-this-together/.

638. No Planeta B. Undated. "Schools Can Act On Climate." *Cut the Red Tape Project*. Accessed October 5, 2016. http://bit.ly/1PCYDBg.

639. No Planeta B. Undated. "Climate Change is Threatening Our Kids." *Cut the Red Tape Project*. Accessed October 5, 2016. http://bit.ly/1PD82c0.

640. Moyer, Ellen. 2015. "Elders Take Action on Climate Change." *The Huffington Post*. http://www. huffingtonpost.com/ellen-moyer-phd/elders-take-action-on-climate-change-_b_7309578.html.

641. Pope Francis. 2015. "Encyclical Letter Laudato Si' of the Holy Father Francis On Care for Our Common Home." http://w2.vatican.va/content/francesco/en/encyclicals/documents/papa-francesco_20150524_enciclica-laudato-si.html.

642. Foundation for Conscious Evolution. Undated. "Interview: The Department of Peace." Accessed October 5, 2016. http://barbaramarxhubbard.com/interview-the-department-of-peace/.

643. Houston, Jean. 2004. *Jump Time: Shaping Your Future in World of Radical Change*. Second edition. Boulder CO: Sentient Publications.

644. Bucknell Environmental Center. Undated. "Sunbury: A History." Accessed October 5, 2016. http://www.departments.bucknell.edu/environmental_center/sunbury/website/ HistoryofIroquoisIndians.shtml.

645. Houston, Jean. 2004. *Jump Time: Shaping Your Future in World of Radical Change*. Second edition. Boulder CO: Sentient Publications.

646. National Priorities Project. Undated. "Military Spending in the United States." Accessed October 5, 2016. https://www.nationalpriorities.org/campaigns/military-spending-united-states/.

647. Houston, Jean. 2004. *Jump Time: Shaping Your Future in World of Radical Change*. Second edition. Boulder CO: Sentient Publications.

648. Weaver, Matther. 2013. "Al Gore: US Democracy Has Been Hacked." *The Guardian*. http://www. theguardian.com/world/2013/feb/03/al-gore-us-democracy-hacked.

649. Public Affairs Television. 2012. "Inequality for All." *Moyers & Company*. http://billmoyers.com/ episode/full-show-inequality-for-all/.

650. Frank, Robert H. 2012. *The Darwin Economy: Liberty, Competition, and the Common Good*. Princeton, NJ: Princeton University Press.

651. Cienfuegos, Paul. 2010. "Corporations vs. People." *Alternative Radio*. http://www.alternativeradio. org/products/ciep001.

652. Hoback, Cullen. 2013. *Terms and Conditions May Apply*. Produced by Cullen Hoback, Nitin Khanna, and John Ramos. https://freedocumentaries.org/documentary/terms-and-conditions -may-apply.

653. Gore, Al. 1992. *Earth in the Balance: Ecology and the Human Spirit*. New York: Houghton Mifflin.

654. Jose, Coleen. 2014. "Good News: The World is More Democratic Than Ever." https://mic.com/ articles/103294/good-news-the-world-is-becoming-more-democratic-than-ever.

655. Public Affairs Television. 2012. "Inequality for All." *Moyers & Company.* http://billmoyers.com/episode/full-show-inequality-for-all/.

656. Vossen, Lois. 2013. "The Revolutionary Optimists." *Independent Lens.* http://www.pbs.org/independentlens/films/revolutionary-optimists/.

657. The World Bank. 2015. "Girls' Education." https://declara.com/content/V5WevBl1.

658. Williamson, Marianne. 2012. "Marianne Williamson on Love and Fear." https://www.youtube.com/watch?v=PQ9tAwEYO4k.

659. Pope Francis. 2015. "Encyclical Letter Laudato Si' of the Holy Father Francis On Care for Our Common Home." http://w2.vatican.va/content/francesco/en/encyclicals/documents/papa-francesco_20150524_enciclica-laudato-si.html.

660. Democker, Mary. 2012. "If Your House Is On Fire: Kathleen Dean Moore On The Moral Urgency of Climate Change." *The Sun.* http://thesunmagazine.org/issues/444/if_your_house_is_on_fire.

661. Orcutt, Mike. 2015. "The U.S. and Europe Are Mostly to Blame for the Climate Conundrum." *MIT Technology Review.* https://www.technologyreview.com/s/544116/the-us-and-europe-are-mostly-to-blame-for-the-climate-conundrum/.

662. Macy, Joanna. 2014. "Five Ways of Being that Can Change the World." *The Center Post.* Spring/Summer 2014.

663. Hawkens, Paul. 2007. *Blessed Unrest.* New York: Viking Press.

664. Lipton, Bruce, and Steve Bhaerman. 2010. *Spontaneous Evolution: Our Positive Future and a Way to Get There From Here.* Carlsbad, CA: Hay House, Inc.

665. UN News Service. 2011. "New Industrial Revolution Needed to Avert 'Planetary Catastrophe'—UN Report." *UN Daily News.* http://www.un.org/news/dh/pdf/english/2011/05072011.pdf.

666. Wilson, Edward O. 1984. *Biophilia.* Cambridge, MA: Harvard University Press. http://www.amazon.com/Biophilia-Edward-Wilson/dp/0674074424.

667. Gallup. Undated. "Satisfaction With the United States." Accessed September 26, 2016. http://www.gallup.com/poll/1669/general-mood-country.aspx; Gallup. 2016. "Americans' Concerns About Water Pollution Up." http://www.gallup.com/poll/190034/americans-concerns-water-pollution-edge.aspx?g_source=Politics&g_medium=newsfeed&g_campaign=tiles.

668. Jayson, Sharon. 2004. "Power of a Super Attitude." *USA Today.* http://usatoday30.usatoday.com/news/health/2004-10-12-mind-body_x.htm.

669. Clarke, Chris. 2014. "Hundreds of Environmental Activists Killed Worldwide Over Past Decade." *Redefine.* http://www.kcet.org/news/redefine/rewild/commentary/hundreds-of-environmental-activists-killed-over-past-decade.html.

670. Lane, Chief Phil, Jr. 2016. "You Can't Eat Money." *Earth Day Summit 2016.* Interview by Nathan Crane. http://earthdaysummit.com/program/154.

671. Sammon, Alexander. 2016. "A History of Native Americans Protesting the Dakota Access Pipeline." *Mother Jones.* http://www.motherjones.com/environment/2016/09/dakota-access-pipeline-protest-timeline-sioux-standing-rock-jill-stein; teleSUR English. 2016. "Unprecedented Show of Native Unity Against Dakota Pipeline." *Facebook.* https://www.facebook.com/telesurenglish/videos/909477372528999/; Fusion. 2016. "Big Oil Vs. Native Americans." *Facebook.* https://www.facebook.com/fusionmedianetwork/videos/1543459422346697/; PBS. 2016. "Tribes Across North America Converge at Standing Rock, Hoping to Be Heard." *PBS NewsHour.* http://www.pbs.org/newshour/videos/#193037; PRI. 2016. "Standing Rock and The Feds." *Living on Earth.* http://loe.org/shows/segments.html?programID=16-P13-00038&segmentID=1; Cerda, Leo. 2016. "Global Solidarity from the Amazon to Standing Rock." *Amazon Watch.* http://amazonwatch.org/news/2016/0922-global-solidarity-from-the-amazon-to-standing-rock?utm_source=Amazon+Watch+Newsletter+and+Updates&utm_campaign=00b6010c3c-2016-09-22-sr&utm_medium=email&utm_term=0_e6f929728b-00b6010c3c-341599041&mc_cid=00b6010c3c&mc_eid=999cb99985.

672. Moe, Kristin. 2013. "For a Future that Won't Destroy Life on Earth, Look to the Global Indigenous Uprising." *Yes! Magazine.* Summer 2013. http://www.yesmagazine.org/issues/love-and-the-apocalypse/mother-earth-at-the-heart-of-it.

673. Democker, Mary. 2012. "If Your House Is On Fire: Kathleen Dean Moore On The Moral Urgency of Climate Change." *The Sun.* http://thesunmagazine.org/issues/444/if_your_house_is_on_fire.

674. Hyman, Mark. 2009. *The UltraMind Solution.* New York: Scribner.

675. Public Affairs Television. 2012. "On Winner-Take-All Politics." *Moyers & Company.* http://billmoyers.com/episode/on-winner-take-all-politics/.

676. Hessel, Stepháne. 2010. *Time for Outrage: Indignez-vous!* New York: Twelve? Hachette Book Group.

677. Robinson, Sara. 2012. "6 People You Need to Start a Revolution." *AlterNet.* http://www.alternet.org/story/154968/6_people_you_need_to_start_a_revolution.

678. Silver, Nate. 2011. "The Geography of Occupying Wall Street (and Everywhere Else)." *The New York Times.* http://fivethirtyeight.blogs.nytimes.com/2011/10/17/the-geography-of-occupying-wall-street-and-everywhere-else/.

679. Cooper, Matthew. 2011. "Poll: Most Americans Support Occupy Wall Street." *The Atlantic.* http://www.theatlantic.com/politics/archive/2011/10/poll-most-americans-support-occupy-wall-street/246963/.

680. Move to Amend. Undated. "Motion to Amend—Sign the Petition." Accessed October 12, 2016. https://movetoamend.org/petition.

681. Bachelet, Michelle. 2012. "Advancing Women's Rights Worldwide." *UN Women.* http://www.unwomen.org/en/news/stories/2012/1/advancing-women-s-rights-worldwide; Walsh, Bryan. 2012. "Population Studies: Birthrates Are Declining. For the Earth—and a Lot of People—That's Not a Bad Thing." *Time.* http://science.time.com/2012/03/14/population-studies-birth-rates-are-declining-for-the-earth-and-a-lot-of-people-thats-not-a-bad-thing/.

682. The White House Office of the Press Secretary. 2015. "Fact Sheet: White House Announces Commitments to the American Business Act on Climate Pledge." *The White House President Barack Obama.* https://www.whitehouse.gov/the-press-office/2015/10/19/fact-sheet-white-house-announces-commitments-american-business-act.

683. Grover, Sami. 2015. "10 Cities Aiming for 100 Percent Clean Energy." *Mother Nature Network.* http://www.mnn.com/earth-matters/energy/stories/10-cities-aiming-for-100-percent-clean-energy.

684. Linzey, Thomas. 2013. "Corporations, Communities & the Environment." *Alternative Radio.* http://celdf.org/category/news/press-releases-and-updates/.

685. PRI. 2016. "Beyond the Headlines." *Living on Earth.* http://loe.org/shows/segments.html?program ID=16-P13-00015&segmentID=6.

686. Nollyvines. 2014. "Meet Yacouba Sawadogo—The Man Who Stopped the Desert." https://www. youtube.com/watch?v=nSTV-KcAd_0; PBS. 2013. "Using 'Nature as an Asset' to Balance Costa Rica's Farming With Preservation." *PBS NewsHour.* http://www.pbs.org/newshour/bb/world-jan-june13-costarica_06-10/; Gotsch, Agenda. 2015. "Life in Syntropy." https://www.youtube.com/ watch?v=gSPNRu4ZPvE; Byck, Peter. 2013. "Soil Carbon Carboys." https://vimeo.com/80518559.

687. PRI. 2015. "Great Green Wonder of the World." *Living on Earth.* http://loe.org/shows/shows. html?programID=16-P13-00016#feature6; A Tree A Day. 2016. "How Trees Help Create the Fresh Water Supply." https://www.youtube.com/watch?v=LbZvOL0dgyU.

688. BBC. 2013. "Why This Could Be One of the Happiest Countries on Earth?" *BBC World News.* http://www.bbc.co.uk/programmes/p01dmw58.

689. McCarthy, Orion. 2015. "Beyond Carbon Neutral—What the World Should Learn from Bhutan." *Conserve.* http://howtoconserve.org/2015/12/18/bhutan/.

690. NPR. 2016. "Gross National Happiness: Bhutan's Unique Measurement." *All Things Considered.* http://www.npr.org/2016/02/21/467582508/gross-national-happiness-bhutan-s-unique-measurement.

691. BBC. 2013. "Why This Could Be One of the Happiest Countries on Earth?" *BBC World News.* http://www.bbc.co.uk/programmes/p01dmw58.

692. Escape. Undated. "Is This the Happiest Country on Earth?" *Escape.* Accessed September 29, 2016. http://www.escape.com.au/world/is-this-the-happiest-country-on-earth/news-story/3b63d539a995 3ff562e8d522cae67867.

693. Hindy, Joseph. Undated. "10 Things Bhutan People Do Differently That Make Them The Happiest People." *Lifehack.* Accessed September 29, 2016. http://www.lifehack.org/articles/ communication/8-things-bhutan-people-differently-that-make-them-the-happiest-people.html; BBC. 2013. "Why This Could Be One of the Happiest Countries on Earth?" *BBC World News.* http://www.bbc.co.uk/programmes/p01dmw58.

694. WHO. 2014. "Bhutan." http://www.who.int/countryfocus/cooperation_strategy/ ccsbrief_btn_en.pdf.

695. McCarthy, Orion. 2015. "Beyond Carbon Neutral—What the World Should Learn from Bhutan." *Conserve.* http://howtoconserve.org/2015/12/18/bhutan/.

696. BBC. 2013. "Why This Could Be One of the Happiest Countries on Earth?" *BBC World News.* http://www.bbc.co.uk/programmes/p01dmw58.

697. Rosenberg, Matthew. 2008. "King of Bhutan Gives Up His Absolute Monarchy." *The Independent.* http://www.independent.co.uk/news/world/asia/king-of-bhutan-gives-up-his-absolute-monarchy-799881.html.

698. Trading Economics. 2016. "Bhutan GDP Annual Growth Rate 1996-2016." *Trading Economics.* http://www.tradingeconomics.com/bhutan/gdp-growth-annual.

699. Earth Day Network. 2016. "History of Earth Day." http://www.earthday.org/about/ the-history-of-earth-day/.

700. Gore, Al. 1992. *Earth in the Balance: Ecology and the Human Spirit.* New York: Rodale, Inc.

701. Wilson, Edward O. 2016. "Half-Earth." *Aeon.* https://aeon.co/essays/half-of-the-earth-must-be-preserved-for-nature-conservation.

702. Pope Francis. 2015. "Encyclical Letter Laudato Si' of the Holy Father Francis On Care for Our Common Home." http://w2.vatican.va/content/francesco/en/encyclicals/documents/papa-francesco_20150524_enciclica-laudato-si.html.

703. PBS. 2016. "Can Environmentalism Become a Bipartisan Movement Again?" *PBS NewsHour.* http://www.pbs.org/newshour/videos/#178840; Rich, Frederic C. 2016. *Getting to Green: Saving Nature: A Bipartisan Solution.* New York: W.W. Norton & Company.

704. Mayer, Gerald. 2014. "The Increased Supply of Underutilized Labor from 2006 to 2014." *Bureau of Labor Statistics.* http://www.bls.gov/opub/mlr/2014/article/the-increased-supply-of-underutilized-labor-from-2006-to-2014.htm.

705. Clifton, Jim. 2011. *The Coming Jobs War.* New York: Gallup Press.

706. Democker, Mary. 2012. "If Your House Is On Fire: Kathleen Dean Moore On The Moral Urgency of Climate Change." *The Sun.* http://thesunmagazine.org/issues/444/if_your_house_is_on_fire.

707. Blue, Laura. 2010. "Is Exercise the Best Drug for Depression?" *Time.* http://content.time.com/time/health/article/0,8599,1998021,00.html.

708. Moyer, Ellen. 2013. "Telling the Truth About Food Ingredients Helps the Consumer, the Environment, and the Economy." *The Huffington Post.* http://www.huffingtonpost.com/ellen-moyer-phd/gmo-labeling_b_2619074.html.

709. Public Affairs Television. 2012. "Inequality for All." *Moyers & Company.* http://billmoyers.com/episode/full-show-inequality-for-all/.

710. Ibid.

711. Klein, Naomi. 2014. *This Changes Everything: Capitalism vs. the Climate.* New York: Simon & Schuster.

712. Ibid.

713. Raskin, Paul. 2013. "Game On: The Basis for Hope in a Time of Despair." *GTI Perspectives on Critical Issues.* http://www.greattransition.org/archives/perspectives/Perspective_Game_On.pdf.

ACKNOWLEDGMENTS

First, thank *you* for your interest and for taking the time to read part or all of *Our Earth, Our Species, Our Selves.* You are the whole point.

Thank you, Paul Dryfoos, Kate Ewald, Evan Johnson, Betsy Moyer, and Bill Moyer, for blazing my trail by generously reading a draft manuscript and providing numerous thoughtful suggestions that strengthened the book enormously.

Thank you, Jean Zimmer, for editing the manuscript and providing sage advice and encouragement throughout the entire process, from outline to finished manuscript. Thank you, Chris Kennedy, for expertly shepherding the book from manuscript to hard copy, e-book, and audiobook. Thank you, Geoffrey Berwind, Martha Bullen, Jack Canfield, Debra Englander, Steve Harrison, Patricia Lee Lewis, and Lisa Tener, for sharing your writing expertise and coaching.

Thank you, Jean Houston and Mark Hyman, MD, for your interest in my work and your wise advice and assistance.

Thanks to other authors for your generous help and encouragement: Janet Bray Attwood, Joel Fuhrman, MD, Jacob Hacker, Ian Hanington, James Hansen, Frances Moore Lappé, Amory Lovins, Joan Maloof, Joel Pett, Paul Pierson, Dan Piraro, Debra Poneman, Marci Shimoff, Marion Stoddart, David Suzuki, and Ellen Tadd.

Thank you for your kind assistance in providing graphics: Leo Cerda, Brady Couvillion, John Dearie, Jenni Harris, Will Harris, Christy Higgins, Angela Huffman, David Iraya, Chris Matera, Lynne Merchant, Bob Monroe, Paul Paz y Miño, Stefan Smith, Hugh Stoddart, and Dave Williams.

Finally, thanks to the countless people who provided information and insights that I incorporated into this book.

INDEX

ABOUT THE AUTHOR

Ellen Moyer is an environmental consultant with a bachelor's degree in anthropology, a master's degree in environmental engineering, and a doctorate in civil engineering. She is a registered professional engineer as well as a US Green Building Council Leadership in Energy and Environmental Design Accredited Professional.

For three decades, her work has focused mainly on the assessment and cleanup of contaminated soil and groundwater, protection of drinking water supplies, and sustainability. She has copresented more than 100 seminars in North America and Europe. Her publications include numerous articles and three books, and she is a regular contributor to *The Huffington Post*.

When she is not advocating for her clients and the environment, Ellen enjoys creating art in many forms, including drawings, paintings, ceramics, photographs, and fabric designs. She makes her home in western Massachusetts.

For more information, to sign up for updates, or to get in touch with Ellen, please visit her website at www.ellenmoyerphd.com.

Made in the USA
Lexington, KY
29 October 2018